Physiology of the Heart

Arnold M. Katz, M.D.

Philip J. and Harriet L. Goodhart
Professor of Medicine (Cardiology)
Mount Sinai School of Medicine
of the City University of New York
New York, New York

Raven Press ■ New York

LaL k

Raven Press, 1140 Avenue of the Americas, New York, New York 10036

Made in the United States of America

Library of Congress Cataloging in Publication Data

Katz, Arnold M
    Physiology and biophysics of the heart

    Includes bibliographies and index.
    1. Heart- -Diseases. 2. Heart. 3. Biological
physics. I. Title. [DNLM: 1. Heart- -Physiology.
2. Biophysics. WG202 K19p]
RC683.K27   612'.17   75-14580
ISBN 0-89004-053-2

To my father
Louis N. Katz
1898–1973

Preface

Why write a textbook about the biophysical basis of cardiac function? Of what importance are the energetics and chemistry of myocardial contraction to anyone but a physical chemist or a biochemist? Why should electrical potentials at the surface of the myocardial cell concern those who are not basic electrophysiologists? The answers to all of these questions lie in the fact that *virtually every important physiological, pharmacological, or pathological change in cardiac function arises from alterations in the physical and chemical processes that are responsible for the heartbeat.*

Although it remains fashionable to consider the heart as a muscular pump, this organ is much more than a hollow viscus that provides mechanical energy to propel blood through the vasculature. It is an intricate biological machine that contains, within each cell, a complex of control and effector mechanisms. Both the strength of cardiac contraction and its electrical control are modulated by alterations in one or more of these cellular mechanisms, which are involved in the fundamental processes of excitability, excitation-contraction coupling, and contraction.

This text is written for medical students and graduate students in the biological sciences, and for the physician who would like to find a simplified exposition of our current understanding of the physiological and biophysical basis of cardiac function. Therefore, this book is intended to provide a synoptic view of our present knowledge in this rapidly expanding area. The major emphasis is on the relationships between the biochemical properties of individual constituents of the myocardial cell, the biophysics of cardiac muscle function, and the performance of the intact heart.

The task of relating these different aspects of cardiac function to each other has required much selectivity and, undoubtedly, an excess of simplification and speculation. There can be no doubt that much of this conceptual material will become invalid as our knowledge of cardiac function advances. This is, after all, the lesson taught to us by the history of science. The early neurophysiologists who tried to understand nerve conduction as the passage of fluid down hollow tubes were trying to explain physiological phenomena in terms of the limited biophysical knowledge of their time. With the development of an understanding of animal electricity, the focus in neurophysiology shifted to studies of the electrical properties of the nervous system, and attempts were made to explain phenomena such as neuron-to-neuron communication and memory in terms of electrical circuitry. More recently the enormous advances in our knowledge of chemical transmitters and the potential for information storage as newly synthesized macromolecules have cast doubt on many of the theories of the great neurophysiologists of the last century. Yet these were not unintelligent scientists. They were, however, required to interpret their observations within the framework of knowledge that existed during their lifetime. It would be presumptuous indeed for us now to assume that the evolution of new principles of science has ended. For this reason no apology is made for the misconceptions and faulty interpretation that will inevitably accompany the present attempt to organize our knowledge of cardiac function in terms of the broad principles that are understood today.

The only true "facts" in biology are the results of individual experiments carried out under controlled conditions by a carefully defined methodology. Yet it is not the purpose of this book to catalogue and discuss these biological "facts"; for this the reader is referred to the large number of reviews, symposia, multiauthored texts, and, most important, individual scientific papers. Instead, the present text attempts to identify and describe the unifying themes that connect different lines of investigation of the function of the heart and, in so doing, to set out interpretations of these biological "facts." The bibliographies to each chapter are intentionally brief and generally include one or more recent reviews to which the interested student may refer for more complete lists of references. In some cases "classic" articles are also cited.

Every effort has been made to keep this book simple—suitable for use as a text for graduate and undergraduate teaching. Achievement of this goal, however, requires the resolution, more or less arbitrarily as the case may require, of many serious conflicts, as well as the addition of speculative material to connect important biochemical, biophysical, physiological, and pathophysiological observations. It is the author's intention that these departures into the realm of speculation be clearly identified in the text. Yet the expert in these fields will undoubtedly be troubled by this attempt to provide a coherent and unified text. While the author is not laboring under the illusion that all of his interpretations will prove correct, it seems especially important to provide the student with an indication of the significance of the many biological "facts" describing the heart and its function rather than just to catalogue specific experimental findings. It is, after all, the pattern on the fabric that holds the interest of most of us, rather than the threads. For this reason, though with apologies to the protagonists of opposing viewpoints, the author has chosen the present format for this text.

Arnold M. Katz

Acknowledgments

This text was to have been co-authored by my late father, Louis N. Katz, whose life ended before we were able to launch this venture. To him, and to his teachers whose wisdom he transmitted to me, I am dedicating this book.

This book was written while the author was a Philip J. and Harriet L. Goodhart Professor of Medicine (Cardiology) at Mount Sinai School of Medicine of the City University of New York. The Bundeschrepublik Deutschland, through the Alexander von Humboldt Stiftung, provided a generous Senior U.S. Scientist Award that allowed this text to be completed in the stimulating and serene atmosphere of Heidelberg. I am grateful to Professor W. Hasselbach and the Max-Planck-Institut für Medizinische Forschung, Heidelberg, for providing me with a quiet but inspiring setting in which to write.

I am greatly indebted to Mrs. Jo-Anna Iorio Finegan, Miss Priscilla Nash, and Mrs. Dianne Gaffield, who carried for me many of the burdens of producing this manuscript. I would like to thank Mrs. Lorraine Moseley for assistance in preparing much of the original art. The cooperation of Mrs. Judy Upshaw Early and Dr. Ernest Page, who provided unpublished electron microphotographs for Chapter 1, and Dr. Alfred Pick for allowing me access to the illustrations from the Book *Clinical Electrocardiography. Part I. The Arrhythmias,* which he co-authored with my father, is acknowledged. I am grateful to Lea and Febiger, Philadelphia, who permitted me to quote almost verbatim Professor Wiggers' classic description of the cardiac cycle for the benefit of the younger scholars who will probably find Wiggers' *Physiology in Health and Disease* available only in libraries. Many individuals and publishers kindly allowed me to use published figures, as will be apparent throughout the text. I thank Dr. David Littmann for the use of many illustrations from his book *Textbook of Electrocardiography.* To my friends and colleagues Gary Bailin, Howard Morgan, Katherine LaNoue, Gerald Pollack, Harald Reuter, and Hasso Scholz, who read many of these chapters and corrected numerous errors and clarified many obscurities, much thanks is due. These individuals are to be credited only with correct statements in this text—the errors are mine alone.

To Raven Press, its President Dr. Alan Edelson, and especially Miss Laura Kosden who spent countless hours working with me to polish this text, I owe many thanks. The personal care and attention I received from all of the staff at Raven Press has contributed in large measure to the attractive format of this book.

Acknowledgment is warmly given to the students I have taught at Columbia University, The University of Chicago, and The Mount Sinai School of Medicine. These students are largely responsible for my writing this text; many have read these chapters as syllabus material for their lectures. Their firm, though usually kindly, disagreements with my efforts to explain things has contributed much to my attempt to achieve clarity in presentation in this text, and no small number of errors have been corrected by their searching and open minds.

Arnold M. Katz

Contents

Glossary

Calcium: Calcium in any form: free, bound, or ionized.
Ca^{2+}: Ionized calcium.
Sodium: Sodium in any form: free, bound, or ionized.
Na^+: Ionized sodium.
Potassium: Potassium in any form: free, bound, or ionized.
K^+: Ionized potassium.
Chloride: Chloride in any form: free, bound, or ionized.
Cl^-: Ionized chloride.
ATP: Adenosine triphosphate.
ADP: Adenosine diphosphate.
AMP: Adenosine monophosphate (adenylic acid).
P_i: Inorganic phosphate.
PP_i: Pyrophosphate.
CoA: Coenzyme A.
CoA-SH: Reduced coenzyme A.
NAD: Nicotinamide adenine nucleotide (formerly DPN).
NADH: Reduced nicotinamide adenine nucleotide (formerly DPNH).
FAD: Flavine adenine dinucleotide.
FFA: Free fatty acids, i.e., not esterified.
Acyl-CoA: Fatty acid esters with CoA.
Acetyl-CoA: Acetate (2-carbon fragment) ester with CoA.
[ ]: Concentration; e.g., $[K^+]$ = potassium concentration.
$[ ]_o$: Concentration outside the cell (serum concentration).
$[ ]_i$: Concentration inside the cell.
EGTA: Ethylene glycol bis (β-amino ethyl ether)-N,N^1-tetraacetic acid, a chelator of Ca^{2+}.
Ⓘ: First heart sound.
ⒾⒾ : Second heart sound.
ⒾⒾ Ⓘ : Third heart sound.
Ⓐ : Atrial heart sound.

1

Structure and Function of Cardiac Muscle

It has been shown by reason and experiment that blood by the beat of the ventricles flows through the lungs and heart and is pumped to the whole body . . . the blood in the animal body moves around in a circle continuously, and . . . the action or function of the heart is to accomplish this by pumping. This is the only reason for the motion and beat of the heart.

William Harvey
Exercitatio Anatomica de Moto Cordis et Sanguinis in Animalibus, 1628

The heart, by virtue of the contractile activity of its muscular walls, propels blood throughout the body so as to deliver nutrients to and remove wastes from each of the organs. The heart also provides for the transport of hormones and other regulatory substances between various regions of the body. All these transport functions are made possible by the fact that the heart is a hollow muscular pump that is provided with valves and so is able to move blood "around in a circle continuously."

In both structure and function, cardiac muscle is much more complex than skeletal muscle. Control of the contractile properties of the myocardium, for example, is quite different from the mechanisms which regulate contractile performance in skeletal muscle. In the latter, each fiber contracts in a relatively stereotyped manner when stimuli reach the muscle via motoneurons from the central nervous system (CNS). The cardiac muscle cells, on the other hand, contain a complex control system which is able to modulate the pumping action of the heart to meet the constantly changing demands of the body. Furthermore, the excitatory impulse that activates the myocardium is neither initiated by nor conducted through nervous tissue. Instead, specialized muscle cells in the heart initiate an action potential which is then propagated to all regions of the myocardium by other muscle cells that are specialized for conduction. The innervation of the heart does not participate directly in either the initiation or the propagation of the stimulus to contractile activity in the heart. Instead, the nerves supplying the heart play only a modulatory role, serving to increase or decrease various aspects of cardiac function.

GROSS STRUCTURE

The heart is divided into four pumping chambers: the *right* and *left atria* and the *right* and *left ventricles* (Fig. 1.1). Between the cavities of the atria and

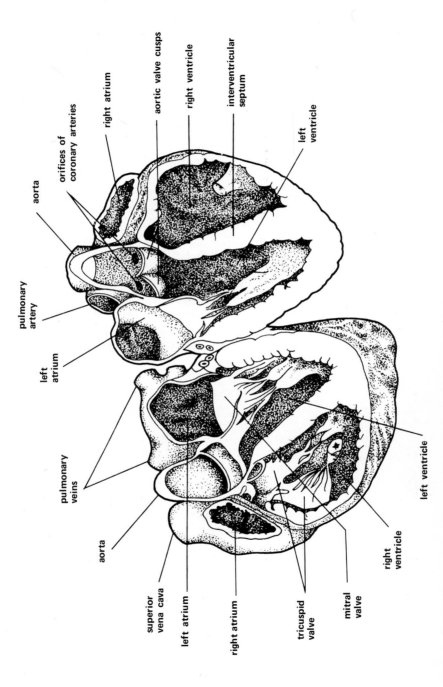

FIG. 1.1. The heart transected slightly anterior to its midline. Note the more elongated left ventricle, which has thicker walls than the right ventricle. (Modified from Berne and Levy: *Cardiovascular Physiology*, 1967. Mosby, St Louis.)

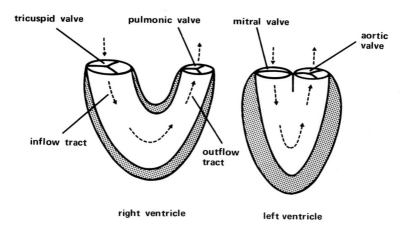

ANTERIOR VIEW

FIG. 1.2. Right and left ventricular chambers, showing the more "tubular" right ventricular pump and the narrower pumping chamber of the left ventricle.

ventricles lie the *atrioventricular valves:* on the right the *tricuspid valve,* and on the left the *mitral* or *bicuspid valve.* Between the outflow tracts of each ventricle and the great arteries to which they give rise are the *semilunar valves:* between the right ventricle and pulmonary artery lies the *pulmonic valve,* and between the left ventricle and aorta lies the *aortic valve.*

Both atria are thin-walled muscular chambers. The thinness of their walls reflects the low pressures normally developed in the atrial cavities. The ventricles, on the other hand, have thick muscular walls—especially the left ventricle, which has approximately three times the mass and twice the thickness of the right ventricle. The cavity of the left ventricle resembles an elongated cone in which both the inflow and outflow tracts are placed adjacent to each other at the wider end (Fig. 1.2). The right ventricle, in contrast, is crescentic in cross section, and its inflow and outflow tracts are separated so that the right ventricular cavity forms a shallow U (Fig. 1.2). The inner surfaces of both the atria and ventricles are lined with connective tissue, the *endocardium,* which also covers the valves. Over the outer surface of the heart lies another layer of connective tissue, the *epicardium.*

The *ventricular myocardium,* which lies between epicardium and endocardium, consists of a series of overlapping sheets of muscle bundles which arise from the fibrous base of the heart (Fig. 1.3). These sheets of myocardium, which follow spiral paths as they sweep from the base of the heart to its apex, can be considered to represent a series of "bulbospiral" and "sinuspiral" muscles. As one examines the epicardial surface of the left ventricle, the muscle fibers tend to be oriented perpendicularly to the base-apex axis of the heart, whereas at the endocardial surface the muscle fibers tend to be more circumferentially oriented (Fig. 1.4).

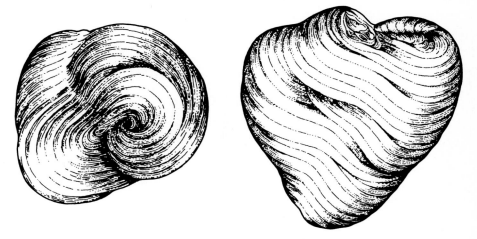

FIG. 1.3. Spiral musculature of the ventricular walls. These helical muscle bundles have been classified as bulbospiral and sinuspiral muscles.

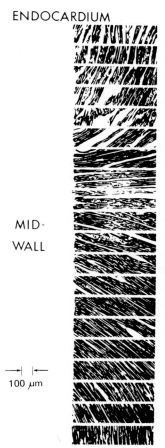

ENDOCARDIUM

MID-
WALL

100 μm

EPICARDIUM

FIG. 1.4. Reconstruction of the left ventricular wall, prepared from a series of microphotographs, showing changing fiber angles at different depths. Compare with Fig. 1.3 to obtain a concept of nonparallel forces generated during systole. (From Streeter et al.: *Circ. Res.*, 24:339, 1969, by permission of the American Heart Association.)

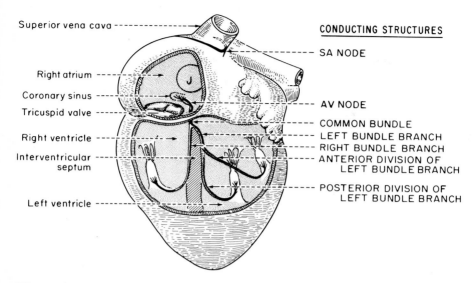

Superior vena cava

Right atrium

Coronary sinus

Tricuspid valve

Right ventricle

Interventricular septum

Left ventricle

CONDUCTING STRUCTURES

SA NODE

AV NODE

COMMON BUNDLE
LEFT BUNDLE BRANCH
RIGHT BUNDLE BRANCH
ANTERIOR DIVISION OF
 LEFT BUNDLE BRANCH

POSTERIOR DIVISION OF
 LEFT BUNDLE BRANCH

FIG. 1.5. Conducting system of the human heart, showing anatomical features of the heart *(labels at left)* and the conducting structures *(labels at right)*. (Modified from Benninghoff: *Lehrbuch der Anatomie des Menschen,* 1944. J. F. Lehmanns Verlag, Munich.)

Activation of the heart normally begins in the *sinoatrial (SA) node* (Fig. 1.5), which lies in the sulcus between the superior vena cava and the right atrium. The pacemaker cells of the SA node normally initiate the wave of depolarization that is propagated through the myocardium to excite all the rest of the heart. For this reason, the SA node is recognized as the primary cardiac pacemaker. Because of the proximity of the SA node to the atria, the first structures to contract in the normal activation sequence of heart are the atria. After a delay, due to the slow passage of the wave of depolarization from atria to ventricles by way of slowly conducting tissue of the *atrioventricular (AV) node,* the wave of electrical activation reaches the ventricles via the *atrioventricular bundle (bundle of His)* and its divisions, the *right* and *left bundle branches.* These structures then ramify, giving rise to an endocardial network of *Purkinje fibers,* specialized conduction tissue that carries the electrical impulses to all portions of the ventricular myocardium. Additional details of the anatomy of the conduction system of the ventricles and the physiology of these activation processes are in Chapter 15.

The blood supply of the heart arises from the *right* and *left coronary arteries* and their branches, which course over the epicardial surface of the heart (Fig. 1.6). Nutrient blood flow reaches the myocardium by way of small arteries which enter the walls of the ventricles at right angles to the larger arteries at the epicardial surface (Fig. 1.7). The venous effluent from the ventricles is collected in small intramyocardial veins, which carry venous blood to the larger veins that parallel the coronary arteries on the epicardial surface of the heart. A very small portion of the endocardial surface of the ventricles is nourished by blood passing

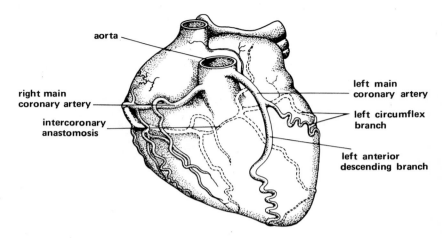

FIG. 1.6. The major coronary arteries.

into the myocardium from the ventricular cavity via *arterioluminal vessels.* Most of the venous drainage from the left ventricle reaches the right atrium by way of the *coronary sinus,* which enters the posterior wall of the right atrium immediately above the tricuspid valve. A smaller portion of this venous drainage, including much of that derived from the right ventricle, reaches the right atrium and

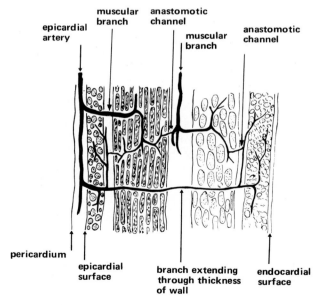

FIG. 1.7. Distribution of the coronary arteries which enter the myocardium from the epicardial surface *(left)* and reach the endocardium *(right)* after penetrating the various layers of muscle bundles. (Modified from Lowe: *Am. Heart J.,* 21:326, 1941.)

right ventricle by way of the *anterior cardiac veins.* A small fraction of the venous drainage of the ventricular myocardium drains directly into the cavities of the right and left ventricles by way of *Thebesian veins.*

The heart is *innervated* by both sympathetic and parasympathetic fibers. The former arise mainly from the fourth and fifth segments of the thoracic spinal cord and reach the heart by way of synaptic connections in the cervical and thoracic cervical ganglia and cardiac plexus. Sympathetic fibers are distributed to all regions of the heart. No specialized sympathetic nerve endings have been identified in the heart; instead, these nerves terminate in depressions in the sarcolemma of the cells they innervate. The parasympathetic innervation of the heart originates in the medulla oblongata, where parasympathetic fibers arising in the vagal nuclei reach the heart by the cardiac branches of the vagus nerve. Parasympathetic nerves impinge on ganglion cells located mainly within the heart. The parasympathetic innervation of the heart supplies mainly the SA and AV nodes and the atria. Some parasympathetic fibers innervate the ventricular blood vessels, and there is functional evidence for limited parasympathetic innervation of the ventricular myocardium.

MICROSCOPIC STRUCTURE

Several cell types are found within the myocardium, all of which represent functionally specialized striated muscle cells (Fig. 1.8). Most important are the *working myocardial cells* of the atria and ventricles, which are specialized for contraction: the *Purkinje fibers,* which effect rapid conduction of the electrical impulse through the heart; and the *nodal cells* of the SA and AV nodes, which are responsible for pacemaker activity and atrioventricular impulse conduction, respectively.

The cells of the *working myocardium* (Fig. 1.8A) stain darkly and are filled with cross-striated myofibers. The cells of the atria are smaller in diameter than those of the ventricles. These cells usually contain a single centrally located nucleus. The *Purkinje fibers* (Fig. 1.8B) are large, pale cells containing more glycogen and many fewer contractile filaments than the cells of the working myocardium, while the SA (Fig. 1.8C) and AV nodes (Fig. 1.8D) are made up of small, glycogen-rich *nodal cells,* which, like the Purkinje fibers, contain very few contractile filaments. There are, in addition, cells in the atria and ventricles that are intermediate in appearance between the Purkinje fibers and the ordinary working myocardial cells. These are often called "transition cells" (Fig. 1.8E). In the ventricle, transition cells are found where the Purkinje network communicates with the myocardium. Similar cells are also found in the atria, where they are scattered in a pattern that may account for preferential conduction pathways (the "internodal tracts"; Chapter 15).

All of these cell types make up a branched network that for many years was thought to represent a true anatomical syncytium. However, the *intercalated discs,* which are densely staining transverse bands that characteristically appear

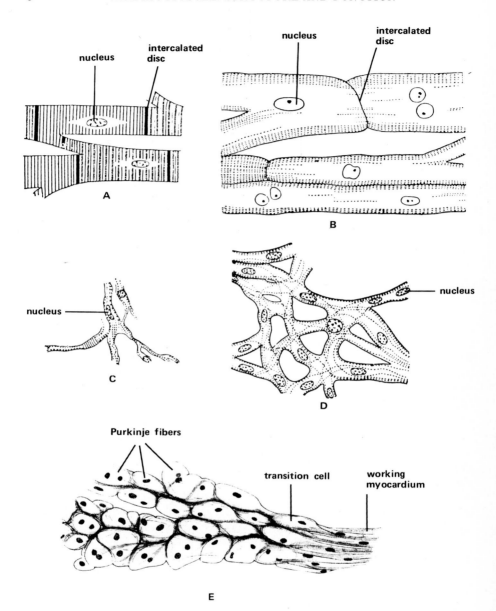

FIG. 1.8. Cells comprising the human heart. **A:** Working myocardial cell of the ventricle, showing intensely staining cross striations, central nuclei, and intercalated discs. **B:** Purkinje fiber, showing large, faintly staining cells with sparse cross striation. **C:** SA node. **D:** AV node. Both nodes have a network of small, sparsely cross-striated cells. **E:** Point of impingement of Purkinje fibers *(left)* on the working myocardium *(right),* showing transition cells. The scale for **E** is about half that of **A–D.** (Modified from Benninghoff: *Lehrbuch der Anatomie des Menschen,* 1944. J. F. Lehmanns Verlag, Munich.)

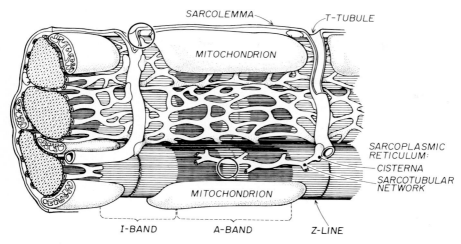

SARCOLEMMA

T-TUBULE

MITOCHONDRION

SARCOPLASMIC
RETICULUM:
–CISTERNA
SARCOTUBULAR
NETWORK

MITOCHONDRION

I-BAND   A-BAND   Z-LINE

FIG. 1.9. Ultrastructure of the working myocardial cell. Contractile proteins are arranged in a regular array of thick and thin filaments (seen in cross section at the left). The A-band represents the region of the sarcomere occupied by the thick filaments into which thin filaments extend from either side. The I-band is the region of the sarcomere occupied only by thin filaments; these extend toward the center of the sarcomere from the Z-lines, which bisect each I-band. The sarcomere, the functional unit of the contractile apparatus, is the region between each pair of Z-lines; it contains two half I-bands and one A-band. The sarcoplasmic reticulum, a membrane network that surrounds the contractile proteins, consists of the sarcotubular network at the center of the sarcomere and the cisternae, which abut on the t-tubules and the sarcolemma. The transverse tubular system (t-tubule) is lined by a membrane that extends from the sarcolemma and carries the extracellular space into the myocardial cell. In contrast to the t-tubules of skeletal muscle, those of the myocardium can run in a longitudinal as well as a transverse direction. Mitochondria are shown in the central sarcomere and in cross section at the left. (From Katz: *N. Engl. J. Med.,* 293:1184, 1975.)

at right angles to the long axis of the cardiac myofibers, are now known to represent true cell-cell junctions. With the recognition that the intercalated discs delimit individual cardiac muscle cells, the concept of the myocardium as a true anatomical syncytium became untenable. Because these discs represent regions of low electrical resistance, however, the heart can be considered to be a syncytium from a functional, although not an anatomical, standpoint (Chapter 15).

ULTRASTRUCTURE

The cells of the working myocardium (Fig. 1.9) contain large numbers of *myofibrils* and *mitochondria* (Fig. 1.10). In addition to the *sarcolemma,* which delimits the cell contents, these cells contain two distinct intracellular membrane systems: the *transverse tubular system* (t-system) and the *sarcoplasmic reticulum.* Together these structures occupy almost 90% of the myocardial cell volume, the remainder consisting mainly of the cytosol and nuclei (Table 1.1).

The cells of the heart's conduction system have a relatively larger amount of cytoplasm that contains many fewer mitochondria and myofibrils. This tissue,

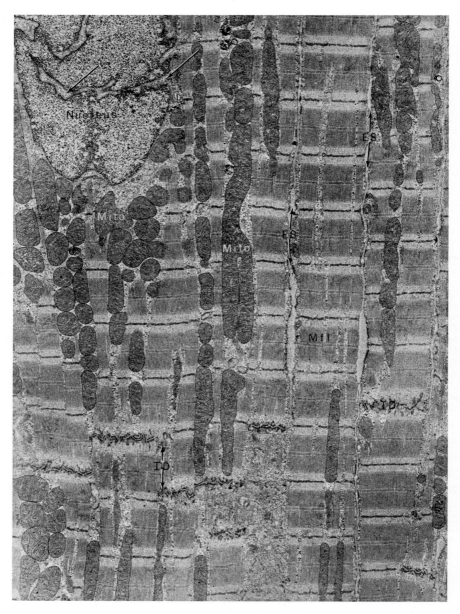

FIG. 1.10. Electron microphotograph of working myocardial cells of the cat, showing the nucleus (*arrows,* invagination of nuclear envelope), myofibrils (Mfl), and mitochondria (Mito), the latter occupying approximately 40% of the cell volume. The sarcolemma lies immediately adjacent to the extracellular space (ES) and merges with the intercalated discs (ID), which represent a specialized cell-cell junction. (From McNutt and Fawcett: In: *The Mammalian Myocardium,* 1974, edited by Langer and Brady. Wiley, New York.)

TABLE 1.1. *Composition of the working myocardium*

Organelle	Percent of cell volume
Myofibrils	48
Mitochondria	36
t-System	1
Sarcoplasmic reticulum	
Subsarcolemmal cisternae	0.35
Sarcotubular network	0.15
Other (cytosol, nuclei, etc.)	14

From Page and McCallister: *Am. J. Cardiol.,* 31:172–181, 1973.

which from a biochemical standpoint is adapted more for anaerobic than oxidative metabolism (Chapter 2), has only 10% of its volume occupied by mitochondria. The fact that the contractile activity of the conduction tissue is much less than in the working myocardium is reflected in the low content of myofibrils, which occupy approximately 20% of the cell volume.

The myofibrils of the working myocardium, like those of mammalian skeletal muscle, are striated and exhibit a characteristic repeating pattern of light and dark transverse bands (Fig. 1.11). When viewed through crossed polaroids, the more darkly staining bands are brightly illuminated; i.e., they rotate the polarized light and so are birefringent. These birefringent bands are thus *anisotropic*—hence their designation *A-bands.* The ability of the A-bands to rotate polarized light indicates that they contain a highly ordered parallel array of macromolecules. The more lightly staining of the striations are less birefringent and so are named *I-bands* because of their more isotropic nature. Each I-band is bisected by a narrow, darkly staining *Z-line;* and a broad, dense *M-band* is found in the center

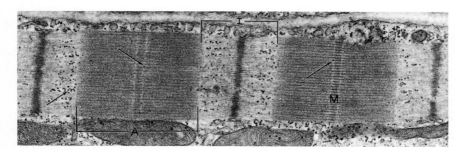

FIG. 1.11. Longitudinal section of a myofiber of cat atrial myocardium, showing the characteristic cross striations. Closely arrayed thick filaments make up the A-band (A) in the center of which is a region of increased electron density, the M-band (M). Very thin filaments running transversely to the long axis of the myofiber are visible in the region of the M-band. The I-band (I) is made up of the thin filaments and is bisected by the Z-line. Glycogen granules are present in the cytoplasm and between the myofilaments *(arrows),* while mitochondria are seen below. (From McNutt and Fawcett: In: *The Mammalian Myocardium,* 1974, edited by Langer and Brady. Wiley, New York.)

FIG. 1.12. Cross section of myofilaments at different levels of the sarcomere. **A:** The A-band, where thin filaments lie at the trigonal points in the hexagonal array of thick filaments. **I:** The I-band, where thick filaments are absent and the thin filaments are less highly ordered. **M:** The M-band in the middle of the thick filament, where thin radial filaments connect adjacent thick filaments.

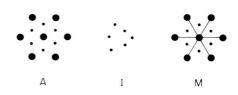

A   I   M

of the A-band. The sarcomere, the fundamental morphological unit of striated muscle, is defined as the region between two Z-lines and thus consists of a single A-band plus the two adjacent half I-bands (Fig. 1.9).

The elaboration of the filamentous nature of the sarcomere and the sliding filament model of muscular contraction during the mid-1950s by H. E. Huxley and Hanson was one of the most elegant electron microscopic studies of muscle. These investigators demonstrated that the cross striations of vertebrate skeletal muscle arise from the characteristic way in which the contractile proteins are organized into *thick* and *thin filaments.* The *thick filaments,* which are composed largely of the protein *myosin,* extend throughout the length of the A-band to which they contribute both its darkly staining characteristics and high birefringence. The two half I-bands at either side of the A-band contain *thin filaments,* which extend into the A-band in the center of the sarcomere from their origin in the Z-lines. The thin filaments are composed largely of *actin* but also contain the regulatory proteins *tropomyosin* and *troponin.*

The lightly staining I-band is occupied only by thin filaments, whereas the A-band contains not only thick filaments but also the ends of the thin filaments, which extend toward the center of the A-band. The extent to which the thin filaments overlap the thick filaments depends on the length of the sarcomere, which in turn is determined by the length of the muscle. As a result, the degree of overlapping between the thin and thick filaments in the central portion of the sarcomere is variable. At physiological sarcomere lengths in cardiac muscle, the thin filaments extend almost to the center of the A-band (Chapter 8). In cross section the A-band contains a hexagonal array of thick filaments, each of which is surrounded by six thin filaments which lie at the trigonal points between adjacent thick filaments (Fig. 1.12). In the I-band, on the other hand, only the thin filaments are seen. Here the array of thin filaments is less orderly than in the A-band. In cross section the M-band (at the center of the A-band) contains thick filaments held together in a hexagonal array of radial cross links. These structures, as seen in a cross section of the myocardial cell, are shown in Fig. 1.13.

The structure of the Z-line remains incompletely understood. It is clear that the thin filaments are interconnected at the Z-line, but the means by which these connections are established remains in dispute. One attractive hypothesis is that each of the two strands of actin, the protein which makes up the backbone of the thin filaments, becomes separated from its partner and loops through the

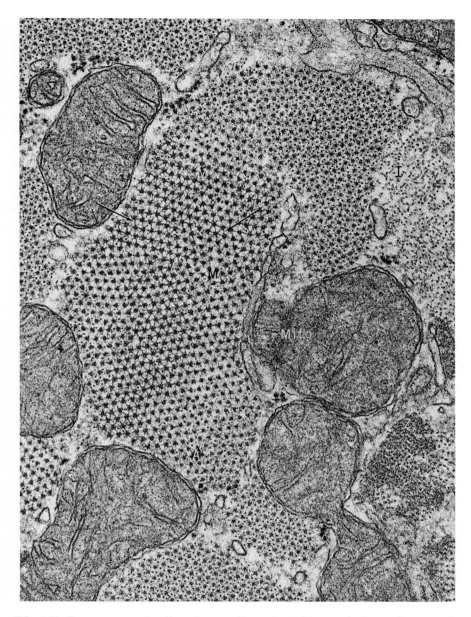

FIG. 1.13. Transverse section through a myofiber of cat right ventricular papillary muscle, showing mitochondria (Mito) and myofilaments cut at the level of the M-band (M), A-band (A), and I-band (I). Arrows point to the radial filaments between the thick filaments in the center of the A-band. Compare with Fig. 1.12. Also shown is the Z-line (Z, *lower right*), which appears as a dense meshwork. (From McNutt and Fawcett: In: *The Mammalian Myocardium,* 1974, edited by Langer and Brady. Wiley, New York.)

Z-line to return to the center of the sarcomere in one of the adjacent thin filaments.

The sliding filament hypothesis of muscular contraction is based on the observation that as a muscle shortens the lengths of both the thick and thin filaments remain constant. Thus as sarcomere length decreases, the I-bands become narrower while the widths of the A-bands remain constant (Chapter 8). This finding, which was predicted from X-ray diffraction studies by H. E. Huxley and subsequently confirmed by electron microscopic findings, effectively disproved the earlier view that muscular contraction was produced by the folding of the large macromolecules. Instead, sarcomere shortening occurs when the thin filaments "slide" by the thick filaments. During contraction the thin filaments are pulled toward the center of the sarcomere, causing the I-band to narrow without changing the length of either the thick or thin filaments. This contractile process is believed to be effected by the *cross-bridges,* which project from the thick filaments to establish links with adjacent thin filaments (Fig. 1.14). Motion of the cross-bridges, which resembles the rowing motion of the oars of a racing shell, may sweep the thin filament toward the center of the sarcomere, thereby causing the muscle to contract (Fig. 1.14).

At shorter sarcomere lengths, the thin filaments from the two half I-bands at either side of the sarcomere can pass through the M-line, giving rise to a so-called "double overlap." The significance of the double overlap between thick and thin filaments arises from the finding that in each of the two halves of the sarcomere both the thick and thin filaments have an opposite polarity. Thus the thin filament penetrating the A-band from the left side of a sarcomere can interact only with the cross-bridges of the left half of the thick filament to develop tension and to shorten. Similarly, the thin filament that enters the A-band from the right side

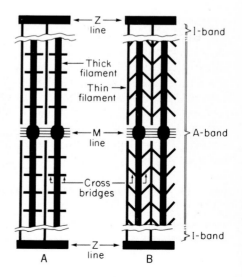

FIG. 1.14. A single sarcomere during diastole **(A)** and systole **(B).** This illustration, based on data from insect flight muscle, shows a shift in cross-bridge orientation that accompanies their attachment to the thin filaments. This shift, which occurs during systole, causes shortening and the development of tension. (Modified from Reedy: *Am. Zool.,* 7:465, 1967.)

can interact only with the right half of the thick filament. Where there is double overlap, therefore, there can be no tension-producing interactions between the portion of the thin filament from the left side of the sarcomere which has passed into the "domain" of the right half of the thick filament, and vice versa (Chapter 8).

The *mitochondria,* which are largely responsible for the aerobic production of chemical energy in the myocardium, are located immediately adjacent to the myofilaments (Fig. 1.10). Mitochondria are complex membranous structures that contain the enzymes responsible for oxidative phosphorylation (Chapter 4). The surface of the inner mitochondrial membrane is markedly increased by a series of infoldings, the *cristae.* The electron microscopic configuration of the cristae is now recognized to be determined by the functional state of the mitochondria at the time the muscle is fixed for electron microscopy. If the cells are fixed under conditions which do not allow active oxidative phosphorylation (e.g., low oxygen tension or low substrate concentration), the cristae appear as stacks of flat membrane sheets. If the mitochondria are actively performing oxidative phosphorylation at the time of fixation, the cristae are angulated and often form a network, giving rise to the so-called "energized" configuration. Phase contrast studies of living cardiac muscle have shown that the shape of the mitochondria is constantly changing: These structures can enlarge or contract, as well as branch or fuse with each other. The volume of the myocardial cell occupied by the mitochondria is correlated with the rate of energy utilization, being greatest in rapidly beating hearts and less in larger mammals with slower heart rates.

The myocardial cell is enclosed by the *sarcolemma,* a membrane which defines the boundary between intra- and extracellular spaces (Fig. 1.10). Portions of the extracellular space, however, are carried into the interior of the cell within the *transverse tubular* or *t-system.* The t-system, which in the myocardium not only extends in a transverse direction but also can turn and run longitudinally between adjacent sarcomeres (Fig. 1.9), opens freely to the extracellular space as evidenced by the ready penetration of large molecules such as ferritin into the space enclosed by the t-system. The t-system is much larger in diameter in mammalian cardiac muscle than in skeletal muscle, and the points at which the tubules open through the sarcolemma into the extracellular space are clearly seen. The sarcolemma and the membranes of the t-system act as a barrier that permits maintenance of an intracellular environment which is different from that of the extracellular fluid. In addition, these membranes contain ion pumps that establish a number of important chemical and charge differences between the intra- and extracellular environments (Chapter 9), as well as a number of ionic channels which effect transient changes in membrane potential (Chapter 14). Several regulatory enzymes, such as that which synthesizes cyclic AMP, are also present on the sarcolemma and possibly on the membranes of the t-system.

It is important to recognize that the "static" image of the sarcolemma of fixed and stained cells, such as is illustrated in Fig. 1.10, is probably an oversimplification of the dynamic state of this membrane in the living myocardium. Motion pictures of the living sarcolemma demonstrate hectic activity, including rapid motion by pinocytotic vesicles that traverse the cell membrane. Thus even though subsequent discussions of ion selective channels and ion pumps focus on fluxes across a fixed membrane, it must not be forgotten that the dynamic state of these membranes allows for other mechanisms by which substances can be transferred between the intra- and extracellular environments.

In addition to the sarcolemma and the membranes of the t-system, which define the limits of the intracellular space, other intracellular membrane systems divide the cell interior into separate regions or "compartments." One of these is represented by the mitochondria, which have already been mentioned in terms of their ability to carry out aerobic energy production. The functional significance of the intramitochondrial compartment, the ionic composition of which is different from that of the remainder of the cytosol, is probably related to the ability of the mitochondrial membrane to transduce the energy made available when ions move along their electrochemical gradients into the synthesis of adenosine triphosphate (ATP) (Chapter 4). In this way the osmotic energy potentially available from the concentration differences of ions between the intramitochondrial compartment and the remainder of the cytosol can be converted to chemical energy. This energy then becomes available, as ATP, for metabolic processes elsewhere in the cell (Chapter 2). Most other intracellular membranes, however, are like the sarcolemma in that they effect the opposite process; i.e., they utilize the chemical energy of ATP for the active transport of substances, including ions, against an electrochemical gradient.

The *sarcoplasmic reticulum* is a system of intracellular membranes that contains two morphologically distinct membrane systems. In a small portion of these membranes, the *rough sarcoplasmic reticulum,* the outer surface is studded with ribosomes. It is probable that, like the endoplasmic reticulum of other cells, the rough sarcoplasmic reticulum is involved primarily in protein synthesis. By far the majority of the sarcoplasmic reticulum lacks ribosomes and so is smooth in appearance. Unlike the rough sarcoplasmic reticulum, the *smooth sarcoplasmic reticulum* does not participate in protein synthesis; instead, it plays a major role in controlling the fluxes of ions, especially of calcium, within the myocardium.

The *smooth sarcoplasmic reticulum* (which is designated simply *sarcoplasmic reticulum* in the remainder of this text) consists of a network of intracellular tubules called the *sarcotubular network* that surrounds the bundles of contractile proteins. (Figs. 1.9 and 1.15). The sarcoplasmic reticulum forms specialized structures where it comes in contact with the sarcolemma and t-system. Here the tubules of the sarcoplasmic reticulum flatten to form the *subsarcolemmal cisternae* (Fig. 1.9). The latter, which represent functionally specialized regions of the sarcoplasmic reticulum, are analogous to the terminal cisternae of skeletal muscle. The term "subsarcolemmal cisternae" is to some extent a misnomer in that these structures are found adjacent to the membranes of the t-system as well as the sarcolemma. However, if one remembers that the composition of the fluid within the t-tubule is probably similar to that in the extracellular space, the subsarcolemmal cisternae can be considered to have similar functions in both

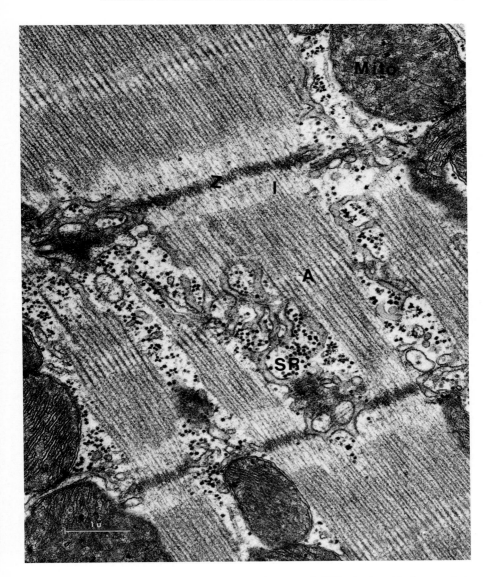

FIG. 1.15. Electron micrograph showing sarcotubular network (SR) of rat ventricular muscle in a "grazing" section over the sarcomeres *(center)*. The dark granules near this structure are glycogen. Mito, mitochondria. A, A-band. I, I-band. Z, Z-line. Scale = 1 μm. (Courtesy of Mrs. Judy Upshaw-Early and Dr. Ernest Page.)

locations. The composite structure formed by the subsarcolemmal cisternae and the adjacent region of either the sarcolemma or t-tubule is called the *dyad* (Fig. 1.16). The membranes of the sarcoplasmic reticulum approach those of either the sarcolemma or t-system, but the two membranes neither fuse nor establish intimate contact. Instead, a narrow space remains between these membranes that

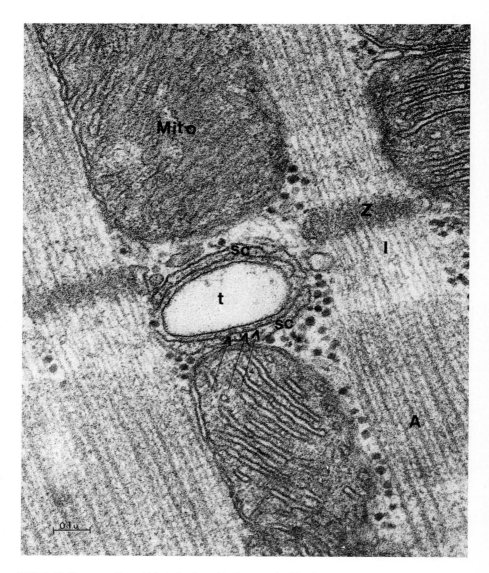

FIG. 1.16. Cross section of triad of rat ventricular muscle. The large central structure represents a portion of the transverse tubular system (t) surrounded by two subsarcolemmal cisternae (sc), each of which partially envelops the transverse tubule. The membrane of the subsarcolemmal cisterna fails to establish intimate contact with that of the t-tubule; instead, electron-dense "foot processes" lie between these two membranes *(arrows)*. Mito, mitochondria. A, A-band. I, I-band. Z, Z-line. Scale = 0.1 μm. (Courtesy of Mrs. Judy Upshaw-Early and Dr. Ernest Page.)

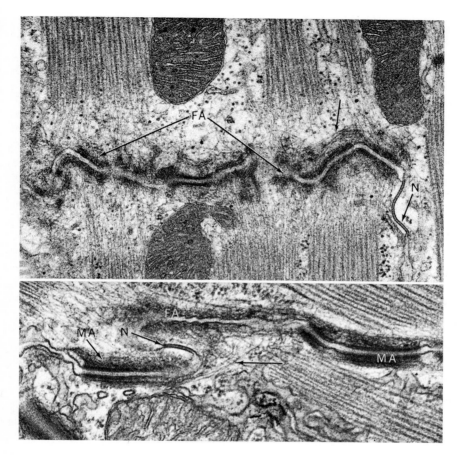

FIG. 1.17. Electron micrographs of the intercalated disc. **Top:** Transverse section in cat ventricular myocardium, showing insertion of thin filaments into filamentous mats *(arrows)*, which bind to the intercalated disc to form the fascia adherens (FA). This intracellular junction changes form at the right of the figure, where the two cells come into contact at a nexus or "gap" junction (N). **Bottom:** Oblique section of intercalated disc in mouse ventricular myocardium, showing filaments *(arrow)* joining fascia adherens (FA) and a nexus (N). In addition, two maculae adherens (MA), or desmosomes, are shown. All of these structures represent specialized cell-cell junctions. (From McNutt and Fawcett: In: *The Mammalian Myocardium,* 1974, edited by Langer and Brady. Wiley, New York.)

contain electron-dense material called "foot processes." This space, and the foot processes that it contains, appear to play an important, although not yet fully understood, role in the initiation of contraction in the heart.

The *intercalated disc* (Fig. 1.17), as stated earlier, represents a specialized region made up of the sarcolemmae of adjacent cells and thus constitutes a true cell–cell junction. Three types of specialized areas are found along the intercalated disc: *fascia adherens, macula densa,* and *nexus.* The *fascia adherens,* which is the predominant form of the intercalated disc, is made up of the two plasma membranes which parallel each other, separated by a distance of 200–300 Å. Extensions from the thin filaments of the myofibrils appear to bind tightly to the plasma membrane at either side of the fascia adherens in a manner similar to their interweaving at the Z-line. The *macula densa,* or *desmosome,* represents a more complex, almost laminated structure made up of the two plasma membranes. The *nexus,* or *gap junction,* is a region of close contact between the plasma membranes of adjacent cells that is freely permeable to many ions. It is this latter structure, with its high ionic permeability, that accounts for the low electrical resistance of the intercalated disc. A regular array of particles found between the two membranes of the nexus may represent the ion channels that account for the low electrical resistance and high ionic permeability of the intercalated disc.

CARDIAC CYCLE

The structural characteristics of the heart, and especially the pathway followed by the wave of excitation which activates all regions of the myocardium, underlie the characteristic manner in which event follows event during every heartbeat. Each time the heart contracts, a series of electrical and mechanical events takes place. These in turn govern the flow of blood into and out of the heart. They determine the opening and closing of the cardiac valves and thus account for the characteristic timing of the heart sounds. This sequence of events is also manifest at the body surfaces as changes in electrical potential: the electrocardiogram, which is discussed in Chapter 15. All together, this sequence of events is called the *cardiac cycle.*

The description that follows, including Fig. 1.18, are modified only slightly from the last edition of the late Dr. Carl J. Wiggers' classic text *Physiology in Health and Disease.* This eloquent description and the "Wiggers diagram," once of interest mainly to the basic scientist, are now an integral part of modern cardiology and must be understood fully by all who wish to know the basis for the pumping action of the heart.

The series of superimposed curves which are reproduced in Fig. 1.18 unfold at a glance the story of cardiodynamic events which may be briefly summarized as follows:

At the onset of ventricular systole (I) the pressures are approximately equal in the atrium and ventricle, and the AV valves are in the act of floating into apposition. After the pressure has risen slightly within the ventricle, the AV valves close completely giving rise to the first heart sound [encircled I]. Since the semilunar valves are still closed, the ventricle contracts isovolumically, and the intraventricular pressure rises rapidly (I–II). The abrupt elevation of pressure causes a bulging of both the semilunar and AV valves which accounts for the small positive oscillations in the aorta and atrium during this period. The descent of the ventricular base and the consequent traction on the aorta and atria cause the sharp oscillations—which are not, however, synchronous. The semilunar valves open at II, i.e., when the ventricular pressure exceeds the aortic. As a

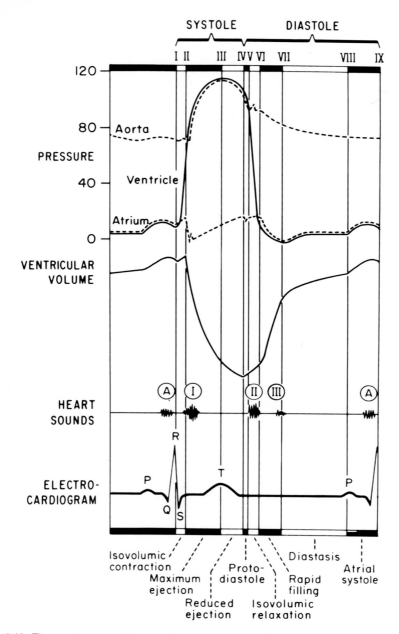

FIG. 1.18. The cardiac cycle (Wiggers diagram), showing nine phases. The top three curves represent the aortic pressure *(dashed line)*, left ventricular pressure *(solid line)*, and left atrial pressure *(dashed line)*. The units of pressure are millimeters of mercury. The middle curve *(solid line)* represents the left ventricular volume, below which is a representation of the heart sounds. These are depicted as phonocardiographically documented vibrations: Ⓐ, atrial sound. ①, first heart sound. ⑪, second heart sound. ⑪⑪, third heart sound. The bottom line represents the ECG with its P, Q, R, S, and T waves.

result, aorta and ventricle become a common cavity, and the two pressure curves follow one another closely.

With the rapid expulsion of blood during early moments of ejection—indicated by volume changes of the ventricles—the pressures in the left ventricle and aorta rise to a summit (III), because the rate at which blood is expelled into the aorta exceeds that at which it flows from its branches through the arterioles. As seen in Fig. 1.18, the rise is rounded (II–III) chiefly because, with rather constant ejection rate, the runoff increases gradually with progressive rise of aortic pressure. The rounded summit (III) is reached when ejection and runoff become equal. Since the rate of ejection diminishes during the latter part of systole (III–IV) while the flow from aortic branches continues high, aortic and ventricular pressures gradually decline. On the basis of pressure curves, it is therefore possible to separate the period of ejection into two phases, viz., maximum ejection (II–III) and reduced ejection (III–IV). Summarizing, the rise and fall of aortic and ventricular pressures always represent a balance between the rate at which blood is ejected into the aorta and the rate at which it leaves by its branches. However, the changes in rate of ventricular ejection normally dominate the shape of the curves during ejection.

At the onset of ventricular diastole (IV), aorta and ventricle are still in communication. The first effect of relaxation consists in a sharp drop in pressure in the ventricle and aorta, the latter being quickly terminated by the closure of the semilunar valves at V, after which a few vibrations occur, and the aortic curve declines very gradually for the remainder of diastole. The closure of the semilunar valves is associated with the second heart sound [encircled II]. The rate of diastolic decline is determined chiefly by the rate at which blood flows out of the aorta, but is affected to a variable extent by the increasing distensibility of arteries at different pressure levels.

Within the ventricle, the decline continues rapidly until VI, at which point the AV valves open, and the phase of isovolumic relaxation terminates. During this phase of ventricular relaxation the intra-atrial pressure usually continues to rise slowly; occasionally, however, a more marked positive elevation occurs, which must be assigned to a compression effect produced by the upward movement of the ventricular base. As soon as intraventricular pressure has declined to a level lower than that in the atrium (VI), the AV valves are opened again by the difference of pressure and a rapid inflow of blood into the ventricle begins. While this continues (VI–VII), pressures in the atrium and ventricle decline together, but the atrial pressure remains a trifle higher than the ventricular. In long cycles this is followed by a diastasis phase (VII–VIII), during which ventricular inflow is exceedingly slow, and the pressure rises very gradually both in the atrium and ventricle. In young normal individuals, and in some pathological states, the rapid inflow of blood into the ventricle is associated with an audible sound, the third heart sound [encircled III]. Occasionally, atrial systole also produces a sound [encircled A] sometimes called the fourth heart sound.

The Phases of the Cardiac Cycle. The succession of atrial and ventricular events constitutes the cardiac cycle. Since ventricular contraction is dynamically the most important it is fitting to start the cycle with this event. Accordingly, the cardiac cycle can be divided advantageously into ventricular systole and diastole, but each of these periods must be further subdivided. For the sake of clarity these subdivisions are designated as phases of systole and diastole. The vertical lines of Fig. 1.18 serve to demarcate the successive periods and phases of systole and diastole. I–IV indicates the period of *systole,* IV–IX the period of *diastole.* The first phase of systole, I–II, is called the *isovolumic contraction phase,* for the ventricle contracts essentially in this manner with all valves closed.

The second phase, II–IV, is best referred to as the *ejection phase*. It can be further subdivided by reference to the aortic pressure curve alone or with the aid of the ventricular volume curve into the phase of *maximum ejection*, II–III, and the phase of *reduced ejection*, III–IV.

The *protodiastolic phase*, IV–V, which constitutes the first interval of diastole, ends with closure of the semilunar valves. It is followed by the *isovolumic relaxation* phase, V–VI, which ends as soon as atrial pressure exceeds that in the ventricle, viz., at VI. With opening of the AV valves at VI, the *rapid filling phase* supervenes, VI–VII, and this is followed by a variable phase of *diastasis*, VII–VIII. Finally, *atrial systole*, VIII–IX, terminates the period of ventricular diastole.

The durations of these successive phases have been repeatedly studied but with varying degrees of accuracy. The average values in seconds (Table 1.2) derived from an analysis of many pressure pulses, are sufficient to give an idea as to the relative duration in man of the most commonly used phases.

TABLE 1.2. *Durations of the phases of the cardiac cycle in adult man*

Isovolumic contraction	0.05
Maximum ejection	0.09
Reduced ejection	0.13
Total systole	0.27
Protodiastole	0.04
Isovolumic relaxation	0.08
Rapid inflow	0.11
Diastasis	0.19
Atrial systole	0.11
Total diastole	0.53

A schematic electrocardiographic recording of the changing electrical potential differences at the body surface and their relation to the cardiac cycle is also shown in Fig. 1.18. As is discussed at length in Chapter 15, the P wave reflects the electrical depolarization of the atria; the QRS complex that of the ventricles. The T wave is produced by potential differences set up within the ventricle during repolarization.

In the chapters that follow, our current understanding of the biochemical and biophysical bases of the mechanical and electrical events that produce the cardiac cycle are described. In these discussions, however, the reader should always keep the "Wiggers diagram" in mind, for this classic view of the electrical and mechanical properties of the heart remains the focal point of modern cardiology. It is hoped that the molecular mechanisms to be described provide a basis for understanding the normal physiology of the pumping action of the heart and facilitate the understanding of newer findings regarding the causation and therapy of some of the many forms of clinical heart disease.

BIBLIOGRAPHY

Gregg, D., and Fischer, L. C. (1963): Blood supply to the heart. In: *Handbook of Physiology*, Vol. II, pp. 1517–1584. American Physiological Society, Washington, D.C.

Hawthorne, E. W., et al. (1969): Physiology Society symposium: Dynamic geometry of the left ventricle. *Fed. Proc.,* 28:1323–1367.

Levy, M. N., et al. (1972): Physiology Society symposium: Neural regulation of the cardiovascular system. *Fed. Proc.,* 31:1197–1252.

McNutt, N. S., and Fawcett, D. W. (1974): Myocardial ultrastructure. In: *The Mammalian Myocardium,* edited by G. A. Langer and A. J. Brady, pp. 1–49. Wiley, New York.

Page, E., and McAllister, L. P. (1973): Quantitative electron-microscopic description of heart muscle cells: Application to normal, hypertrophied and thyroxin-stimulated hearts. *Am. J. Cardiol.,* 31:-172–181.

Streeter, D. D., Spotnitz, H. M., Patel, D. P., Ross, J. Jr., and Sonnenblick, E. H. (1969): Fiber orientation in the canine left ventricle during systole and diastole. *Circ. Res.,* 24:339–347.

Wiggers, C. J. (1949): *Physiology in Health and Disease,* 5th ed. Lea & Febiger, Philadelphia.

2

Energetics of Muscle

The pumping action of the heart results from the contractile activity of its muscular walls, so that for the ventricles to eject blood under pressure into the aorta and pulmonary artery the individual muscle fibers must shorten under load. The product of force times distance, which represents the *work* performed by each element of the myocardium, is a measure of the mechanical energy liberated during systole. According to the First Law of Thermodynamics, energy cannot be created *de novo,* so the mechanical energy that appears during the muscular work of the ventricular walls must be matched by the disappearance of energy elsewhere. In the case of the heart, this energy is lost by utilization of the energy contained in a variety of chemical compounds. Thus like all muscles, the heart can be regarded as a *mechanochemical transducer* in that during contraction chemical energy is transformed into mechanical energy. The present chapter examines the chemical processes responsible for energy production in the heart and their relationship to both the liberation of mechanical energy and the physiological constraints under which the mammalian heart is required to function.

If a strand of muscle is isolated in a closed, insulated box and arranged so that it lifts a load when stimulated (Fig. 2.1), two kinds of energy appear after stimulation: *mechanical energy,* which is equal to the product of the load and

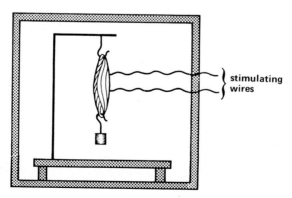

FIG. 2.1. A muscle within an insulated box, the only communication with the outside environment being the two stimulating wires. Delivery of a minute amount of electrical energy causes the muscle to contract. The accompanying appearance of energy, as work and heat, must be matched by the disappearance of chemical energy within the muscle because the sum of the energies within the box must remain constant.

the distance shortened, and *heat.* According to the First Law of Thermodynamics, the sum of all energies in a closed system must remain constant, so that the appearance of energy (as work and as heat) must be matched by the disappearance of energy elsewhere. As already indicated, a loss of *chemical* (or internal) *energy* accompanies muscular contraction, so it is both theoretically and experimentally possible to measure changes in the chemical composition of contracting muscle.

In thermodynamic terminology the change in internal energy during muscle contraction can be defined as $-\Delta E$, which is equal to E_2 (the chemical energy at the end of the contraction) minus E_1 (the chemical energy at the beginning of contraction). One can therefore describe the net change in chemical energy during contraction by the following equation:

$$-\Delta E = E_2 - E_1 \qquad (2.1)$$

The change in external energy, which in a closed system is also ΔE, is the sum of energies liberated as heat *(q)* and as work $(-W)$.[1] Thus the net change in external energy during muscular contraction can be described by the equation:

$$\Delta E = q - W \qquad (2.2)$$

With the use of modern recording and analytical methods, it is possible to measure all the parameters in Eq. (2.1) and (2.2). The terms E_2 and E_1 can be evaluated by chemical determination of the concentrations of key metabolic compounds at the beginning and end of the contractile cycle. The net changes in these concentrations are then multiplied by the enthalpy changes (ΔH) in the chemical reactions to approximate the free energy made available. These enthalpy changes, which represent the heat produced or absorbed during the individual chemical reactions, provide a useful index of the energy changes accompanying each reaction. The relationship between ΔE and ΔH is given by the equation:

$$\Delta E = \Delta H + P\Delta V \qquad (2.3)$$

where P is the pressure at which the reaction takes place and ΔV is the change in volume that accompanies the reaction. Because muscular contraction takes place with little or no volume change, it can be taken that $\Delta E \cong \Delta H$.

More precise estimates for E_2 and E_1 require knowledge of the free energy changes (ΔG) which accompany each chemical reaction. The relationship between ΔH and ΔG is given by the equation:

$$\Delta H = \Delta G + T\Delta S \qquad (2.4)$$

where T is the absolute temperature and ΔS the entropy change, a measurement directly proportional to the "disorder" or randomness of the system at the beginning and end of the reaction. Because of the difficulties in measuring these entropy changes, it is most convenient to relate the change in internal energy ($-\Delta E$) to the enthalpy change ($-\Delta H$), although this evaluation of $-\Delta E$ clearly requires that certain assumptions be made regarding the relationship between changes in metabolite concentration and the energy made available.

---

[1] The use of the negative sign for the work term $(-W)$ is a convention of thermodynamics that can be confusing if the reader is not warned that the conventions of muscle physiology reverse this sign (Chapter 5).

Accurate measurements of heat liberation *(q)* in active muscle have been made possible by the use of the *thermopile,* which is a series of *thermocouples.* Each thermocouple represents a pair of junctions between two dissimilar metals, in which the appearance of a temperature gradient generates a small electrical potential. Finally, the liberation of energy as work $(-W)$ can be calculated by multiplying the force, or load, by the distance over which the muscle shortens. In Chapter 5 we examine Eq. (2.2) to define more precisely the characteristics of energy liberation, and as work and heat; Chapters 3 and 4 focus on the reactions that provide the chemical energy for contraction, i.e., those encompassed by Eq. (2.1).

PROVISION OF CHEMICAL ENERGY FOR MUSCULAR CONTRACTION

It is appropriate here to review how our present understanding grew concerning the provision of chemical energy for muscular contraction; this historical evolution not only facilitates an understanding of this important topic but illustrates some of the pitfalls encountered in scientific investigation. The early observations by Fletcher and Hopkins in 1907 that lactic acid was produced in muscle which went into rigor after death, and the subsequent demonstration that this lactic acid came from glycogen metabolism, led Myerhof during the 1920s to examine the relationship between lactic acid formation and muscular work. Experiments carried out under anaerobic conditions, in which oxidation of lactic acid was blocked, showed that the amount of carbohydrate metabolized was proportional to the work done during muscular contraction. This led to the view that glycolysis, measured as lactic acid formation from glycogen, was directly coupled to muscular contraction by a reaction that could be described as:

$$\text{Glycogen} \longrightarrow \text{lactic acid} + \text{mechanical energy}$$

This attractive formulation, which was consistent with and explained a large body of experimental data, collapsed with the publication of a single, but well-documented observation: that exposure of muscle to iodoacetic acid could stop lactic acid production under conditions where the ability to contract was preserved. Lundsgaard, who reported this observation in 1930, found that in the presence of iodoacetic acid muscular work could take place under conditions where neither glycogen was metabolized nor lactic acid produced. It was soon found, instead, that liberation of mechanical energy by the muscle was accompanied by the breakdown of phosphocreatine, a labile compound of creatine and phosphoric acid. At this time, Eggleton and Eggleton showed that during muscular contraction the decrease in phosphocreatine content was proportional to the work done. It thus seemed reasonable to postulate that energy was provided for muscular contraction by the breakdown of phosphocreatine according to the reaction:

$$\text{Phosphocreatine} \longrightarrow \text{creatine} + P_i + \text{mechanical energy}$$

The energy derived from the metabolism of glycogen to form lactic acid was recognized, therefore, not to provide energy directly to the contractile machinery, but instead to provide for the resynthesis of phosphocreatine from creatine and P_i.

The view that phosphocreatine was the direct source of energy for muscular contraction lasted only a few years. Another substance, discovered independently by Lohman and by Fiske and Subbarow, was found to be synthesized during glycolysis and to release energy on hydrolysis. This substance, the adenine nucleotide *ATP,* was found to be necessary for the hydrolysis of phosphocreatine in that cell-free extracts were unable to catalyze the breakdown of phosphocreatine to form creatine and P_i, and thus to liberate energy, unless adenine nucleotides were present. This function of the adenine nucleotides could be shown to reflect their ability to transfer P_i, and thus chemical energy, from phosphocreatine to a number of energy-consuming reactions. The role of phosphocreatine therefore is to phosphorylate ADP to form ATP, which then can be hydrolyzed to yield ADP, P_i, and energy. The overall reactions that describe the adenine nucleotide requirement for phosphocreatine breakdown can be written:

$$\text{Phosphocreatine} + \text{ADP} \rightleftharpoons \text{creatine} + \text{ATP}$$
$$\text{ATP} \longrightarrow \text{ADP} + P_i$$

These equations explain the finding that phosphocreatine is not itself hydrolyzed to creatine unless compounds like the adenine nucleotides are present.

Since their discovery, the adenine nucleotides have been found to participate in a number of chemical reactions within the cell. In these reactions ADP accepts chemical energy by incorporating P_i to form a high-energy bond in ATP, while ATP is able to donate chemical energy through the hydrolysis of this phosphate bond. This function of ATP has been likened by A. Szent-Györgyi to that of money, ATP being the "chemical currency" of the cell. Thus like money, ATP can be obtained (synthesized) in exchange for the energy derived from a number of different chemical processes (e.g., the metabolism of fats and carbohydrates); and like money, ATP can be used for a variety of energy-consuming processes (e.g., muscular contraction, biosynthesis, membrane transport). In the process of muscular contraction, therefore, it is proposed that ATP carries the chemical energy from phosphocreatine stores, which in this context serve as a reserve of "ready cash." In addition, the energy obtained from intermediary metabolism must first be converted to ATP to provide for the performance of mechanical work by the muscle.

Although ATP has been thought since the mid-1930s to provide the energy for muscular contraction, it was not until the early 1960s that a decrease in ATP concentration could be shown to accompany muscular contraction. Prior to that time, it had been impossible to inhibit selectively the transfer of phosphate from phosphocreatine to ADP, so that all that could be detected to accompany muscular work was a decrease in phosphocreatine. It was not until 1962 that Davies found that fluorodinitrobenzene (Sanger's reagent, an early tool of the protein chemist used to determine the amino acid sequence of insulin) could be used to poison specifically the enzyme creatine phosphokinase, which catalyzes the transfer of P_i from phosphocreatine to ADP. This finding made it possible to demonstrate a proportionality between ATP hydrolysis and muscular work:

$$ATP \longrightarrow ADP + P_i + \text{mechanical energy}$$

Our situation today is different, however, from that of our scientific forebears—who during the 1920s demonstrated the proportionality between lactic acid production from glycogen and the liberation of mechanical energy—because the direct participation of ATP in the chemical processes responsible for contraction has now been shown experimentally (Chapter 6).

GENERATION OF CHEMICAL ENERGY FOR CONTRACTION

The metabolic pathways by which ATP is regenerated are not the same in all types of muscle. With functional specialization, different muscle types have been found to employ different pathways of energy production; and as we shall see, this biochemical specialization is closely related to the functional needs of the individual muscles. In considering these differences, it will be more illuminating if we examine first the physiological requirements of different muscle types and then consider the biochemical specializations and their functional significance. A useful approach is to compare the life habits of two long-eared mammals, the rabbit and the hare [2] (Fig. 2.2).

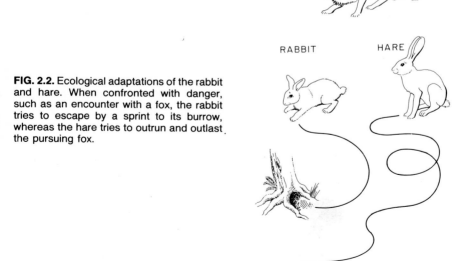

FIG. 2.2. Ecological adaptations of the rabbit and hare. When confronted with danger, such as an encounter with a fox, the rabbit tries to escape by a sprint to its burrow, whereas the hare tries to outrun and outlast the pursuing fox.

RABBIT   HARE

---

[2] The description in the next paragraphs is valid for the European rabbit and hare but not their American counterparts as was first pointed out to the author by a cardiology resident from Texas.

In Europe the *rabbit* lives in a burrow from which it ventures short distances in search of food and adventure. Such animals rely on a sprint to their burrow in order to escape predators, for it is in their ability to accelerate and run rapidly for short distances that they survive in nature. The rabbit is thus an excellent sprinter but a poor distance runner as can be attested to by anyone who has allowed a rabbit to escape in the laboratory. Many species of European *hare,* on the other hand, have no burrow but range widely in their habitat. Such hares are excellent distance runners, relying on their staying power to escape pursuers —indeed the coursing of hares has been known since antiquity.

Early in this century it became clear to scientists, although this information must already have been well known to hunters and cooks, that the muscles used for locomotion by rabbits and hares differ grossly in appearance. Those in the rabbit are pale pink, almost white in color, whereas the back and leg muscles of the hare are deep red. Similar differences in muscle color are found in other vertebrate species; i.e., "white" is generally found where the muscle is called on for short bursts of intense activity, and "red" is present in muscles where activity is sustained. In common culinary experience, for example, the chicken breast, which powers wings that are used only intermittently, is white meat, whereas the dark meat of the chicken leg represents a muscle that is used for the more continuous activity of walking. In birds capable of sustained flight, on the other hand, the breast muscles are "red" (e.g., the dark meat of duck or goose breast).

In the following discussion we focus on these two "extremes" of muscle specialization: red and white. Intermediate fiber types exist, and there are exceptions to the general patterns described below, but for the sake of clarity these are not considered further in this attempt to describe the means by which Nature can adapt biochemical specialization to meet the physiological needs of the organism.

BIOCHEMICAL DIFFERENCES BETWEEN RED AND WHITE MUSCLE

In *red muscle* (Table 2.1), which is specialized for sustained activity without rest periods, it is essential that the rate of energy production not exceed that of energy utilization. In these muscles therefore, ATP is produced in large quantities

TABLE 2.1. *Biochemical differences between red and white muscle*

Biochemical characteristic	Red muscle	White muscle
Pathways of energy production	Aerobic	Anaerobic
Substrates	Lipid, carbohydrate	Carbohydrate
Metabolites	CO_2, H_2O	Lactic acid
Glycolytic enzymes	Sparse	Abundant
Mitochondria	Abundant	Sparse
Phosphocreatine stores	Minor	Significant
Dependence on oxygen	Marked	Little
Intrinsic ATPase of contractile proteins	Low	High

by the efficient pathways of oxidative metabolism. The red color of these muscles is due largely to a high myoglobin content, which serves to facilitate the diffusion of oxygen through the muscle fibers. The most important substrates for aerobic energy production are lipids, although carbohydrates including lactate are oxidized when delivered in appropriate concentrations via the arterial blood supply (Chapter 4). Red muscles are capable of carrying out anaerobic glycolysis (Chapter 3) and have some high-energy phosphate (phosphocreatine) reserves, but these factors are of lesser functional significance in that neither can provide the large amounts of ATP needed for sustained contraction. Thus if aerobic ATP production is brought to a halt (e.g., when blood flow is interrupted, or under conditions of anoxia), the phosphocreatine stores are quickly exhausted. Acceleration of glycolysis can provide only a very limited increase in the rate of ATP production. Furthermore, under anaerobic conditions the increased production of lactate is accompanied by hydrogen ion liberation, so that a state of intracellular acidosis develops which inhibits key regulatory enzymes that control the rate of glycolysis. For this reason accelerated glycolysis is not only limited in its ability to generate ATP under anaerobic conditions, it is also transient and cannot be sustained, especially when the anaerobic state results from interrupted blood flow to the muscle (Chapter 22).

The apparent luxury of a high rate of ATP production in red muscle is not without cost to the muscle. The price that such a muscle must pay is threefold: First, the muscle becomes absolutely dependent on an uninterrupted supply of oxygen without which ATP cannot be generated for contraction. Second, these muscles must contain large numbers of bulky mitochondria that occupy space otherwise available for the contractile machinery. This, as we shall see (Chapter 9), makes the muscle intrinsically weaker. The third price for this biochemical specialization is that the intrinsic rate of ATP hydrolysis by the contractile proteins is generally lower than that of the contractile proteins of white muscle. This low intrinsic rate of chemical energy utilization aids in maintaining a balance between energy utilization and energy production. While not all red muscles contain low ATPase contractile proteins, where this adaption is found the intrinsic speed of shortening is reduced and muscular contractility is lessened (Chapter 7).

In *white muscle* (Table 2.1), where specialization is for brief but intense activity, periods of rest allow the rate of energy expenditure temporarily to exceed that of energy production. Thus there is no need for these muscles to be provided with the highly efficient mechanisms of oxidative metabolism. Instead, the volume of muscle otherwise needed for mitochondria is occupied by contractile proteins, thereby adding to the strength of the muscle. During their brief bursts of activity, white muscles utilize primarily energy stored as phosphocreatine and the limited supply of energy available from anaerobic glycolysis. The lactate produced during activity is oxidized largely during the periods of rest, either within the muscle or in the liver to which lactate is transported by the circulation. This delayed requirement for oxidative metabolism of lactate represents an "oxygen debt," in that anaerobic glycolysis during the period of contraction leaves behind a quantity of this metabolite, which must subsequently be oxidized to CO_2 and water by aerobic processes. Freed of the need to balance the rates of energy production and energy utilization during normal activity, most white muscles contain contractile proteins that have a high intrinsic rate of ATP hydrolysis. This specialization, as we shall see later (Chapter 7), permits these muscles to achieve a high velocity of shortening, so that these white muscles are properly called "fast" muscles. This specialization is clearly in accord with the functional requirement for speed (in the rabbit, for example, to facilitate escape to the burrow).

Returning to the physiological—and ecological—consequences of these biochemical differences, we can see how the rabbit escapes pursuit by a rapid dash to its burrow (the "jackrabbit" start), which utilizes a limited supply of energy stored as phosphocreatine and derived from anaerobic glycolysis. If far from the burrow, the rabbit quickly tires because the phosphocreatine stores are soon depleted and lactic acid accumulation causes the muscle cells to become acidotic, thereby arresting anaerobic glycolysis. If it reaches the safety of its burrow, the rabbit must rest in order to replenish its phosphocreatine reserves and to repay the "oxygen debt" by oxidation of lactate. The hare, on the other hand, relies on its staying power to elude pursuit. It can run long distances because during activity its red muscle regenerates ATP at the same rate at which it is being consumed. The muscle of the hare, however, requires a continuing supply of oxygen and substrate that must be delivered via the bloodstream. Furthermore, the hare muscle is both slower and weaker than that of the rabbit owing to the lower intrinsic ATPase of the contractile proteins and the large volume of muscle occupied by the mitochondria. In this context it is clear that the myocardium functions like and so has biochemical properties similar to those of red muscle. These differences between white and red muscle were summarized concisely by Mommaerts, who said that white muscle operates on a "twitch now, pay later" basis, whereas the modus operandi of red muscle is "pay as you go."

> With few exceptions, human skeletal muscles are of a mixed type and contain three types of fibers. These are *slow oxidative,* which are similar to the red muscles described above, *fast glycolytic,* which are like white muscle (although they are pink in color), and *fast oxidative-glycolytic,* which have high ATPase contractile proteins but also contain numerous mitochondria and therefore are able to produce ATP by oxidative reactions.
>
> It is possible by physical training to alter the metabolic properties of human skeletal muscle. Where emphasis is placed on sustained exercise (e.g., distance running), the capacity for aerobic energy production increases. Where training is in short bursts (e.g. sprinting), the glycolytic enzymes become more prevalent. There is currently no convincing evidence that training alters the characteristics of the contractile proteins.

MUSCULAR EFFICIENCY

The term efficiency has many meanings, the most precise of which is that used in thermodynamics: that fraction of the free energy change associated with the chemical reactions that take place during a cycle of contraction and relaxation which appears as mechanical work. *Thermodynamic efficiency* therefore equals $W/-\Delta G$. Because the many chemical reactions taking place during the contractile cycle are incompletely described and because the free energy changes of most individual reactions are not precisely known, a rigorous definition of thermodynamic efficiency cannot be achieved. Instead it is customary to measure the ratio between useful work and the enthalpy change that accompanies the chemical reactions which occur during contraction. Expressed in this way, *mechanical efficiency* equals $W/-\Delta H$. In the heart, which derives its energy almost entirely by oxidative metabolism, enthalpy changes can be closely approximated by measuring the oxygen consumption. This is true because even though the amount of heat energy liberated per gram of fat oxidized (~ 9 kcal) is more than twice that per gram of either carbohydrate or protein (~ 4 kcal), the enthalpies when expressed per liter of oxygen consumed are quite similar (fat 4.69 kcal, carbohydrate 5.05 kcal, protein 4.60 kcal). This follows because more oxygen is needed to metabolize a gram of fat than a gram of either carbohydrate or protein. Regardless of the substrate being oxidized, therefore, the enthalpies of the metabolic reactions responsible for ATP production can be estimated quite well from measurements of oxygen consumption. This fact permits cardiovascular physiologists to estimate the mechanical efficiency of the heart from the ratio between useful work performed and oxygen consumed. The proportion of the energy that does not appear as useful work (i.e., that contributing to the "inefficiency" of the muscle) is liberated largely as heat [Eq. (2.2)] or contributes to "internal work" (Chapter 13).

Studies of different skeletal muscles have shown that the efficiency with which a muscle performs a given type of work is determined in part by the intrinsic rate of ATP hydrolysis by the contractile proteins. The amount of energy utilized by a fast white muscle to shorten rapidly in the face of a light load is less than that of a slow red muscle, which has contractile proteins that hydrolyze ATP at a slower intrinsic rate (Table 2.1). Conversely, tension is maintained at lesser energy cost by a slow red muscle than by a fast white muscle. Thus rapidly contracting muscles, the contractile proteins of which have a high intrinsic rate of ATP hydrolysis, work most efficiently when shortening rapidly against light loads, whereas more slowly contracting muscles, with contractile proteins that have low intrinsic rates of ATP hydrolysis, function at highest efficiency when developing tension. These differences may be significant in the adaptive response of the myocardium to sustained hemodynamic overloading (Chapters 11 and 21).

Actual values for the efficiency of muscular contraction, as would be expected from the preceding discussion, depend on whether one is considering mechanical or thermodynamic efficiency. Based on measurements of external work and oxygen consumption in the working heart, mechanical efficiency ranges up to 20–25%. In skeletal muscle—in which a decline in high-energy phosphate, or ATP levels, can be used to calculate the denominator in the expression $W/-\Delta H$ for mechanical efficiency—values of efficiency up to 40% can be recorded. As up to 25% of the total energy consumed during muscular activity is used not for the contractile process itself but for the release and reuptake of activator calcium (Chapter 9), the true mechanical efficiency of the contractile process is significantly higher (over 50%). The thermodynamic efficiency of the contractile process itself is probably much higher because the hydrolysis of the high-energy phosphate bond of ATP is accompanied by the release of a hydrogen ion. Neutralization of this proton by the buffer systems of the muscle liberates energy that, while it probably does not contribute to the energy available to the contractile proteins, has a significant enthalpy. As a result, almost 40% of the energy available from ATP hydrolysis can be utilized when this neutralization takes place. Thus if the energy for muscular contraction comes only from the remainder of the energy available from ATP hydrolysis, the true thermodynamic efficiency of muscle may be higher than 90%, a value which compares favorably with those of manmade machines, e.g., the gasoline engine with an efficiency of only approximately 30%.

BIBLIOGRAPHY

Engels, W. K. (1966): The multiplicity of pathologic reactions of human skeletal muscle. In: *Proceedings of the 5th International Congress on Neuropathology,* edited by F. Lüthy and A. Bischoff, pp. 613–624. Excerpta Medica Foundation, Amsterdam.

Gibbs, C. L. (1974): Cardiac energetics. In: *The Mammalian Myocardium,* edited by G. A. Langer and A. J. Brady, pp. 105–133. Wiley, New York.

Katz, A. M. (1967): Patterns of energy production and energy utilization in cardiac and skeletal muscle. In: *Factors Influencing Myocardial Contractility,* edited by R. Tanz, F. Kavaler, and J. Roberts, pp. 401–416. Academic Press, New York.

Needham, D. M. (1960): Biochemistry of muscular action. In: *Structure and Function of Muscle,* Vol. II, edited by G. H. Bourne, pp. 55–104. Academic Press, New York.

3

Anaerobic and Aerobic Glycolysis

ATP can be generated in the myocardium by two metabolic pathways: glycolysis and oxidative phosphorylation (Chapter 2). Although the latter represents the major energy-producing reaction in the heart, the glycolytic reactions are also essential for the aerobic breakdown of carbohydrates to CO_2 and H_2O. Furthermore, under abnormal conditions (e.g., in the hypoxic or ischemic heart) ATP production can take place anaerobically by way of the glycolytic pathways so as to compensate, although only in part, for the cessation of aerobic ATP production. The discussion that follows focuses on the overall scheme of glycolysis, and especially on the mechanisms by which this process is controlled. The many individual steps in this series of reactions are not described here, nor are structural formulae written for most of the metabolites, as this material is readily available in many excellent textbooks of biochemistry.

Control of glycolysis is extremely complex. Yet certain overall patterns of regulation emerge from the many details of this process (see also Chapter 4 and Table 4.4). One of these is that at least three distinct types of regulatory influences can modify the rate of glycolysis. The first, exemplified by the mechanisms controlling glycogen metabolism, is *hormonal*. The same hormones that increase energy utilization during contraction also increase the breakdown of glycogen to glucose. This type of control allows the same signal that increases the work of the heart to increase concomitantly the provision of substrates for energy production. A second type of control—seen clearly in the reaction catalyzed by phosphofructokinase—is exerted by factors related to the *energy requirements of the cell*. In the phosphofructokinase reaction, glycolysis is accelerated when high-energy phosphates are depleted, and inhibited when ATP concentrations are high. This second type of control is also extremely important in the regulation of oxidative metabolism (Chapter 4). A third type of control, seen with the enzyme glyceraldehyde-3-phosphate dehydrogenase, permits the rate of glycolysis to respond to changes in the *supply of essential cofactors for oxidation*. This latter type of control inhibits glycolysis when excessive reliance on anaerobic energy production has shifted the cell milieu to a reduced state and so has exceeded both the supply of oxidized coenzymes and the ability of other cellular reactions to provide them.

The initial metabolic reactions of glycolysis, which provide substrate for energy production, are under *hormonal control;* those toward the middle of these pathways are regulated mainly by *energy requirements,* whereas the latter steps in this pathway are responsive to the ability of the cell to supply cofactors that are essential for substrate *oxidation*. In terms of the monetary analogy cited in Chapter 2, these control mechanisms are like those which regulate the flow of capital through a bank account. The latter is determined first by the wish to spend (hormones), secondly by the balance in the account (high-energy phosphates), and ultimately by the earning capacity (supply of oxidized coenzymes). This analogy is of course oversimplified; for example, most of the enzymatic reactions mentioned above are subject to more than one of these principles of control. Yet the monetary analogy may be helpful in understanding the principles by which energy production is regulated in the myocardial cells.

THE GLYCOLYTIC PATHWAY

The major glycolytic pathway of the heart is outlined in Fig. 3.1. In the overall reaction, one molecule of glucose is broken down to form two molecules of lactate. Although 4 moles of ATP are synthesized, net ATP synthesis is only 2 moles because the myocardial cell must "invest" 2 moles of ATP to phosphorylate each mole of 6-carbon sugar. Four moles of ATP are then recovered through the metabolism of each of two 3-carbon sugars when dihydroxyacetone phosphate and glyceraldehyde-3-phosphate are metabolized to pyruvate.

The initial investment of phosphate-bond energy, which may seem somewhat wasteful to the cell, is necessary for two reasons. First, the fact that glycolysis occurs through the action of soluble enzymes on soluble substrates in the cytosol requires that neither leak out of the cell in appreciable amounts. While the glycolytic enzymes are large proteins and so do not pass readily through the sarcolemma, the permeability properties of the cell membrane would not prevent the loss of soluble 3- and 6-carbon sugars. When these glycolytic intermediates are phosphorylated, however, the nonpolar sugars are converted into negatively charged ions to which the sarcolemma is impermeable. In this way phosphorylation of the glycolytic intermediates reduces their ability to leak out of the cell. Second, this phosphorylation is necessary to provide the intramolecular forces that permit high-energy phosphate bonds to be formed in 1, 3-diphosphoglycerate and phosphoenolpyruvate.

The glycolytic pathway contains one oxidative step (*4, Fig. 3.1). Where glyceraldehyde-3-phosphate is oxidized (at the same time that inorganic phosphate is incorporated into the molecule) to form 1,3-diphosphoglycerate, NAD (nicotinamide adenine dinucleotide, the coenzyme formerly called DPN) is reduced to NADH. This reaction cannot proceed in the absence of oxidized NAD, so that the reduced NADH must be reoxidized if glycolysis is to continue. Normally the reoxidation of NADH to NAD takes place by aerobic reactions in the mitochondria (Chapter 4). In the heart functioning under anaerobic conditions, limited oxidation of NADH can occur through coupling to the reduction of pyruvate, although this reaction causes large quantities of lactate to be produced in the ischemic or anoxic myocardium (Chapter 22).

Under normal, aerobic conditions NADH is not oxidized by the glycolytic pathway, so that pyruvate is not reduced to form lactate. Instead, in the normally

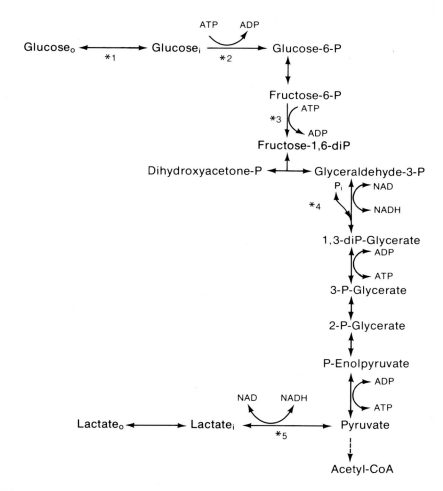

FIG. 3.1. Overall reaction scheme of glycolysis. Major control points are: (*1) glucose transport; (*2) the hexokinase reaction (glucose phosphorylation); (*3) the phosphofructokinase reaction (fructose-6-phosphate phosphorylation); (*4) the glyceraldehyde-3-phosphate dehydrogenase reaction (glyceraldehyde-3-phosphate oxidation); and (*5) the lactate dehydrogenase reaction (pyruvate reduction). ATP is utilized at two steps at the beginning of the scheme. Two moles of ATP are generated at each of two steps toward the end of the scheme, giving a net yield of 2 moles of ATP per mole of glucose. (Two moles of ATP are produced per mole of glucose at each of the reactions involving 3-carbon metabolites, whereas only 1 mole of ATP is needed to phosphorylate each mole of the 6-carbon sugars.) Glycolysis involves a single oxidative step, where NAD is reduced to NADH. Under anaerobic conditions limited amounts of NADH can be oxized to NAD at the step where pyruvate is reduced to lactate.

oxygenated heart pyruvate is converted to a 2-carbon fragment that is subsequently oxidized in the tricarboxylic acid cycle (see below). Oxidation of NADH in the mitochondria generates large quantities of ATP, whereas the oxidation of NADH that accompanies conversion of pyruvate to lactate contributes no energy for cell function. Thus even though glycolysis is able to provide limited amounts of ATP under anaerobic conditions, the breakdown of carbohydrate to lactate by the reactions shown in Fig. 3.1 is far from optimal in terms of ATP production.

CONTROL OF GLYCOLYSIS

The glycolytic pathway is controlled primarily by four enzymes and by the transport of glucose into the cell (Fig. 3.1). At each of these control points, however, the mechanisms of regulation differ.

Glucose Transport

The entry of glucose into the myocardial cell (*1, Fig. 3.1) is carrier-mediated but does not require energy as the sugar moves from a region of high concentration outside the cell to one of lower concentration in the cytosol. In this process, however, glucose must combine with a glucose carrier in the sarcolemma to gain rapid entry into the cell.

The carrier-mediated transport of glucose into the cell can be accelerated by a number of factors, including the hormones insulin and epinephrine, as well as oxygen lack. The fact that epinephrine can accelerate glucose transport accounts in part for its ability to increase the glycolytic rate. The resulting increase in energy production can be considered to complement the action of this hormone in accelerating energy utilization through its effects to increase both the strength (Chapter 11) and frequency (Chapter 19) of cardiac contraction. Stimulation of glucose transport in the hypoxic myocardium serves to increase the availability of the carbohydrate substrate for anaerobic glycolysis under conditions where oxidative metabolism is inhibited (Chapter 22). Unfortunately the mechanism by which these factors govern the rate of glucose transport remains incompletely understood.

Hexokinase

The enzyme hexokinase catalyzes glucose phosphorylation (*2, Fig. 3.1), which, as was already pointed out, involves investment by the cell of one molecule of ATP per molecule of glucose. Variations in the intracellular levels of glucose-6-phosphate, ATP, ADP, AMP, and P_i are of considerable importance in regulating the rate of hexokinase-catalyzed glucose phosphorylation. Most important of these control mechanisms is that mediated by glucose-6-phosphate, which at high concentrations inhibits the ability of hexokinase to catalyze glucose phosphorylation. This inhibition is not simply due to the operation of the law of mass action (i.e., by increasing the reverse of the hexokinase reaction, Fig. 3.1) because this reaction is essentially irreversible. Instead, high concentrations of glucose-6-phosphate modify the structure of the enzyme hexokinase, reducing its ability to phosphorylate glucose.

The effect of glucose-6-phosphate to inhibit the enzymatic action of hexokinase can be modulated by changing concentrations of other phosphate compounds in the cell: ATP, ADP, AMP, and P_i. The high-energy compound ATP exerts an inhibitory effect, whereas the products of ATP utilization stimulate glucose phosphorylation. In this way the rate of the hexokinase reaction is controlled by the availability of phosphate-bond energy in the cell. The importance of this control system can be seen, for example, when the work of the heart is suddenly increased, which causes ATP levels to fall and those of P_i and the other adenine nucleotides to rise. The ability of these phosphate compounds to modify the hexokinase reaction causes glucose phosphorylation to be accelerated by a declining level of ATP and concomitantly rising levels of the products of ATP hydrolysis. The ability of the phosphate compounds to control the hexokinase reaction is due to *amplification* of the controlling influence of glucose-6-phosphate on this enzyme, much as an amplifying radio circuit increases the strength of an electromagnetic signal. The process of amplification is described further in the following discussion of the control exerted at the step catalyzed by phosphofructokinase.

Control of the hexokinase reaction by glucose-6-phosphate permits the glucose phosphorylation rate to be matched to the rate at which glucose-6-phosphate is consumed in the subsequent reactions of glycolysis (Fig. 3.1). In this way an accelerated flux of substrates through the subsequent reactions of this metabolic pathway, by consuming glucose-6-phosphate, increases the rate at which this phosphosugar is produced from glucose.

Phosphofructokinase

The major point of control of the glycolytic pathway is at the step where phosphofructokinase catalyzes the formation of fructose-1,6-diphosphate (*3, Fig. 3.1). This reaction is thus the most important of the rate-limiting steps in glycolysis. A number of substances can regulate this process, which is probably due to the fact that they influence complex allosteric interactions that take place between six subunits which, when aggregated, form the fully active form of the enzyme.

Both *high-* and *low-energy phosphate compounds* modulate the catalytic activity of this enzyme (Table 3.1). As is the case for the hexokinase reaction, the former are inhibitory and the latter stimulatory (Table 3.1). As a result, phosphofructo-

TABLE 3.1. *Factors controlling phosphofructokinase activity*

Increased activity	Decreased activity
ADP	H+ (acidosis)
AMP	ATP
P_i	Phosphocreatine
Fructose-1,6-diphosphate	Citrate
Cyclic AMP	
NH_4^+	

kinase activity is increased under conditions where high-energy phosphates are depleted. The marked acceleration of glycolysis that constitutes the initial response to hypoxia and ischemia can be attributed to both the increased cellular concentrations of ADP, AMP, and P_i, and the declining concentration of ATP and (especially) phosphocreatine. *Acidosis,* on the other hand, exerts a powerful inhibitory effect on this enzyme. This inhibition contributes to an eventual slowing of glycolysis, which in the ischemic myocardium follows a transient acceleration described above (see also Chapter 22). The reaction product, *fructose-1,6-diphosphate,* also activates phosphofructokinase. The importance of this activating effect arises not because fructose-1,6-diphosphate is the product of the reaction catalyzed by phosphofructokinase (Fig. 3.1) but because of its role in yet another complex of regulatory mechanisms (which for the sake of simplicity is omitted from the present discussion). An action of NH_4^+ to stimulate phosphofructokinase may represent a part of the mechanism responsible for providing substrates for additional metabolic reactions.

Phosphofructokinase is also under *hormonal control* in that cyclic AMP, which is produced in the cell under the influence of epinephrine, stimulates the enzyme. The activating effect of cyclic AMP appears to be due to an interaction between the enzyme and the nucleotide itself (and not to a cyclic AMP-catalyzed phosphorylation) (Chapter 9) and probably represents a part of the complex mechanism that mediates the effect of catecholamines to stimulate anaerobic glycolysis.

Citrate, one of the intermediates of *oxidative metabolism,* has a well-documented and important ability to inhibit phosphofructokinase. This aspect of regulating the catalytic activity of phosphofructokinase represents a very important mechanism by which increased aerobic metabolism, which produces citrate, can slow glycolysis. Thus the inhibitory effect of citrate probably plays an essential role in integrating the glycolytic rate with that of oxidative metabolism (Chapter 4).

A full discussion of the mechanisms by which glycolytic flux is regulated by phosphofructokinase is beyond the scope of this book. One feature of this control point, however, warrants some elaboration. This is a phenomenon called *amplification.* For the usual enzymatic reaction that does not show amplification, an increase in enzyme activity from 10% to 90% of its maximum would require a more than 80-fold increase in substrate concentration. (This value is readily calculated from classic saturation kinetics.) The existence of cooperative (allosteric) interactions within an enzyme can reduce such enormous fluctuations in substrate concentration. However, even if there are four interacting binding sites for the substrate, to go from 10% to 90% of maximal activity would require an approximately fourfold increase in substrate concentration. In the case of cellular levels of ATP, such changes are not observed; nor are they practical to the cell in view of thermodynamic considerations that would reduce the ability of ATP to transfer energy as its concentration is decreased—a fourfold decrease in ATP concentration with a concomitant increase in ADP concentration would reduce the energy released during ATP hydrolysis by approximately one-third. For this reason the response of cellular regulatory systems to changing ATP concentrations must be amplified so as to respond to much smaller changes in ATP concentration.

In the case of the phosphofructokinase reaction, amplification is achieved by an interplay between the concentrations of ATP, ADP, and AMP. Both of the latter overcome the inhibitory effects of ATP. The concentrations of ATP, ADP, and AMP are maintained in equilibrium by the enzyme adenylate kinase (or myokinase), which catalyzes the reaction

$$ATP + AMP \longleftrightarrow 2ADP$$

The equilibrium constant for this enzyme is such that the AMP concentration is at an extremely low level in the resting myocardium. For example, at the physiological ATP/ADP ratio of approximately 9:1, the ATP concentration is 4.48 mM, ADP 0.5 mM, and AMP 0.02 mM according to the equilibrium constant for adenylate kinase and assuming a total adenine nucleotide concentration of 5 mM. According to the equilibrium constant for adenylate kinase, a fall in ATP concentration of approximately 15% to 3.89 mM doubles the ADP concentration to 1.0 mM (i.e., twofold) and increases the AMP concentration more than fivefold to 0.11 mM. In this way a slight change in ATP concentration can be amplified manyfold as increases in AMP and ADP concentrations. Thus increased utilization of high-energy phosphate can increase phosphofructokinase activity through a stimulatory effect of decreased ATP level that is amplified by the more marked increases in ADP and AMP concentrations. When energy demands are suddenly increased in the heart, these interlocking reactions can translate a small reduction in ATP level into a powerful stimulus to accelerate glycolysis. The advantages of this amplification are clear; the cell is able to call effectively for replacement of ATP, the major substrate for its energy-consuming reactions, without having to suffer more than a minor fall in ATP concentration.

Glyceraldehyde-3-Phosphate Dehydrogenase

Oxidation of glyceraldehyde-3-phosphate and the resulting formation of 1,3-diphosphoglycerate (*4, Fig. 3.1) couples an oxidative reaction (in which NAD is reduced to NADH) (Fig. 3.1) to the formation of a diphosphosugar containing one high-energy phosphate bond. This reaction, which is catalyzed by glyceraldehyde-3-phosphate dehydrogenase, is normally not of major importance in regulating glycolysis. However, under conditions of hypoxia or ischemia, where phosphofructokinase becomes strongly activated in the heart, control of the glycolytic rate shifts to later reactions in the glycolytic pathway, notably that catalyzed by glyceraldehyde-3-phosphate dehydrogenase. This enzyme is regulated largely by product inhibition in that it is extremely sensitive to the inhibitory effects of 1,3-diphosphoglycerate and NADH accumulation. Where the ability of the cell to oxidize NADH is markedly impaired, as it is under anaerobic conditions, the accumulation of reduced NADH therefore slows glycolysis. In this way glycolysis in the anaerobic heart comes to be regulated by a different set of metabolites than those which in the well-oxygenated heart control the phosphofructokinase reaction.

When there is an abundant supply of oxygen, glycolysis is regulated mainly by high-energy phosphate compounds at the step catalyzed by phosphofructokinase, this enzyme allowing glycolysis to be accelerated when ATP is being consumed more rapidly than it is being generated. In the hypoxic heart, where glycolytic flux becomes markedly accelerated at the step catalyzed by phosphofructokinase (see above), regulation of glycolysis shifts to the later step catalyzed by glyceraldehyde-3-phosphate dehydrogenase. This latter enzyme, unlike phosphofructokinase, is sensitive to factors related to the state of oxidation within the cell, i.e., to the level of reduced NADH. For this reason glycolytic control in the ischemic heart (Chapter 22) shifts from a step that is governed by energy needs (high-energy phosphate) to one at which control is exerted by the ability of the cell to oxidize substrates and coenzymes.

Lactate Dehydrogenase

The reduction of pyruvate to lactate (*5, Fig. 3.1), which allows the cell to regenerate oxidized NAD, is catalyzed by the enzyme lactate dehydrogenase. In white skeletal muscles, which depend heavily on anaerobic glycolysis for energy production (Chapter 2), this enzyme is of major importance in providing a supply of NAD for the earlier steps in glycolysis. In the well-oxygenated heart this reaction is not utilized; instead, NAD is normally regenerated from NADH by the mitochondria (Chapter 4). These differences in the fate of pyruvate in different muscle types are reflected in the isozymes of lactate dehydrogenase (LDH) that are found in cardiac and white skeletal muscle. In the latter, which is more dependent on glycolysis for its energy supply (Table 2.1), the LDH isozyme has a high affinity for pyruvate. As a result, pyruvate is preferentially reduced to lactate in white skeletal muscles. The myocardium, on the other hand, contains an LDH isozyme which has a low affinity for pyruvate. As a result, little or no pyruvate is normally reduced to lactate unless, as in the ischemic heart, pyruvate levels become very high. Instead, pyruvate is converted to acetyl coenzyme A (acetyl-CoA), the 2-carbon fragment which is subsequently oxidized in the tricarboxylic acid cycle. In the myocardium, therefore, the reaction catalyzed by LDH plays little role in determining the metabolic fate of pyruvate; instead, pyruvate metabolism is controlled by pyruvate dehydrogenase, which catalyzes the formation of acetyl-CoA (see below).

GLYCOGEN FORMATION AND BREAKDOWN

In the preceding discussion of anaerobic glycolysis, three regulatory mechanisms were described that can control the glycolytic rate. The first, a hormonal mechanism, controls glucose transport. The second, control by the availability

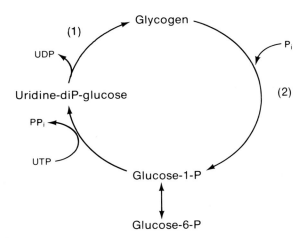

FIG. 3.2. Pathways of glycogen synthesis (*left,* reading upward) differ from those of glycogenolysis (*right,* reading downward). Glycogen synthesis is controlled mainly by glycogen synthetase, which catalyzes reaction 1; and glycogenolysis is regulated by phosphorylase, which catalyzes reaction 2.

of high-energy phosphate, is manifest most strikingly by the enzyme phosphofructokinase. The third, regulation by the cell's ability to reoxidize reduced coenzymes, is apparent in the control exerted by glyceraldehyde-3-phosphate dehydrogenase. The first principle of regulation is also apparent in the control of glycogen formation and breakdown. This type of control, exerted by circulating hormones and neurotransmitters, acts by chemical modification of key metabolic enzymes.

The synthesis and breakdown of glycogen do not occur by forward and reverse fluxes through a single series of reactions but by way of two separate pathways (Fig. 3.2). Each pathway is controlled by an enzyme which can exist physiologically in an active or an inactive form whose interconversion is regulated by a series of hormonally determined reactions.

The transfer of glucose units to glycogen involves two reactions (Fig. 3.2). The first, in which uridine diphosphoglucose is formed by the condensation of glucose-1-phosphate with uridine triphosphate (UTP), does not control the rate of glycogen synthesis. The second reaction, in which addition of the 6-carbon sugar to glycogen is accompanied by the release of uridine diphosphate (UDP)—reaction (1) in Fig. 3.2—is rate-limiting. For this reason the rate of glycogen synthesis is determined by the catalytic activity of glycogen synthetase, the enzyme which catalyzes this rate-limiting step.

Glycogen synthetase can exist in two forms. The *a* (dephospho) form, which is the more active, is converted to the less active *b* (phospho) form when the level of cyclic AMP in the cell is increased. This action of cyclic AMP occurs through acceleration of the reaction shown in Fig. 3.3, in which the terminal phosphate of ATP is transferred to a covalent linkage on glycogen synthetase. The latter

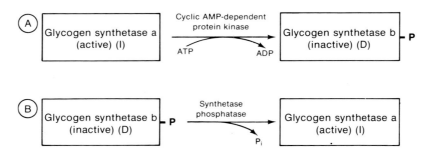

FIG. 3.3. Phosphorylation **(A)** and dephosphorylation **(B)** reactions that modulate glycogen synthetase activity. **A:** Phosphorylation by a cyclic AMP-dependent protein kinase converts the active, dephosphorylated glycogen synthetase a to the inactive, phosphorylated glycogen synthetase b. **B:** Dephosphorylation by synthetase phosphatase converts the inactive, phosphorylated glycogen synthetase b to the active, dephosphorylated glycogen synthetase a.

reaction is catalyzed by a cyclic AMP-dependent protein kinase. The activity of this enzyme is in turn controlled by the level of cyclic AMP within the cell, which stimulates this enzyme to phosphorylate glycogen synthetase a (see below). Glycogen formation can be returned to its high, basal rate by synthetase phosphatase, an enzyme which dephosphorylates glycogen synthetase b.

   The terms *a* and *b* for the active and inactive forms of glycogen synthetase are used here to indicate their similarity to the two forms of phosphorylase, which are described in the following section of this chapter. The older terms "I" (for the active a-form) and "D" (for the inactive b-form) remain useful in understanding how phosphorylation or dephosphorylation of this enzyme alters its activity. The dephosphorylated a-form is independent (I) of the control exerted by several regulatory substances that in the case of the phosphorylated, inactive b-form of glycogen synthetase markedly inhibit activity. The latter, in contrast, is dependent (D) for its activity on other factors that must reverse the inhibitory effects of many of the substrates and metabolites found normally in the myocardium. Thus the ability of the synthetase phosphatase to convert inactive glycogen synthetase b to its active a-form does not reflect a true "activation" of the enzyme. Instead, the dephosphorylation of glycogen synthetase b accelerates glycogen synthesis by allowing the enzyme to become independent of the inhibiting effects of a number of regulatory influences within the cell. Conversely, glycogen synthesis is slowed when phosphorylation by the cyclic AMP-dependent protein kinase converts the enzyme to its dependent b-form, thereby re-establishing its sensitivity to these inhibitory effects.

Phosphorylase

   Phosphorylase, the enzyme responsible for the formation of glucose-1-phosphate through the breakdown of glycogen—reaction (2) in Fig. 3.2—also exists in phosphorylated and dephosphorylated forms (Fig. 3.4). In contrast to the two forms of glycogen synthetase, the phosphorylated form of phosphorylase is the active a-form whereas the dephosphorylated form of the enzyme is the less active b-form of the enzyme. The interconversions of phosphorylase are, from the standpoint of the substrates that are phosphorylated and dephosphorylated, chemically similar to those of glycogen synthetase (Fig. 3.4), but the way in which the phosphorylating enzymes are controlled differs (see below).

> Phosphorylase b, like the less active b form of glycogen synthetase, is not really inactive. Instead, the activity of phosphorylase b is normally less than that of phosphorylase a because the conditions normally present in the cell do not permit full expression of its activity. Thus the hormonal regulation of both glycogen synthetase and phosphorylase does not convert an inactive enzyme to an active enzyme or vice versa. Instead, phosphorylation of these enzymes alters their sensitivity to control by other cell metabolites. In the case of glycogen synthetase, phosphorylation increases inhibitory control, whereas phosphorylation of phosphorylase causes inhibitory control to be reduced.

The enzyme that catalyzes the phosphorylation of phosphorylase b, *phosphorylase kinase,* is subject to a different type of control than that of the cyclic AMP-dependent protein kinase which catalyzes the phosphorylation of glycogen synthetase. The activity of phosphorylase kinase, and thus the conversion of phosphorylase b to phosphorylase a, is markedly dependent on Ca^{2+} but independent of cyclic AMP. At the low levels of Ca^{2+} that are found in the resting myocardium (< 1 μM), phosphorylase kinase is inactive, activity being markedly increased at Ca^{2+} concentrations above 1 μM, such as are found in the heart during systole. The physiological significance of this control by Ca^{2+}, which is readily demonstrated in studies of the enzyme *in vitro,* remains uncertain. There is a tendency now to classify phosphorylase kinase as a *calcium-dependent protein kinase* to contrast it with the *cyclic AMP-dependent protein kinase* which converts glycogen synthetase a to glycogen synthetase b.

In spite of the fact that phosphorylase kinase is not *directly* controlled by cyclic

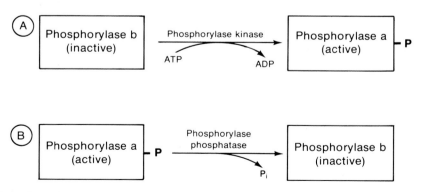

FIG. 3.4. Phosphorylation **(A)** and dephosphorylation **(B)** reactions that modulate phosphorylase activity. **A:** Phosphorylation by phosphorylase kinase, a Ca^{2+}-dependent protein kinase, converts the inactive, dephosphorylated phosphorylase b to the active, phosphorylated phosphorylase a. **B:** Dephosphorylation by phosphorylase phosphatase converts the active, phosphorylated phosphorylase a to the inactive, dephosphorylated phosphorylase b.

AMP, this nucleotide has in fact a major *indirect* effect on phosphorylase kinase. This effect is described below, when the overall actions of cyclic AMP on glycogen metabolism are discussed.

Interplay Between Glycogen Synthetase and Phosphorylase

Taken together, the effects of protein phosphorylation and dephosphorylation provide an interlocking system by which hormones such as epinephrine can control the net flux of glucose-1-phosphate into and out of the intracellular

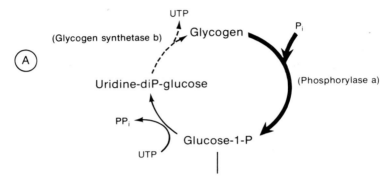

PHOSPHORYLATED ENZYMES

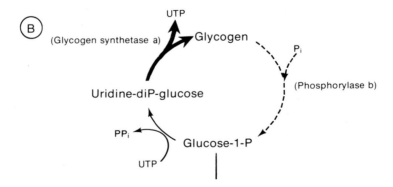

DEPHOSPHORYLATED ENZYMES

FIG. 3.5. Interlocking control of glycogen formation and breakdown by phosphorylation-dephosphorylation of the regulatory enzymes glycogen synthetase and phosphorylase. **A:** When both enzymes are phosphorylated, glycogen synthetase is in the inactive b form, and phosphorylase is in the active a form. Hence glycogen synthesis is inhibited and glycogen breakdown accelerated. **B:** When both enzymes are dephosphorylated, glycogen synthetase is in the active a form and phosphorylase is in the inactive b form. Hence glycogen synthesis is accelerated and glycogen breakdown inhibited.

glycogen stores (Fig. 3.2). Hormone-induced promotion of protein phosphorylation both inhibits glycogen synthesis (Fig. 3.3) and stimulates glycogen breakdown (Fig. 3.4), whereas stimulation of protein dephosphorylation (Figs. 3.3 and
3.4) shifts the balance toward glycogen synthesis (Fig. 3.5). Before describing Fig.
3.5, however, it is necessary to compare and contrast the control exerted by cyclic
AMP on glycogen synthesis with that exerted on glycogen breakdown.

In the case of glycogen synthetase, cyclic AMP is *directly* involved in the
conversion of the dephosphorylated (active) form of the enzyme to the phosphorylated (inactive) form (Fig. 3.3). This control results from the cyclic AMP
requirement of the protein kinase which catalyzes this phosphorylation. In contrast, conversion of the dephosphorylated (inactive) form of phosphorylase into
the phosphorylated (active) form is not *directly* dependent on cyclic AMP because
there is no effect of this nucleotide on the catalytic properties of the Ca^{2+}-
dependent phosphorylase kinase (Fig. 3.4). Yet cyclic AMP does have an important *indirect* role in regulating the phosphorylation of phosphorylase b and thus
the rate of glycogen breakdown. This indirect control by cyclic AMP is exerted
through its ability to catalyze yet another reaction which increases the activity
of the Ca^{2+}-dependent phosphorylase kinase. Like glycogen synthetase and
phosphorylase, phosphorylase kinase can exist in two forms: phosphorylated and
dephosphorylated (Fig. 3.6). The ability of cyclic AMP to promote the phosphorylation of phosphorylase kinase is mediated by a special cyclic AMP-dependent protein kinase (different from that shown in Fig. 3.4). In the case of phosphorylase kinase, the cyclic AMP-dependent protein kinase converts the inactive
dephospho form of phosphorylase kinase to the active phospho form (Fig. 3.6).
Inactivation of phosphorylase kinase occurs when it is dephosphorylated by a
phosphatase. The enzymes which regulate the activity of phosphorylase kinase
are called phosphorylase kinase kinase, and phosphorylase kinase phosphatase,
respectively (Fig. 3.6).

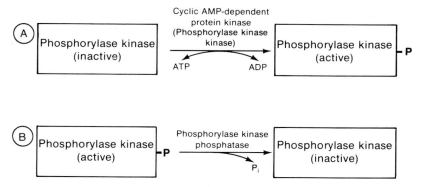

FIG. 3.6. Phosphorylation **(A)** and dephosphorylation **(B)** reactions that mediate the activity of
phosphorylase kinase. **A:** Phosphorylation by a cyclic AMP-dependent protein kinase (phosphorylase kinase kinase) converts the inactive, dephosphorylated form of phosphorylase to the
active, phosphorylated form. **B:** Dephosphorylation by phosphorylase kinase phosphatase converts the active, phosphorylated phosphorylase kinase to the inactive, dephosphorylated form.

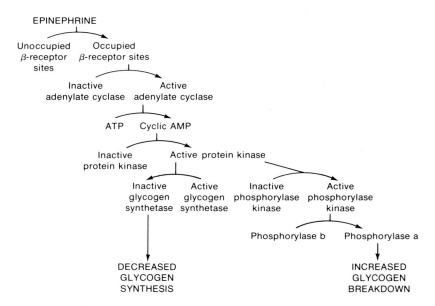

FIG 3.7. Cascade of reactions that allows rates of glycogen synthesis and breakdown to respond to catecholamines (e.g., epinephrine). The reactions in this cascade are depicted as they mediate a decrease in glycogen synthesis and an increase in glycogen breakdown in response to a hormonal influence that leads to increased cyclic AMP production. The earlier steps in this cascade—those which lead to cyclic AMP formation—are discussed in Chapter 9.

In the last analysis, therefore, both glycogen synthesis and breakdown *are* controlled by cyclic AMP, so that agents which stimulate cyclic AMP formation in the heart act at both sides of the cycle shown in Fig. 3.5. The only essential difference between the control exerted by cyclic AMP on glycogen synthesis and that seen for glycogen breakdown is the specific point in the series of enzymatic steps at which the cyclic AMP-dependent phosphorylation is effected. This is seen in a drawing of the "cascade" of reactions which mediate the response of glycogen metabolism to epinephrine (Fig. 3.7). Several additional steps in the earlier portions of this cascade are introduced in this figure and are discussed more extensively in subsequent chapters. At this point attention should be directed to two major features of the figure: (a) that a complex cascade of chemical reactions mediates the action of catecholamines on glycogen metabolism; and, (b) that glycogen synthesis and glycogen breakdown are subject to a reciprocating control by this system in that hormonal stimulation leads to reactions which stimulate glycogen breakdown and inhibit glycogen synthesis (Fig. 3.5).

AEROBIC GLYCOLYSIS

Normally in the well-oxygenated heart glycolysis is an aerobic process. While the endproduct of anaerobic glycolysis is lactate (see above), that of aerobic glycolysis is acetate, a 2-carbon fragment that can be oxidized further within the mitochondria. The final step in aerobic glycolysis is therefore the conversion of pyruvate to acetate. Similar 2-carbon fragments are split off from the long-chain fatty acids during the successive steps of fatty acid oxidation (Chapter 4).

The 2-carbon fragments which enter the tricarboxylic acid cycle do so not as free acetate but bound in a complex with coenzyme A (abbreviated CoA-SH because the coenzyme contains a sulfhydryl group). In the complex between acetate and CoA-SH, the acetate is attached to the sulfhydryl group of CoA by a high-energy thioester bond, much as the terminal phosphate group is attached to ATP by a high-energy phosphoester bond. Acetyl-CoA is like ATP in another way: both serve within the cell as carriers—ATP as a carrier of chemical energy (see Chapter 2), and acetyl-CoA as a carrier of substrate for oxidation.

The formation of acetyl-CoA, both from the carbohydrate metabolites produced during glycolysis and as the result of β-oxidation of fatty acids (Chapter 4), takes place in the mitochondria. These reactions, which generate the 2-carbon fragments that are subsequently oxidized within the mitochondria, represent yet another major site at which energy production in the heart can be regulated.

Pyruvate Dehydrogenase

The conversion of pyruvate to acetyl-CoA (Fig. 3.8), which is accompanied by the liberation of CO_2, involves an extremely complicated series of reactions that are catalyzed by a huge multienzyme compound with a molecular weight of approximately 4 million. This enzyme complex contains five enzymes that act on each other as well as on the substrates. Furthermore, the overall reaction involves (and so can be controlled by) not only CoA-SH but also lipoic acid, thiamine pyrophosphate, NAD, and ATP. In addition, the pyruvate dehydro-

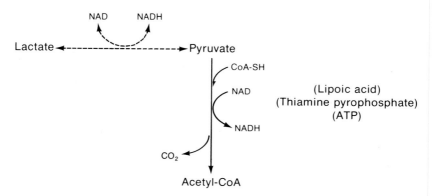

FIG. 3.8. Production of 2-carbon fragments as the final step in aerobic glycolysis. Decarboxylation of pyruvate leads to formation of acetyl-CoA, the 2-carbon fragment that is subsequently oxidized in the tricarboxylic acid. Acetyl-CoA formation is an extremely complex process that requires coenzyme A, oxidized NAD, lipoic acid, thiamine pyrophosphate, and ATP.

genase reaction may be subject to control by changing Ca^{2+} and Mg^{2+} concentrations. Finally, this reaction is modulated by a phosphorylation-dephosphorylation reaction similar to that shown in Fig. 3.4. In the case of the pyruvate dehydrogenase reaction, the formation of acetyl-CoA is inhibited when the enzyme is phosphorylated.

The extreme complexity of the regulation of this step in carbohydrate metabolism is not surprising when it is recognized that the metabolic fate of pyruvate stands at the crossroads between anaerobic and aerobic metabolism. Pyruvate can be converted to lactate (Fig. 3.1), thereby regenerating oxidized NAD for continuing glycolysis as in the heart under anaerobic conditions (see Chapter 22 and above). On the other hand, in the well-oxygenated heart pyruvate is "prepared" for entry into oxidative metabolism by conversion to acetyl-CoA (Fig. 3.8).

The existence of multiple, interacting control mechanisms at this important step in intermediary metabolism is in accord with the general rule that the more critical the reaction, the more checks and balances are provided by nature. The operation of this rule is apparent throughout this text. Nature is neither simple nor an adherent of the famous precept of William of Ockham, who during the early fourteenth century wrote: "Essentials ought not to be multiplied" ("Ockham's razor"). The survival of our complex biological machinery in the hostile natural environment is attributable to the great wisdom of our bodies, which provides layer upon layer of checks and balances for the protection of every important regulatory process that governs our bodily function. The words of Stephen Hales, written in 1733, seem especially appropriate in this regard: "So curiously are we wrought, so fearfully and wonderfully are we made."

BIBLIOGRAPHY

Neely, J. R., and Morgan, H. E. (1974): Relationship between carbohydrate and lipid metabolism and the energy balance of heart muscle. *Annu. Rev. Physiol.,* 31:413–459.

Newsholme, E. A. (1971–1972): The regulation of phosphofructokinase in muscle. *Cardiology,* 56:22–34.

Wildenthal, K., Morgan, H. E., Opie, L. H., and Srere, P. A. (1976): Regulation of cardiac metabolism (symposium). *Circ. Res. (Suppl. I),* 38:I-1–I-160.

4

Oxidative Metabolism

The concluding sentences in the preceding chapter on the principles of glycolytic control are equally well suited to serve as an introduction to the discussion of oxidative metabolism. This most important of the energy-producing processes in the heart is considerably more complex than that of glycolysis, the latter from an evolutionary standpoint being almost certainly the more primitive. Whereas glycolysis is catalyzed by soluble enzymes distributed widely throughout the cytosol, oxidative metabolism takes place almost entirely within specialized membranous structures, the *mitochondria*. This fact in itself increases the complexity of oxidative metabolism because all of the substrates, metabolites, and cofactors that move between the mitochondrial matrix and the cytosol must traverse a membrane barrier that exists between two aqueous compartments—the *cytosol* and the *mitochondrial matrix*. The existence of this barrier between cellular compartments permits changing permeability of the mitochondrial membrane to modulate the transfer between the cytosol and mitochondrial matrix of key substances that participate in oxidative metabolism. Thus an entirely new dimension for the control of oxidative metabolism is added to those already described for glycolysis.

Variations in the catalytic properties of individual enzymes, which in the case of glycolysis have already been seen to represent an extraordinarily complex set of interwoven control mechanisms, also participate in the control of oxidative metabolism. Oxidative metabolism differs fundamentally from glycolysis, however, in that many of the oxidative enzymes are bound to the mitochondrial membrane in a highly ordered structure which allows changes in enzyme-membrane and enzyme-enzyme interactions to participate in the control of oxidative energy production.

It is of interest that mitochondria contain a small number of DNA molecules that resemble in size the genetic material of small bacterial viruses, rather than that of mammalian cell nuclei. This finding has led to the suggestion that the mitochondria might be welcome passengers in our cells, having wandered fairly late in evolution to establish a symbiotic relationship with mammalian cells, which they provide with large quantities of chemical energy in return for a warm, moist, compositionally satisfying environment. If this hypothesis is correct, it is apparent that the mitochondrial membrane plays a major role in the communications between the "symbiote" and the "host."

Both carbohydrates and fats can be oxidized in the mitochondria (Chapter 2). Oxidation of some of the amino acids is also theoretically possible in the heart, although in fact proteins make up virtually none of the substrate for normal cardiac function. Both fats and carbohydrates enter the final reactions of oxidative metabolism as 2-carbon fragments, which are then broken down to form CO_2 and H_2O. The pathways by which carbohydrates are converted to acetate were described in Chapter 3. The following section describes the processes by which this 2-carbon fragment is derived from fats.

FATTY ACID METABOLISM

Fats are found in the blood mostly in the form of free fatty acids (FFA) and triglycerides. The FFA are free only in that they are not bound as esters; they are in fact bound to the plasma proteins, mainly to albumin. The triglycerides represent complexes of fatty acids and phospholipids that are esterified to glycerol, a 3-carbon sugar. The oxidation of fats therefore requires first that FFA be taken up by the cell and that triglycerides be broken down to liberate FFA. The latter are then "activated" and transported into the mitochondria where they are oxidized to form acetate. The overall scheme of fatty acid metabolism is shown in Fig. 4.1.

Uptake of Fatty Acids by the Cell

Fatty acids are made available to the cell both as FFA and as triglycerides, in which the fatty acids are esterified to the hydroxyl groups of glycerol. Increas-

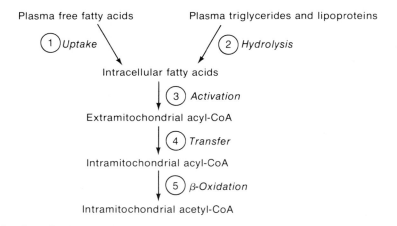

FIG. 4.1. Overall scheme of fatty acid metabolism. The conversion of circulating lipids to the 2-carbon fragments that are oxidized within the cell involves five key reactions: (1) uptake of plasma free fatty acids; (2) liberation of esterified fatty acids by hydrolysis of plasma triglycerides and lipoproteins; (3) fatty acid activation, i.e., binding to CoA; (4) transfer of activated fatty acids (acyl-CoA) from the cytosol to the mitochondrial matrix; and (5) β-oxidation to yield the 2-carbon fragment acetyl-CoA.

ing the plasma concentration of FFA leads to increased fatty acid uptake. This effect is due partly to the law of mass action and partly to the fact that high concentrations of fatty acids in the plasma saturate the high-affinity fatty acid binding sites of albumin. As a result of the latter, when blood levels of fatty acids are increased a greater portion of the fatty acids comes to be bound to albumin at sites of lower affinity, which are less able than the high-affinity binding sites to restrain fatty acid diffusion into the cells.

The movement of fatty acids across the cell membrane appears to be due to passive diffusion, possibly involving fatty acid-binding proteins in the sarcolemma.

Hydrolysis of Plasma Triglycerides and Lipoproteins

The regulation of fatty acid transport from plasma triglycerides and lipoproteins into the cell is more complex than that from FFA because esterified fatty acids (in triglycerides and lipoproteins) do not enter the cell. In some ways the mechanisms controlling fatty acid transport from triglycerides into the cell are similar to those controlling glucose transport, which were described in Chapter 3. The esterified fatty acids are first released from their complex with glycerol by the enzyme *lipoprotein lipase,* which is located on the capillary endothelium. This enzyme is controlled by circulating hormones (notably epinephrine) which increase triglyceride hydrolysis. The ability of epinephrine to activate lipoprotein lipase in the heart probably results from phosphorylation of the enzyme, which is effected by a cyclic AMP-dependent protein kinase. The net result of this action of epinephrine is similar in its functional consequences to the epinephrine-induced stimulation of both glucose transport and glycogen breakdown: All increase the availability of substrate within the cell. In this way, when epinephrine increases the rate of energy expenditure by the heart, there is a concomitant increase in the supply of glucose and fatty acids for energy production.

Fatty Acid Activation

The term fatty acid activation describes the processes responsible for the formation of a fatty acid complex with coenzyme A (CoA). The resulting fatty acid esters, *acyl-CoA,* represent precursors for the acyl carnitine derivatives which cross mitochondrial membranes from the cytosol to the mitochondrial matrix, where fats are subsequently oxidized. Like the entry of glucose into the glycolytic pathway, the formation of acyl-CoA, and thus the entry of fatty acids into the mitochondria, requires the initial "investment" of ATP. The high-energy bond of ATP is used to form an enzyme-bound fatty acyl adenylate complex according to the reaction:

$$\text{Fatty acid} + \text{E} + \text{ATP} \rightleftharpoons \underset{\textit{Fatty acyl adenylate}}{\text{E} \cdot \text{fatty acid} \sim \text{AMP}} + \text{PP}_i$$
$$\underset{\textit{Enzyme}}{}$$

Coenzyme A then replaces the AMP that is bound to the fatty acid, liberating acyl-CoA according to the reaction

$$E \cdot \text{fatty acid} \sim AMP + CoA\text{-}SH \rightleftharpoons E + \text{acyl-CoA} + AMP$$

The overall process of fatty acid activation can thus be written:

$$CH_3\text{---}(CH_2)_n\text{---}COOH + ATP + CoA\text{-}SH \rightleftharpoons$$
$$\underset{\textit{Fatty acid}}{} \qquad \underset{\textit{Reduced CoA}}{}$$

$$\underset{\textit{Acyl-CoA}}{CH_3\text{---}(CH_2)_n\text{---}\overset{\overset{\displaystyle O}{\|}}{C}\text{---}SCoA} + AMP + PP_i$$

Acyl-CoA, the main product of this reaction, is the "activated" fatty acid. The mechanisms controlling fatty acid activation, aside from the effects of changing concentrations of the reactants depicted above, remain poorly understood.

Different fatty acids are activated in different regions of the myocardial cell. A large portion of the acyl-CoA produced by this process takes place outside the mitochondria, so that regulation of the transport of acyl-CoA into the mitochondrial matrix may play an additional role in controlling the rate of oxidative energy production.

Transfer of Acyl-CoA

The transfer of activated fatty acids into the mitochondria cannot take place unless the acyl groups are first linked to carnitine, a 7-carbon organic acid that can replace the coenzyme A to which the fatty acid is esterified. The formation of *acyl carnitine* is therefore an essential step in this transport process. Fatty acid transfer can be described by the overall reaction

$$\text{Acyl-CoA}_o + \text{carnitine} \rightleftharpoons \text{acyl carnitine} + CoASH$$

$$\text{Acyl carnitine} + CoASH \rightleftharpoons \text{acyl-CoA}_i + \text{carnitine}$$

where acyl-CoA$_o$ is the activated fatty acid outside the mitochondrial matrix and acyl-CoA$_i$ is the activated fatty acid within the mitochondria.

The role of carnitine in this transport process is probably that of a "carrier;" i.e., the acyl carnitine derivative is the form in which the fatty acids are transported into the mitochondria. The transport of fatty acids into the mitochondria requires the participation of two membrane-bound transferring enzymes, or transferases. One is associated with the mitochondrial outer membrane and the other with the inner membrane, so that together the two transferases "pass" the fatty acid into the mitochondria. The factors that govern the overall rate of transfer of the activated fatty acids into the mitochondria remain poorly understood.

β-Oxidation

The entry of fatty acids into the tricarboxylic acid cycle, which is the major oxidative pathway of the myocardium, occurs through the formation of acetyl-

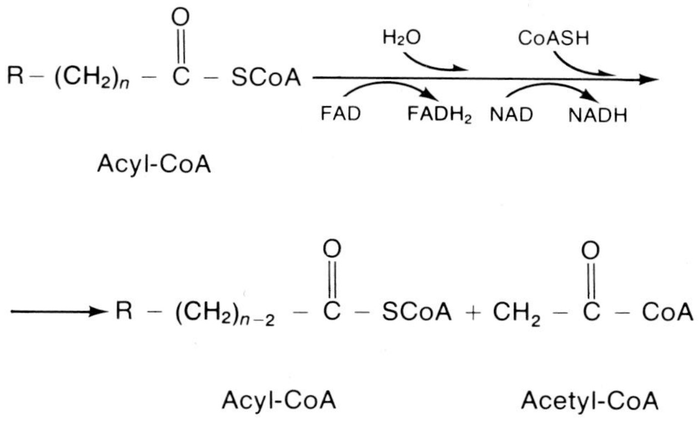

$$R - (CH_2)_n - \overset{\overset{\displaystyle O}{\|}}{C} - SCoA \xrightarrow{\quad \underset{\text{FAD} \quad \text{FADH}_2 \quad \text{NAD} \quad \text{NADH}}{\text{H}_2\text{O} \qquad \text{CoASH}} \quad}$$

Acyl-CoA

$$\longrightarrow R - (CH_2)_{n-2} - \overset{\overset{\displaystyle O}{\|}}{C} - SCoA + CH_2 - \overset{\overset{\displaystyle O}{\|}}{C} - CoA$$

Acyl-CoA   Acetyl-CoA

FIG. 4.2. Overall reaction of β-oxidation by which activated fatty acids (acyl-CoA) are broken down to form the 2-carbon fragment acetyl-CoA.

CoA. In this way fatty acid metabolism, like that of carbohydrates, leads to the formation of a common 2-carbon endproduct, acetyl-CoA. This general similarity between these two metabolic pathways, however, is only superficial. In the case of carbohydrate metabolism, there is an alternative pathway for pyruvate metabolism that can proceed in the absence of oxygen, i.e., the formation of lactate. Fat metabolism, on the other hand, is absolutely dependent on a continuing supply of oxygen so that, for example, when coronary flow is interrupted ATP cannot be produced from fats.

The breakdown of acyl-CoA to acetyl-CoA occurs within the mitochondria and involves four steps, each of which is catalyzed by a different enzyme. The overall reaction is shown in Fig. 4.2. The cofactors for β-oxidation include not only CoA, but also flavine adenine dinucleotide (FAD) and NAD, which are reduced to $FADH_2$ and NADH, respectively, in this process. FAD is a coenzyme much like NAD, both of which serve as reducing agents for substrate oxidation. β-oxidation allows fatty acids to be degraded in a stepwise fashion to form acetyl-CoA, the 2-carbon fragment (identical to that produced by carbohydrate metabolism) that is subsequently oxidized in the tricarboxylic acid cycle.

The rate of β-oxidation is regulated by both the concentrations of fatty acids within the cell and the availability of oxidized FAD and NAD. The requirement for oxidized coenzymes means that this process cannot proceed in the ischemic or anoxic heart. Regulation of β-oxidation by the availability of oxidized coenzymes is similar to that seen for the glyceraldehyde-3-phosphate dehydrogenase reaction in controlling the rate of glycolysis so that fat metabolism, like glucose metabolism, is inhibited when the interior of the cell shifts toward a reduced state. The FAD used in β-oxidation also participates in the oxidation of succinate by the tricarboxylic acid cycle, a dual role for FAD that allows an increased carbohydrate flux through the tricarboxylic acid cycle to inhibit fatty acid oxidation.

OXIDATION OF ACETYL-CoA BY THE
TRICARBOXYLIC ACID CYCLE

The preceding section of this chapter, as well as Chapter 3, included some details of the process by which carbohydrates and fats are metabolized to yield acetyl-CoA, which is then oxidized within the mitochondria. This process of oxidation, by which acetyl-CoA is degraded to CO_2 and H_2O, occurs by a cyclic series of reactions, the *tricarboxylic acid cycle.* The enzymes which catalyze this cycle are free within the intramitochondrial matrix, i.e., not bound to the membrane of the mitochondria.

The reactions of the tricarboxylic acid cycle can be described in general terms (Fig. 4.3A) as the condensation of the 2-carbon fragment, acetyl-CoA, with a 4-carbon organic acid, oxaloacetate, to form citrate, a 6-carbon organic acid. Following configurational rearrangements, which yield *cis*-aconitate from citrate, the 6-carbon organic acid is converted to isocitrate, which is then oxidized and decarboxylated to form α-ketoglutaric acid, a 5-carbon organic acid. α-Ketoglutarate is then oxidized and decarboxylated to form the 4-carbon organic acid succinate. Coenzyme A is required for the formation of succinate from α-ketoglutarate, succinyl-CoA being the initial product of a series of reactions that leads to the formation of succinate. As in acetyl-CoA, the ester link between the coenzyme and substrate in succinyl-CoA is a high-energy bond. Thus when succinyl-CoA is hydrolyzed to succinate, the high-energy bond is first transferred to an enzyme (E), to form E $\sim$ CoA (Fig. 4.3B), and then to phosphate to form E $\sim$ P. The high-energy phosphate bond is then used to convert GDP to GTP, eventually being transferred to ADP to form ATP. It should be noted that the series of reactions shown in Fig. 4.3B, which is set into motion by the oxidation of α-ketoglutarate to succinate, represents the only point in the tricarboxylic acid cycle where a high-energy phosphate bond is formed directly by *substrate-level phosphorylation.* As is discussed later in this chapter, by far the greater amount of ATP is formed when NADH and $FADH_2$ are oxidized by *respiratory-chain-linked phosphorylation.*

The succinate produced from α-ketoglutarate is oxidized by an enzyme, E-FAD (Fig. 4.3A), which contains bound FAD. As a result of the oxidation of succinate, the E-FAD complex is reduced to E-$FADH_2$ and fumarate is formed. After water is added to fumarate to form malate, the latter is oxidized by the conversion of NAD to NADH. This latter reaction yields oxaloacetate, thereby completing the cycle.

The overall reaction of the tricarboxylic acid cycle is: addition of two molecules of water to the 2-carbon fragment derived from carbohydrate or fat metabolism, splitting off of two molecules of carbon dioxide, and four steps of oxidation. A high-energy phosphate bond is formed only at one step in this process (see above). By far the greatest portion of the chemical energy released through oxidation of the 2-carbon fragment is trapped in the four oxidation reactions, three of which yield NADH, and the other enzyme-bound $FADH_2$. Thus ATP production by the tricarboxylic acid cycle requires yet another process, the respiratory-chain-

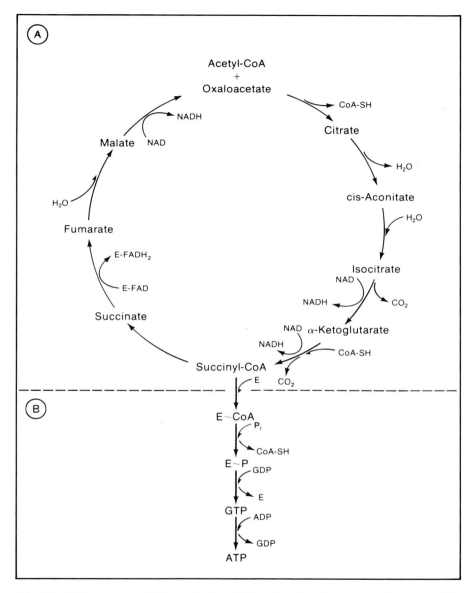

FIG. 4.3. Pathways of acetyl-CoA oxidation. **A:** Tricarboxylic acid cycle. Condensation of the 2-carbon fragment acetyl-CoA with the 4-carbon organic acid oxaloacetate *(top)* yields a 6-carbon organic acid (citrate). The latter, after isomerization to isocitrate, is oxidized and decarboxylated. The resulting 5-carbon organic acid (α-ketoglutarate) is oxidized and decarboxylated in a reaction that yields succinyl-CoA. Oxaloacetate is regenerated after succinyl CoA undergoes two steps of oxidation and one of hydration. **B:** Substrate level phosphorylation. Each mole of enzyme-bound CoA released from succinyl-CoA provides for generation of a single mole of ATP by substrate level phosphorylation.

linked phosphorylation that takes place during oxidative phosphorylation (see below).

The rate of turnover of the tricarboxylic acid cycle is regulated in part by the availability of acetyl-CoA for degradation (see above) and of oxidized NAD and FAD for reduction (see below). The first step in the cycle—condensation of oxaloacetate and acetyl-CoA to form citrate—is regulated by the levels of both of these precursors. The oxaloacetate level in the mitochondria is in turn determined by the redox state. The mechanism by which oxaloacetate level is controlled can be seen in Fig. 4.3A, where the final step in the tricarboxylic acid cycle is shown to be oxidation of malate to oxaloacetate, along with the reduction of NAD to NADH. The ratio between NAD and NADH levels, which reflects the redox state of the mitochondrial matrix, thus plays a key role in determining oxaloacetate levels as the ratio NAD/NADH is proportional to the ratio oxaloacetate/malate. (This follows from the overall equilibrium of the reaction: malate + NAD $\rightleftharpoons$ oxaloacetate + NADH.) In this way a shift in the mitochondria to a more reduced state (e.g., in myocardial hypoxia or ischemia) slows the tricarboxylic acid cycle by decreasing the amount of oxaloacetate available for condensation with acetyl-CoA.

There are many additional regulatory influences within the tricarboxylic acid cycle. Most important of these is that exerted by the enzyme *isocitric dehydrogenase,* which catalyzes the production of α-ketoglutarate from isocitrate. Much like phosphofructokinase in the regulation of glycolysis, isocitric dehydrogenase responds to the high-energy phosphate levels within the cell (in the case of isocitric dehydrogenase, within the mitochondria). The reaction catalyzed by isocitric dehydrogenase is stimulated by ADP and inhibited by ATP, although neither of these nucleotides participates in the reaction catalyzed by this enzyme. This ability of high-energy phosphate compounds to regulate the tricarboxylic acid cycle allows acetyl-CoA oxidation to be accelerated when the energy requirements of the cell are increased, i.e., when ATP levels fall and ADP accumulates. Isocitric dehydrogenase is inhibited by a high NADH/NAD ratio so that the reaction catalyzed by this enzyme represents another point in the tricarboxylic acid cycle, in addition to oxaloacetate formation, that is sensitive to the depletion of oxidized NAD and the accumulation of reduced NADH. A similar control by the availability of oxidized coenzymes is exerted at the next step in the tricarboxylic acid cycle, which is catalyzed by the enzyme α-*ketoglutarate dehydrogenase,* because this latter enzyme is also inhibited by a high NADH/NAD ratio. In this way the rate of oxidation of acetyl-CoA in the mitochondria can be controlled by the energy requirements of the heart (i.e., ATP levels), the availability of oxidized coenzymes, and the supply of substrate.

TRANSPORT OF REDUCED NADH FROM CYTOSOL TO MITOCHONDRIA: THE MALATE-ASPARTATE CYCLE

The reduced NADH formed during oxidation of the acetyl-CoA derived from fats and carbohydrates and during the β-oxidation of fatty acids gains ready access to the enzymes of the respiratory chain because all of these reactions occur within the mitochondria. In the case of NADH produced during glycolysis, however, the coenzyme is reduced in the cytosol and so must be returned to the mitochondria before it can be oxidized. Similarly, under normal aerobic conditions where lactate is not being produced, the NAD essential for glycolysis must be derived from intramitochondrial supplies of the oxidized coenzyme. The exchange between NADH produced in the cytosol and NAD produced in the mitochondria does not take place by simple diffusion because the mitochondrial inner membrane is not permeable to this coenzyme. As a result, the transfer of NADH into the mitochondria in exchange for NAD must be effected by a membrane transport mechanism. In a number of tissues, notably the liver, this exchange is effected by a "shuttle" that involves glycerol phosphate and dihydroxyacetone phosphate. In the heart, however, the more complex malate-aspartate cycle plays an important role in the exchange of reducing equivalents across the mitochondrial membrane. This shuttle involves not only oxidation and reduction reactions but also transaminations, i.e., the transfer of amino groups between the organic acids produced during carbohydrate metabolism and amino acids such as are found in the proteins (Fig. 4.4).

The malate-aspartate cycle is most easily understood by considering first the transfer of reducing equivalents across the mitochondrial membrane, which is a relatively simple process, and then examining the additional reactions necessary

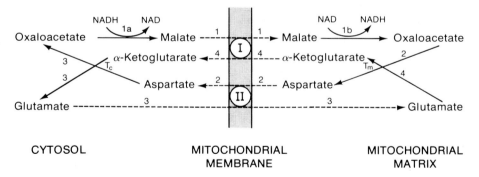

CYTOSOL   MITOCHONDRIAL MEMBRANE   MITOCHONDRIAL MATRIX

FIG. 4.4. Malate-aspartate cycle. This complex series of reactions proceeds by the following sequence: (1) reduction of oxaloacetate in the cytosol and transfer of the 4-carbon acid malate into the mitochondrial matrix by a membrane carrier (I). This step leads to oxidation of NADH in the cytosol (1a), and subsequent oxidation of malate leads to reduction of NAD in the mitochondria (1b). (2) Oxaloacetate, the 4-carbon acid that has appeared in the mitochondrial matrix during reaction 1b, is transferred back to the cytosol as the 4-carbon amino acid aspartate by a second membrane carrier (II) following a transamination (T_m) with mitochondrial glutamate. (3) Oxaloacetate is regenerated in the cytosol by transamination of aspartate with α-ketoglutarate (T_c). This reaction leads to formation of glutamate, which is subsequently transferred to the mitochondrial matrix in exchange for aspartate (produced during reaction 2) by membrane carrier II. (4) The glutamate transferred to the mitochondrial matrix is converted to α-ketoglutarate by transamination with oxaloacetate (T_m) as described in reaction 2. The α-ketoglutarate so produced moves back to the cytosol to replace that utilized in reaction 3, the transport being effected by membrane carrier I in exchange for the malate transported to the mitochondrial matrix (reaction 1).

to restore the two metabolic pools—the cytosol and the mitochondrial matrix—at either side of the mitochondrial membrane to their original states.

The reaction that in effect transfers NADH across the mitochondrial membrane is labeled *1* in Fig. 4.4. The reduced NADH formed in the cytosol during glycolysis is oxidized to NAD by the coupled reduction of oxaloacetate to malate (*1a*, Fig. 4.4). Malate is then transported into the mitochondria by a specific membrane carrier (*I*, Fig. 4.4) rather than by free diffusion. Once inside the mitochondria, malate is oxidized by NAD to produce oxaloacetate and reduced NADH (*1b*, Fig. 4.4). The net effect of this reaction therefore is the same as if NADH from the cytosol were exchanged for NAD in the mitochondria: in the cytosol NADH has been oxidized to NAD; in the mitochondria NAD has been reduced to NADH. This reaction, in effect, resupplies the cytosol with oxidized NAD for further glycolysis, while the mitochondria obtains NADH that serves as a substrate for the energy-yielding processes of oxidative phosphorylation. This "transfer" of NADH from cytosol to mitochondria, however, leaves the cytosol depleted of oxaloacetate, which has appeared within the mitochondria. Thus to complete the malate-aspartate cycle, further reactions are needed to return the excess oxaloacetate from the mitochondria to the cytosol.

A simple transfer of oxaloacetate from mitochondria to cytosol is prevented by the impermeability of the mitochondrial membrane to this organic acid and by the fact that there is no oxaloacetate carrier in heart mitochondria. Instead of moving directly back to the cytosol as oxaloacetate, therefore, this 4-carbon organic acid must first be transaminated in the mitochondrial matrix (Tm) to form aspartate, a 4-carbon amino acid for which a carrier does exist in the mitochondrial membrane (*II*, Fig. 4.4). This carrier-mediated transfer of aspartate (*2*, Fig. 4.4) does not, however, restore the two cell compartments to their original state. If anything, these two compartments are even more different than they were at the start of the process because amino groups have now moved from the mitochondrial matrix to the cytosol. The initial composition of these compartments must therefore be restored by two additional reactions, each of which provide substrates for cotransport by the two membrane carriers already mentioned. The first of these additional reactions (*3*, Fig. 4.4) consists of the transamination of α-ketoglutarate in the cytosolic compartment (Tc) with the amino groups previously carried into this compartment by aspartate. This reaction allows the amino groups to be transferred to glutamate, which can return to the mitochondrial matrix (see below). At the same time, this reaction converts the cytosolic aspartate to oxaloacetate, thereby restoring the initial level of this 4-carbon organic acid in the cytosol. This cytosolic transamination requires the participation of α-ketoglutarate, a 5-carbon organic acid which is transaminated to form glutamate. The latter, a 5-carbon amino acid, is returned to the mitochondrial matrix by the carrier II (which has already been described as the carrier of the 4-carbon amino acid aspartate that was transported to the cytosol).

The malate-aspartate cycle is completed when a 5-carbon organic acid is returned to the cytosol from the mitochondrial matrix. This final step—which both replenishes the α-ketoglutarate utilized in the process labeled *3* in Fig. 4.4 and supplies the amino groups for the initial transamination labeled Tm in Fig. 4.4—is initiated by the transfer of amino groups within the mitochondria from glutamate to oxaloacetate. This transamination, you recall, provided the mechanism by which a 4-carbon acid was returned from the mitochondrial matrix to the cytosol as aspartate. In Fig. 4.4 this final step is depicted by the reactions labeled *4,* which include the second half of the transamination within the mitochondrial matrix, just described, and the transfer of α-ketoglutarate back to the cytosol. This final reaction is coupled to the transfer of malate into the mitochondrial matrix by the carrier labeled *I,* which was involved in the initial step in the transfer of reducing equivalents into the mitochondria.

The complex series of reactions shown in Fig. 4.4 comprises nothing more than a means to "move" NADH from the cytosol to the mitochondrial matrix for subsequent oxidation, and to "move" NAD back to the cytosol in return so as to allow glycolysis to proceed. The complexity of this transfer (why do the mitochondria not simply have a carrier that can transfer NADH in return for NAD?) again illustrates the nonadherence of the myocardium to the precepts of Ockham's razor. Yet this complexity is not without its advantages to the cell, for it provides yet another means by which metabolism can be controlled and by which the many individual catalytic reactions that are responsible for energy production in the heart can be integrated.

The implications of the malate-aspartate cycle in terms of the control of energy production in the heart remain incompletely understood, but a number of features of this cycle appear to be extremely important in integrating the rates of anaerobic and aerobic energy production. Thus in addition to its role in regulating the transport of reducing equivalents, this cycle can regulate the flux of substrates through the tricarboxylic cycle by its ability to modulate the concentrations of oxaloacetate and α-ketoglutarate within the mitochondria. (Recall that both of these are intermediates of the tricarboxylic acid cycle; see above and Fig. 4.3.)

The importance of the control permitted by the malate-aspartate cycle can be seen under conditions where an inability of the mitochondria to oxidize oxaloacetate leads to an increased concentration of this 4-carbon acid within the mitochondria. This in turn promotes the accumulation of oxaloacetate in the cytosol through reactions 2 and 3 shown in Fig. 4.4. Once in the cytosol, oxaloacetate can be reduced to malate (reaction 1a) thereby regenerating oxidized NAD, which in the ischemic heart becomes critical for the production of ATP by anaerobic glycolysis.

Movement of other substances by way of this cycle provides additional means of "communication" between the mitochondrial matrix and the cytosol. In the case of citrate (which has an important regulatory influence on the glycolytic rate by virtue of its effects on the enzyme phosphofructokinase, as discussed in Chapter 3) the movements of this 6-carbon organic acid across the mitochondrial membrane cannot occur by simple diffusion. Instead, citrate is converted in the mitochondrial matrix to α-ketoglutarate, which then is transferred across the mitochondrial membrane by carrier I (Fig. 4.4) to the cytosol where the α-ketoglutarate is reconverted to citrate. The latter reactions and their control by the malate-aspartate cycle are not yet fully understood, but their importance in mediating the control of glycolytic rate by citrate may be related to the likelihood that the glutamate-aspartate carrier (carrier II, Fig. 4.4) is energy-dependent and thus sensitive to changes in cellular energy metabolism.

OXIDATIVE PHOSPHORYLATION

The major reactions of aerobic ATP production occur neither within the tricarboxylic acid cycle nor in fatty acid oxidation. Although both of the latter represent oxidative reactions, only the former is coupled directly to ATP synthesis and yields but 1 mole of high-energy phosphate per "turn" of the cycle (Fig. 4.3B). Instead, virtually all of the ATP generated by aerobic metabolism is obtained from yet another series of oxidative reactions—that catalyzed by the enzymes of the respiratory chain. These enzymes, which are tightly bound to the mitochondrial membrane, couple ATP formation to the oxidation of NADH and FADH$_2$, the reduced coenzymes produced when carbohydrates and fatty acids are oxidized by the tricarboxylic acid cycle and by fatty acid oxidation (see above). The reactions catalyzed by the respiratory chain also provide for oxidation of the NADH produced during aerobic glycolysis (Chapter 3).

The overall reaction catalyzed by the enzymes of the respiratory chain can be described by the equations:

$$NADH + H^+ + \tfrac{1}{2}O_2 \longrightarrow NAD + H_2O$$

and

$$FADH_2 + \tfrac{1}{2}O_2 \longrightarrow FAD + H_2O$$

A large amount of energy is liberated in these reactions, as can readily be appreciated when one remembers the explosive reaction that occurs when molecular hydrogen is ignited in an oxygen-containing environment. It is the function of the respiratory chain to trap this explosive burst of energy in a form that can be used within the cell, i.e., as the high-energy phosphate bonds of ATP.

The reactions of the respiratory chain can be looked on either as the transfer of reducing equivalents, as shown above, or as the transfer of electrons. The relationship between hydrogen (i.e., reducing equivalent) transfer and electron transfer is readily understood because one atom of hydrogen (H) represents a hydrogen ion (H$^+$) plus an electron (e$^-$). The function of the respiratory chain enzymes, and especially the role of the iron-containing heme pigments they contain, is more easily understood if these reactions are described in terms of electron transport. Looked on in this way, the overall reactions described above are:

$$NAD\text{-}2e^- + 2H^+ + \tfrac{1}{2}O_2 \longrightarrow NAD + 2H_2O$$
$$\text{(reduced)} \qquad\qquad\qquad\qquad \text{(oxidized)}$$

and

$$FAD\text{-}2e^- + 2H^+ + \tfrac{1}{2}O_2 \longrightarrow FAD + 2H_2O$$

(reduced)   (oxidized)

where the electrons initially carried by the reduced coenzymes (NAD-$2e^-$ and FAD-$2e^-$) are ultimately transferred to molecular oxygen, thereby leading to the production of O^{2-}, which can then combine with $2H^+$ to form H_2O.

The successive transfer of electrons by the enzymes of the respiratory chain occurs through a series of oxidation and reduction steps. Starting with reduced NAD, the series of reactions can be depicted as shown in Table 4.1. The electrons are "carried" in NAD, FAD, and coenzyme Q through their introduction into complex organic ring structures according to the general reactions:

$$=\overset{|}{N}{}^+- + e^- \rightleftharpoons -\overset{|}{N}-$$

(reduced)   (oxidized)

and

$$=O + e^- \rightleftharpoons -O^-$$

(reduced)   (oxidized)

The electrons carried by the cytochromes reduce the ferric iron of the heme rings according to the general reaction

$$Fe^{3+} + e^- \rightleftharpoons Fe^{2+}$$

(reduced)   (oxidized)

In this way the oxidation of fats and carbohydrates described in the reactions outlined in the preceding sections of this chapter can be viewed as representing the removal of electrons and hydrogen ions from these substrates. The electrons are then transferred through the coenzymes and iron atoms in the respiratory chain, eventually reaching molecular oxygen. At this final step, where the electrons are transferred to oxygen, the hydrogen ions liberated from the substrates are utilized to form water.

The energy set free during the passage of electrons through the respiratory chain is trapped to form ATP at the three steps in the reaction sequence shown

TABLE 4.1. *Passage of electrons through the respiratory chain*

Initial reactants		Final reactants	
Reduced	Oxidized	Reduced	Oxidized
Substrate-2H	NAD	NAD-$2e^-$	Substrate +$2H^+$
*{ NAD-$2e^-$	Flavoprotein	Flavoprotein-$2e^-$	NAD
Flavoprotein-$2e^-$	Coenzyme Q	Coenzyme Q-$2e^-$	Flavoprotein
Coenzyme Q-$2e^-$	2 Cytochrome b	2 Cytochrome b-e^-	Coenzyme Q
* 2 Cytochrome b-e^-	2 Cytochrome c	2 Cytochrome c-e^-	2 Cytochrome b
2 Cytochrome c-e^-	2 Cytochrome a	2 Cytochrome a-e^-	2 Cytochrome c
*{ 2 Cytochrome a-e^-	2 Cytochrome a_3	2 Cytochrome a_3-e^-	2 Cytochrome a
2 Cytochrome a_3-e^-	$\tfrac{1}{2}O_2$ +$2H^+$	H_2O	2 Cytochrome a_3

* One mole of ATP is generated at this step.

in Table 4.1 that are marked with an asterisk. The oxidation of each mole of NAD in the respiratory chain therefore provides for the formation of 3 moles of ATP.

ENERGY BALANCES

The generation of ATP during the metabolic processes described here and in Chapter 3 can be considered in terms of two types of reaction. The first, *substrate-level phosphorylation,* occurs when the substrate itself contains a high-energy phosphate bond that is transferred to ADP, yielding ATP. Much more important from a quantitative standpoint is *respiratory-chain-linked phosphorylation,* in which the high-energy phosphate bonds are formed during oxidative phosphorylation.

The net synthesis of ATP by the reactions of anaerobic glycolysis, where NADH is oxidized through the reduction of pyruvate to lactate (Fig. 3.1), produces 2 moles of ATP per mole of glucose through substrate-level phosphorylation (Table 4.2). Under aerobic conditions more ATP is produced during glycolysis because the NADH that is formed can be oxidized by respiratory-chain-linked phosphorylation to produce ATP. As shown in Fig. 3.1, each mole of glucose yields 2 moles of glyceraldehyde-3-phosphate, so that 2 moles of NAD per mole of glucose can be reduced to NADH during the subsequent oxidation

TABLE 4.2. *Energy balances*

Reaction	ATP (moles generated/mole of glucose)		
	Substrate-level phosphorylation	Respiratory-chain-linked phosphorylation	Total
Anaerobic			
Anaerobic glycolysis			
Glucose → lactate	2	0	2
Oxidative			
Aerobic glycolysis			
Glucose → pyruvate	2	0	
2 NADH → 2 NAD	0	4	
Total	2	4	6
Pyruvate oxidation			
2 Pyruvate → 2 acetyl-CoA + 2CO_2	0	0	
2 NADH → 2 NAD	0	6	
Total	0	6	6
Acetate oxidation			
2 Acetyl-CoA → 4 CO_2	2	0	
6 NADH → 6 NAD	0	18	
2 $FADH_2$ → 2 FAD	0	4	
Total	2	22	24
Glucose oxidation (total)			
Glucose → 6 CO_2	4	32	36

of this 3-carbon compound to 3-phosphoglycerate. Had these 2 moles of NADH been generated inside the mitochondria, they would have provided for the formation of a total of 6 moles of ATP (Table 4.1). Because glycolysis occurs in the cytosol, however, this NADH first must enter the mitochondria. This transport process, which occurs by way of the malate-aspartate shuttle, requires the expenditure of energy so that approximately 2 moles of ATP are recovered per mole of NADH. Aerobic glycolysis thus provides an additional 4 moles of ATP per mole of glucose through oxidation of NADH (Table 4.2), giving a total of 6 moles of ATP generated by metabolism of each mole of glucose.

The oxidation of each mole of pyruvate to acetyl-CoA, which occurs within the mitochondria, is accompanies by the reduction of a mole of NAD (Fig. 3.8). The subsequent oxidation of the NADH formed in this reaction provides an additional 3 moles of ATP per mole of pyruvate oxidized. As each glucose molecule yields two of pyruvate, this reaction yields 6 moles of ATP per mole of glucose (Table 4.2).

The oxidation of acetate by the enzymes of the tricarboxylic acid cycle yields 3 moles of NADH and one of enzyme-bound $FADH_2$ (Fig. 4.3A). Each mole of NADH formed by the oxidation of isocitrate, α-ketoglutarate, and malate yields 3 moles of ATP, so that NADH oxidation yields a total of 9 moles of ATP per mole of acetate. Oxidation of the E-$FADH_2$ complex formed during succinate oxidation yields only 2 moles of ATP. To this total—11 moles of ATP from each mole of acetyl-CoA produced by respiratory-chain-linked phosphorylation— must be added the single mole of ATP produced by the substrate-level phosphorylation that follows the oxidation of α-ketoglutarate (Fig. 4.3B). Acetate oxidation therefore provides 12 moles of ATP from the oxidation of each mole of the 2-carbon fragment. As 2 moles of acetyl-CoA are formed from each mole of glucose, a total of 24 moles of ATP is formed by the oxidation of both of the 2-carbon fragments derived from glucose (Table 4.2).

The "balance sheet" presented in Table 4.2 shows that of the 36 moles of ATP that can be produced by the metabolism of a single mole of glucose all but two require that the cell be provided with oxygen. For this reason anoxia or ischemia halt the pathways responsible for producing almost 95% of the ATP produced during carbohydrate metabolism. In addition, anoxia and ischemia inhibit completely the oxidation of fatty acids, which normally comprise a more important energy source for the heart than carbohydrates. For this reason the devastating effects of anoxia and ischemia on cardiac function are readily understandable.

MECHANISM OF OXIDATIVE PHOSPHORYLATION

The mechanism by which the transfer of electrons along the respiratory chain provides energy for ATP synthesis has long remained a mystery. For a number of years it was thought that this energy was used to form a "phosphorylated intermediate," where high-energy phosphate bonds were generated in one or more proteins associated with the respiratory chain. This process, called *chemical coupling,* would be analogous to the substrate-level phosphorylation shown in Fig. 4.3B, and the two ATP-producing reactions of glycolysis shown in Fig. 3.1. It now appears more likely, however, that the energy transfer to ATP during oxidative phosphorylation takes place instead by a *chemiosmotic* process. In this process the energy released during the three oxidation steps (with asterisks) in Table 4.1 is utilized initially to establish a concentration gradient for some substance, or substances, across the inner mitochondrial membrane. High-energy phosphate bonds are then generated by a process in which this osmotic energy is coupled to the formation of ATP. In other words, the chemiosmotic hypothesis states that the chemical energy obtained by the oxidative reactions of the respiratory chain is converted first to osmotic energy, a form of potential energy, by the establishment of a transmembrane concentration gradient, a charge gradient, or both. This potential energy is then reconverted to chemical energy (the formation of ATP) in a subsequent reaction or reactions.

A number of observations now favor the chemiosmotic hypothesis. Among these is the failure, so far, to find a phosphorylated intermediate such as would be formed if oxidative phosphorylation was a chemically coupled process. Evidence that oxidative phosphorylation requires the structural integrity of the mitochondrial membrane also favors the chemiosmotic hypothesis. The recent discovery of *ionophores*—substances that can render biological membranes permeable to a more or less restricted class of ions—has also contributed to the support of this hypothesis. It has been possible to show that when ionophores allow certain cations to pass freely across the mitochondrial membrane oxidative phosphorylation is "uncoupled." "Uncoupling" of oxidative phosphorylation means that respiration can proceed but no ATP is formed. This is similar to the consequence of depressing the clutch in a car in that this maneuver does not interfere with the turnover of the engine although power is no longer transmitted to the wheels. The aptness of this analogy is reflected in the fact that in the same way that depressing the clutch in an accelerating car allows the engine to "race," so uncoupling agents accelerate respiration. In both cases, however, these processes are uncoupled from their normal function, i.e., transmission of power and ATP formation.

Another feature of mitochondrial behavior compatible with an essential role for ion separation across the mitochondrial membrane in the process of oxidative phosphorylation is the finding that mitochondrial conformation changes during oxidative phosphorylation. Thus the highly ordered array of cristae shown in Fig. 1.10 for resting mitochondria is changed when the mitochondria are actively generating ATP; the picture becomes one in which the space delimited by the inner membrane has shrunk markedly within the outer membrane. These morphological changes are consistent with the chemiosmotic theory since they provide evidence that the highly organized system of respiratory enzymes (which are bound tightly to the inner mitochondrial membrane) can transform the energy obtained from oxidation to changes in the composition and volume of the spaces on either side of this membrane.

The finding that oxidative phosphorylation can be coupled directly to ion transport also supports the chemiosmotic hypothesis. Thus electron transport through the respiratory chain can be shown to be linked stoichiometrically to ion transport, notably that of Ca^{2+} and H^+ without the participation of ADP or ATP. This observation is especially important as it has been clearly shown that another membrane in the heart, the sarcoplasmic reticulum, can transform the energy made available by the "downhill" movement of Ca^{2+} along an electro-chemical gradient into the formation of ATP from ADP and P_i (Chapter 9).

If the chemiosmotic hypothesis in fact accounts for oxidative phosphorylation, it appears likely that the ion whose concentration gradient is initially responsible for the reactions which lead to ATP formation is H^+. If correct, this view of a critical role of hydrogen ion would mean that the protons released during substrate oxidation play more than a passive role in the processes of oxidative phosphorylation. In other words, it might be more appropriate to highlight an energy-linked separation of hydrogen ion as the direct cause of ATP formation, rather than, as in Table 4.1, to focus on the transfer of electrons through the respiratory chain.

CONTROL OF OXIDATIVE PHOSPHORYLATION

The rate of ATP production in the mitochondria is determined primarily by the availability of substrates and oxygen and by the relative concentrations of ADP, P_i, and ATP. Normally, in the well-oxygenated heart substrate and oxygen supplies are not rate-limiting, so that ATP formation is determined primarily by the rate at which ATP is being utilized. This type of control tends to match the rate of energy production to that of energy utilization because ADP and phosphate promote oxidative phosphorylation, whereas ATP inhibits this process.

The most important regulator of ATP formation in the mitochondria is ADP, whose ability to govern the rate of oxidative phosphorylation through its role to accept high-energy bonds is called *acceptor control*. The extreme sensitivity of the mitochondria to changing ADP concentrations allows the rate of ATP production to be closely regulated by the energy needs of the cell. When energy consumption proceeds at a relatively low rate, as for example in the heart under basal conditions, there is relatively little ADP formed because the rate at which the high-energy bonds of ATP are hydrolyzed by the contractile proteins is low (Chapter 6). An intervention that increases the rate of ATP hydrolysis (e.g., any agent that increases myocardial contractility) increases ATP hydrolysis and thus raises ADP concentration. The latter, through acceptor control, causes an immediate acceleration of ATP formation. In this way the rate of oxidative phosphorylation closely matches the rate of energy utilization. This mechanism of acceptor control is in some ways similar to that which controls the glycolytic rate by regulating the enzymes hexokinase and phosphofructokinase, and that which operates on the enzyme isocitric dehydrogenase to regulate the turnover of the tricarboxylic acid cycle (Table 4.4, below). Although these regulatory processes differ from each other in the specific way in which increased ATP utilization promotes ATP production, all share the ability to accelerate energy production to meet increasing rates of energy utilization.

INTEGRATION OF GLYCOLYSIS AND RESPIRATION

A number of the factors that allow the respiratory and glycolytic rates to be interrelated have already been discussed. One clearly evident expression of this integration is the finding that the intact heart normally extracts lactate from the coronary arterial blood, so that lactate is consumed by the myocardium under aerobic conditions. Under hypoxic or ischemic conditions, however, large quantities of this metabolite appear in the coronary venous blood because lactate is produced by the heart. The inhibition of lactate production seen when the heart goes from anaerobic to aerobic conditions is accompanied by a shift from carbohydrate to fatty acid oxidation. Together these represent an expression of the *Pasteur effect,* i.e., inhibition of anaerobic glycolysis when oxidative metabolism is activated.

The regulatory influence of the NAD/NADH ratio plays a major role in the integration of anaerobic glycolysis and oxidative metabolism. Under conditions where NAD is the predominant form of this coenzyme, pyruvate oxidation to form acetyl-CoA is promoted (Fig. 3.8), whereas a preponderance of NADH favors instead the reduction of pyruvate to lactate (Fig. 3.1). This control allows the rapid oxidation of NADH within the mitochondria of the well-oxygenated heart to inhibit the production of lactate almost completely.

The integration of fat and carbohydrate metabolism is of great importance in the heart. Normally the heart is like an omnivore in that it can derive energy from either carbohydrates or lipids. The latter comprise the preferred substrate, however, in that when the well-oxygenated heart is presented with adequate levels of fatty acids glycogenolysis and glycolysis are inhibited. This suppression of carbohydrate metabolism when fatty acids are oxidized is due to a number of factors (Table 4.3). *Glycogen breakdown* is minimized by the inhibition of phosphorylase b (the predominant form of this enzyme in the heart under basal conditions) when high levels of ATP are present during the oxidation of fats. Glycogenolysis is also inhibited by the low levels of AMP and P_i, which also reflect active energy production from lipid oxidation, and by the glucose-6-phosphate that accumulates when glycolysis is inhibited during the oxidation of fats (see below).

The utilization of glucose is inhibited at several steps when fatty acid metabolism is active. A variety of fatty acids inhibit *glucose transport* into the cell directly, although the mechanism for this inhibitory effect is not understood. *Glucose phosphorylation* by hexokinase, like the reaction catalyzed by phosphorylase b, is inhibited by the glucose-6-phosphate that accumulates when the reaction controlled by phosphofructokinase is inhibited. *Fructose-6-phosphate phosphorylation,* which represents a major point at which active fat metabolism is able to

TABLE 4.3. *Inhibition of carbohydrate metabolism during active lipid metabolism*

Reaction in carbohydrate metabolism	Enzyme inhibited	Inhibitory factor
Glycogen breakdown	Phosphorylase b	High ATP, glucose-6-phosphate, low AMP and P_i
Glucose transport	—	Fatty acids
Glucose phosphorylation	Hexokinase	High glucose-6-phosphate
Fructose-6-phosphate phosphorylation	Phosphofructokinase	High citrate, high ATP/ADP ratio
Pyruvate oxidation	Pyruvate dehydrogenase	High acetyl-CoA, NADH

TABLE 4.4. *General features of the control of energy production in the heart*

Hormonal	High-energy phosphates	Redox state (NAD/NADH ratio)	Complex
Glucose uptake	Glycolytic rate Hexokinase Phosphofructokinase	Glycolytic rate Glyceraldehyde-3- phosphate dehydrogenase	Production of Acetyl-CoA Pyruvate dehydrogenase
Glycogen breakdown Phosphorylase Glycogen synthetase	Tricarboxylic acid cycle Isocitric dehydrogenase	Lactate production Pyruvate dehydrogenase	
Fatty acid liberation Lipoprotein lipase	Oxidative phosphorylation Acceptor control	Fatty acid oxidation β-oxidation	
		Tricarboxylic acid cycle Four oxidative steps	

See text for details.

"shut down" that of carbohydrate, is inhibited by citrate, which accumulates when the heart is actively metabolizing fats. A rise in the ATP/ADP ratio due to active ATP production by the mitochondria during active lipid metabolism also plays a role in the inhibition of phosphofructokinase. Finally, a reduced rate of *pyruvate oxidation* can also inhibit carbohydrate metabolism in the heart that is rapidly oxidizing fats. This latter effect, like the inhibition of pyruvate dehydrogenase already described in the case of the Pasteur effect, is attributable to the inhibitory effects of high concentrations of NADH and acetyl-CoA (produced during fatty acid oxidation) on this enzyme.

Another substance that can integrate the rates of fat and carbohydrate metabolism is the coenzyme FAD, which is required both for the tricarboxylic acid cycle (at the step where succinate is oxidized) and for the β-oxidation of fatty acids. In the case of regulation by FAD, however, it may be that the inhibition is of fat metabolism by carbohydrate metabolism, rather than the other way around. This inhibitory effect of active carbohydrate metabolism can be mediated by high levels of the tricarboxylic acid intermediate succinate, which can cause a large proportion of the available FAD to become enzyme-bound and so unable to participate in lipid oxidation (Fig. 4.2). Taken together, these interrelationships between lipid and carbohydrate metabolism provide the myocardium with the means by which to slow the rate of energy production from glycogen and glucose when there is an abundant supply of fats and oxygen.

OVERVIEW OF ENERGY PRODUCTION IN THE HEART

The complex pathways of intermediary metabolism which provide for the supply of the chemical energy utilized during cardiac contraction illustrate the extraordinary extent to which cellular regulation has developed in the myocardium. These many enzymatic reactions are regulated by many different principles of enzymatic control, including *substrate availability, product inhibition,* and dependence on a variety of *cofactors* such as the substrates for phosphorylation and coenzymes for oxidation or reduction. Control of specific enzymes is also affected by *allosteric effects,* which allow substances not directly involved in an enzymatic reaction to affect regulation through changes in the conformation of the enzyme that either increases or decreases catalytic activity. A number of *hormones* can, by certain special types of allosteric regulation, also modulate the rates of several enzymes. The most significant of these appears to be phosphorylation of enzymes through the cascade of reactions involving cyclic AMP (Fig. 3.7). Changes in *membrane transport properties* also participate in controlling intermediary metabolism, e.g., at the sarcolemma by regulating substrate availability, and at the mitochondrial membrane by modulating the transfer of reducing equivalents. Together these regulatory mechanisms allow the rate and pathways of energy production in the heart to be regulated so as to optimize the utilization of substrates under the conditions existing at any moment. Furthermore, these complex regulatory mechanisms fulfill the requirement that ATP be produced at a rate exactly equal to that at which it is being consumed, a mandatory precondition for the continuous beating of the heart in the intact animal (Chapter 2).

Three general types of control which govern the rate of energy production in the heart have been identified (Table 4.4). The first is *hormonal*. This principle of control acts mainly to regulate the entry rates of substrates, both carbohydrate and fat, into the pathways of intermediary metabolism. In this way a hormonal signal is able to augment the availability of chemical energy in the heart at the same time it also increases the rate of energy utilization (by other mechanisms; see Chapter 11). Secondly, there is a control which responds to the cellular requirement for *high-energy phosphates*. The many points at which this type of control operates serve to match the rate of ATP production with that of ATP utilization. In this way the heart fulfills the basic requirement that the cellular levels of this critical source of chemical energy remain virtually constant, and that the rate of energy production not fall behind that of energy utilization. Finally, there is the control exerted by the relative states of *oxidation and reduction* of the coenzymes essential for the critical oxidative steps of intermediary metabolism. This control is largely responsible for integrating oxidative and anaerobic metabolism. At one key point—that at which acetyl-CoA is produced from glucose metabolism—control is extremely complex and probably involves the operation of all these different regulatory mechanisms. This complexity can be understood as reflecting the critical position of this reaction, which is at the "crossroads" between carbohydrate and fat metabolism.

Together these control mechanisms maintain an almost constant level of ATP within the normal myocardium while at the same time allowing the heart to make optimal use of the substrates delivered to it in the coronary arterial blood. The influences of certain disorders of cardiac function on these regulatory systems have already been described, and their functional significance is seen later when the effects of hemodynamic overloading (Chapter 21) and ischemia (Chapter 22) are considered in detail.

BIBLIOGRAPHY

Lehninger, A. L. (1971): *Bioenergetics,* 2nd ed. W. A. Benjamin, Menlo Park, California.
    See also Bibliography to Chapter 3.
Safer, B. (1975): The metabolic significance of the malate-aspartate cycle in the heart. *Circ. Res.,*
    37:527–533.

5

Energetics of Muscle: Energy Utilization (Work and Heat)

The discovery of the relationship between the conditions under which a muscle works and its expenditure of energy as work and as heat represents one of the more fascinating chapters in the history of biology. By defining the link between the *mechanical* expression of the metabolic activity of muscle and the *chemical* processes responsible for contraction, these studies have made an important contribution to our knowledge of the chemistry of muscular contraction.

The internal energy content of muscle becomes reduced during contraction (Chapter 2). This disappearance of internal energy and its conversion to ATP for consumption by the contractile machinery constitutes only half of the energy equation of muscle:

Net energy change = disappearance of internal (chemical) energy
= appearance of external energy (work and heat)

The appearance of external energy, as work and as heat, represents the other half of this equation, which describes in general terms the role of muscle as a mechanochemical transducer. The external energies of muscle are complex and include both tension development and shortening, which contribute to the useful work performed by the muscle. In addition, external energy appears as heat.

The heat produced by a muscle is not entirely "waste"; shivering, for example, can maintain body temperature in cold environments. However, the conversion of chemical energy to heat inevitably reduces muscular efficiency and thus lessens the capacity of the muscle to do useful work [see Eq. (2.2)]. Studies of heat production in muscle therefore provide information to characterize the efficiency or, more directly, the inefficiency of the contractile process. In addition, studies of the dependence of heat production on the conditions under which the muscle contracts have provided a surprisingly detailed insight into the chemistry of the contractile process. In this chapter the influence of loading on the mechanical and energetic behavior of amphibian skeletal muscle is described in order to provide a basis for subsequent examination of the way in which the chemistry of the contractile process is regulated in the heart.

DEPENDENCE OF WORK (MECHANICAL ENERGY LIBERATION) ON LOAD

Variations in *afterload* exert a characteristic effect on the work performance of a muscle. Afterload may be defined as a load that is not apparent to the muscle

FIG. 5.1. A spring, which when stretched by a 10-g load lengthens 10 cm. If this spring obeys Hooke's law, then for each gram of load removed from the spring in its stretched state *(right)* the spring shortens by 1 cm. When the final load is zero, the spring shortens 10 cm *(left)*. If this spring in its stretched state is presented with a series of lighter loads (less than 10 g), the relationship between load and work shown in Table 5.1 and Fig. 5.2 is generated.

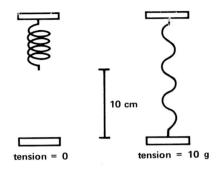

tension = 0   tension = 10 g

when it is in a resting state but which is encountered by the muscle when it begins to contract. In the case of a muscle suspended above a table, for example, an afterload is not supported by the muscle until contraction begins but instead rests on a support such as the tabletop. In contrast, a *preload* is supported by the muscle while it is in a resting state. A preload thus stretches the resting muscle, whereas an afterload does not. Normally the heart behaves as an afterloaded muscle (Chapter 12).

The relationship between loading and the performance of muscular work can be illustrated by considering the properties of a simple spring. Let us assume that when such a spring is stretched 10 cm, it develops a tension equivalent to 10 g (Fig. 5.1), and that as the spring is stretched the force developed is linearly proportional to the increase in length (i.e., the spring obeys Hooke's law). For each centimeter of shortening, therefore, tension decreases by 1 g. Furthermore, if the load is decreased from 10 g in 1-g steps, the spring shortens by 1 cm for each gram removed from the load. Thus if a series of lesser weights is placed on the spring stretched initially to 10 cm by a 10-g weight (column a in Table 5.1),

TABLE 5.1. *Relationship between shortening and work performed by a stretched spring*

(a) Load (g)	(b) Shortening (cm)	(c) Work (g X cm)
10	0	0
9	1	9
8	2	16
7	3	21
6	4	24
5	5	25
4	6	24
3	7	21
2	8	16
1	9	9
0	10	0

FIG. 5.2. Load-work curve of the spring in Fig. 5.1. Starting with the spring in its stretched state, presentation of the series of lighter loads indicated on the abscissa allows the spring to perform the amount of work indicated on the ordinate. The work of the spring is calculated simply as the product of load × distance shortened (Table 5.1).

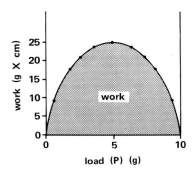

the values for shortening in column b of Table 5.1 are obtained. The work done by shortening of the stretched spring is readily calculated by multiplying the weight on the spring (the force, expressed in grams in column a) by the distance shortened (column b) to give the work performed at each load (column c). In this way the work-load relationship shown in Fig. 5.2 is generated. When the load *(P)* is equal to the maximum tension developed by the spring (P_0), work is zero because the spring cannot shorten. Work is also zero when $P = 0$, as no force is generated during shortening. Work performance is maximal at intermediate levels of both load and shortening (Table 5.1).

Work-load curves such as that in Fig. 5.2 are also produced by active muscle. While this finding provides little information as to the processes responsible for muscular contraction, early muscle physiologists recognized that work-load relationships for muscle resemble that shown in Fig. 5.2, which is compatible with the view that during activity the muscle exists in a state analogous to a stretched spring. As a result, the "new elastic body" theory of muscular contraction was formulated. Although now known to be incorrect, this theory is presented in some detail at this point because recognition of its fundamental errors provides a basis for understanding the significance of the experiments carried out by Wallace Fenn during the early 1920s. These experiments, which led to the definition of the *Fenn effect,* decisively proved the new elastic body theory of muscular contraction to be wrong and are of central importance to our modern understanding of muscular contraction.

NEW ELASTIC BODY THEORY OF MUSCULAR CONTRACTION

Experiments such as that shown in Fig. 5.2 led early workers in the field of muscle physiology to explain the transition from rest to activity in a muscle as the result of new cross links that appeared within the contractile machinery. These new cross links, which were postulated to require chemical energy for their formation, were viewed as giving the muscle a new set of spring-like characteristics.

resting state   active state

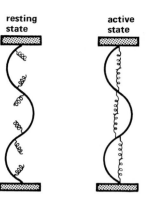

FIG. 5.3. The new elastic body theory of muscle contraction states that transition of a muscle from its resting state *(left)* to its active state *(right)* can be depicted as the acquisition of new "spring-like" characteristics. This theory carries predictions as to muscle energetics, most important of which is that a constant amount of energy is added in the transition from rest to activity.

According to the new elastic body theory of muscular contraction, the transition from rest to activity in a muscle is analogous to that in a spring which at a constant length assumes new elastic characteristics so as to increase its capacity to generate tension. Such a transition could occur, for example, by formation of chemical bonds along the chains of a polymer (Fig. 5.3). In this way the muscle at rest (*a,* Fig. 5.3) develops only a small amount of tension (resting tension). During activity tension increases through the formation of cross links (*b,* Fig. 5.3), which cause the muscle to assume the characteristics of the stretched spring seen in Fig. 5.1. The new elastic body theory predicts, therefore, that a fixed amount of chemical energy is delivered to the contractile machinery to effect this transition from rest to activity. As a result, a *constant amount of energy would be released in each contraction* regardless of the conditions under which the muscle contracts. Because this external energy is released as work and heat, and because the work-load curve (Fig. 5.2) defines the load dependence of work, the dependence of energy release as heat would be as shown in Fig. 5.4. All of the energy added during the transition from rest to activity would appear as heat

FIG. 5.4. Predicted relationship between load during shortening *(P)* and the total energy released during contraction of a muscle which operates according to the new elastic body theory. If a constant amount of total energy is added to the muscle during transition from the resting to the active state (Fig. 5.3), the energy released per contraction—as work plus heat—*(ordinate)* is the same regardless of load *(abscissa).* Because the load-work curve of the muscle is similar to that depicted for the spring in Fig. 5.2, heat production is predicted to decrease at intermediate loads so as to maintain energy release per contraction at a constant level.

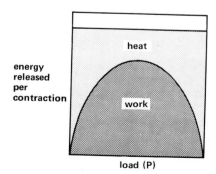

energy released per contraction

heat

work

load (P)

where $P = P_0$ because no work is done. Similarly this energy would appear solely as heat during contraction of the unloaded muscle, where $P = 0$. The release of work energy, as in the spring (Fig. 5.2), would be maximal at intermediate loads, where energy liberation as heat is minimal.

This postulated mechanism of muscular contraction, which was generally accepted until 1922, had to be abandoned with the fundamental discovery by Fenn that *the liberation of energy by contracting muscle is not constant but is influenced by the amount of work done.*

FENN EFFECT

Fenn's decisive contribution to our understanding of the relationship between work and total energy release in muscle is shown in Fig. 5.5. This discovery was that the total energy released in muscular contraction as work and heat varies in proportion to the work performed. Figure 5.5 thus demonstrates that the energy available to active muscle is not predetermined at the time of activation but instead is influenced by the conditions under which contraction takes place. In simple terms, the Fenn effect states that *as muscle does more work, more energy is liberated.* In this way a muscle is like an automobile, rather than a new elastic body, in that the performance of additional work (as in the automobile when it pulls a trailer) causes more energy to be utilized by the contractile machinery.

The existence of the Fenn effect was confirmed in a different way during the early 1960s by Mommaerts and by Carlson, who measured not the change in *external* energy, released as work and heat, but the change in *internal* energy, measured as a decrease in high-energy phosphate compounds. They found that at intermediate loads, where the highest levels of work were performed, the utilization of energy-rich compounds was maximal (Fig. 5.6).

It is a historical curiosity that the Fenn effect was first documented in cardiac muscle almost a decade before Fenn carried out his classic experiments in skeletal muscle. Both C. Lovatt Evans and Starling found that cardiac oxygen consumption, which is a valid index of internal energy release by the heart (Chapter 2), increased when the work of the heart was increased.

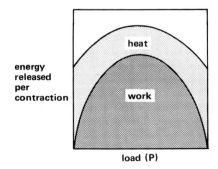

FIG. 5.5. Actual relationship between load during shortening *(P)* and total energy released during contraction of frog sartorius found by Fenn. The total energy released is variable and parallels the total work performed. The ability of a muscle to increase its total energy when performing a greater amount of work constitutes the Fenn effect.

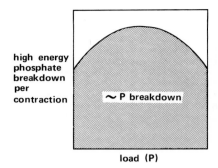

FIG. 5.6. Observed relationship between load during shortening *(P)* and high-energy phosphate breakdown per contraction. An increased amount of chemical energy is used when the muscle shortens at an intermediate load and so is performing a larger amount of work than at heavy or light loads (Fig. 5.2). These data provide an independent demonstration of the Fenn effect shown in Fig. 5.5.

high energy
phosphate
breakdown
per
contraction

~ P breakdown

load (P)

FORCE-VELOCITY RELATIONSHIP

The force-velocity relationship, which defines the influence of load on the velocity of muscle shortening, provides additional evidence that the contracting muscle does not behave like a stretched spring (a new elastic body). The correct shape of the curve relating load and shortening velocity was first shown clearly by Fenn and Marsh in 1935. Prior to that time contracting muscle was looked on as an elastic element which shortened in parallel with a viscous element (Fig. 5.7). If this model was correct and the viscous element had the characteristics of a Newtonian viscosity, then according to the new elastic body theory shortening velocity would increase in a linear manner as the load is decreased (curve A, Fig. 5.8). Fenn and March found instead that the force-velocity relationship was hyperbolic (curve B, Fig. 5.8). While this hyperbolic relationship could be explained within the context of the new elastic body theory by assuming non-Newtonian characteristics for the viscous element of muscle, it is now clear that the hyperbolic force-velocity curve of muscle is instead an expression of fundamental characteristics of the contractile element of muscle.

The relationship between the energetics of muscular contraction and the characteristics of the contractile machinery was greatly clarified by the classic experiments carried out in 1938 by Hill. These experiments demonstrated, among other things, that the hyperbolic force-velocity curve shown in Fig. 5.8 could be pre-

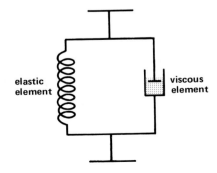

FIG. 5.7. Representation of an active muscle showing an elastic element (depicted at left as a spring) and a viscous element (depicted at right as a "dashpot").

elastic
element

viscous
element

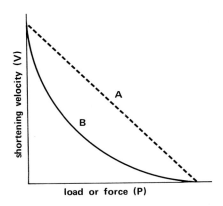

FIG. 5.8. Force-velocity relationship predicted from the model shown in Fig. 5.7 when the elastic element obeys Hooke's law and the viscous element has Newtonian characteristics (A). This predicted relationship differs from the hyperbolic force-velocity relationship actually found for frog sartorius muscle by Fenn and Marsh (B).

dicted from measurements of the influence of load on the rate of energy liberation as work and heat.

HEAT LIBERATION BY ACTIVE MUSCLE

The subject of muscle heat is extremely complex, yet historically its accurate measurement was of central importance in the evolution of our understanding of the processes responsible for muscular contraction. This difficult subject can be simplified to some extent by dismissing for further discussion two of the three general classes of muscle heat (Table 5.2 and Fig. 5.9). *Maintenance heat,* the slow liberation of heat by resting muscle, is unrelated to contraction and thus can be ignored as representing a "background" heat. *Recovery heat,* the heat generated after the end of contraction, can similarly be ignored as being related primarily to those processes that return the chemical state of muscle to that which existed before the contraction. Recovery heat in skeletal muscle is largely aerobic and appears to be related primarily to the oxidation of lactate produced during activity (Chapters 2 and 3). Note in Fig. 5.9 that a large additional quantity of

TABLE 5.2. *Heat liberated by muscle*

Maintenance heat:	Slowly liberated, unrelated to contraction. A "background" heat.
Initial heat:	Extra heat liberated during contraction as a by-product of the chemistry of the contractile process itself.
Activation heat, *A:*	Related to excitation-contraction coupling.
Shortening heat, *ax:*	Related to shortening of muscle.
Tension-time heat, *f(P,t):*	Related to cross-bridge turnover during a time when the muscle is maintaining tension.
Recovery heat:	Generated at end of contraction; related mainly to chemical reactions associated with energy production. If muscle relaxes while bearing a load, it includes degradation of potential energy of lifted load into heat.

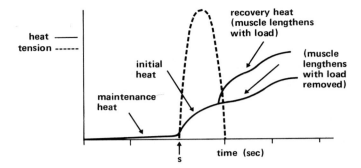

FIG. 5.9. Time course of heat liberation by an active muscle *(solid line)* and, for reference, the time course of tension developed by the muscle *(dashed line)*. Maintenance heat is liberated by the resting muscle. Initial heat is liberated during contraction, and recovery heat is liberated during and immediately after relaxation. Note that recovery heat is considerably greater when the muscle is allowed to lengthen under loaded conditions than when the load is removed from the muscle prior to relaxation.

recovery heat is liberated during relaxation if the muscle is allowed to relax while bearing a load. This extra component of the recovery heat disappears if the load is removed from the muscle at the end of contraction and so is due simply to dissipation of the potential energy of the lifted load as the load returns to a lower position. Although of significance in the generation of muscle heat in the living animal, maintenance heat, recovery heat, and the heat caused by muscle lengthening under load are not directly related to the contractile process. Therefore these forms of muscle heat are ignored in the following discussion.

The third form of muscle heat, somewhat confusingly called *initial heat,* is the extra heat (extra in that it exceeds maintenance heat) liberated immediately after the stimulus (*s,* Fig. 5.9) and during contraction. Initial heat, which immediately precedes and accompanies shortening and generation of tension, occurs during the depolarization and repolarization of the sarcolemma (Chapter 14), the release of activator calcium by the sarcoplasmic reticulum (Chapter 9), and the binding of this calcium to troponin C (Chapter 6). A larger component of the initial heat accompanies the mechanical activity of the activated contractile proteins. The following discussion shows how measurements of initial heat permitted Hill to predict the hyperbolic shape of the force-velocity curve and to define the chemical bssis of muscular contraction even before the discovery of actin and the ATPase activity of myosin (Chapter 6).

LIBERATION OF INITIAL HEAT IN AN ISOMETRIC CONTRACTION

During an *isometric contraction*—in which the ends of the muscle are fixed so that the muscle neither shortens nor performs external work—two components of initial heat are seen (Fig. 5.10). The first component, which appears immedi-

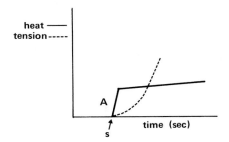

FIG. 5.10. Time course of initial heat liberation by a muscle contracting under isometric conditions *(solid line)* and, for reference, the time course of initial tension development *(dashed line)*. The quantity of heat (A) liberated immediately after stimulation (s) is the activation heat.

ately after stimulation of the muscle (*s*, Fig. 5.10) is the *activation heat (A,* Fig. 5.10). Activation heat is manifest as a brief burst of heat, most of which appears before the development of significant tension at the ends of the muscle. Following the liberation of activation heat, a second and slower rate of heat production accompanies the development of tension. This second phase of heat liberation is relatively small and for simplicity is ignored at this point in the discussion.

The liberation of energy during an isometric contraction can be described as

$$\Delta E = A + W_i \tag{5.1}$$

The change in external energy ΔE is equal to the heat of activation *(A)* plus the internal work which takes place in the isometrically contracting muscle W_i. This term W_i reflects the fact that even though the ends of the muscle are fixed a small amount of internal work is done by the contractile elements because of slight shape changes in the muscle and stretching of the "series elasticity" (Chapter 8).

The conventions used in Eq. (5.1) are those of muscle physiology (Chapter 2). When stated in thermodynamic terms, Eq. (5.1) becomes

$$\Delta E = Q - W \tag{5.2}$$

where Q is the activation heat (plus the small amount of heat liberated during contraction) and W the internal work. The term W_i in Eq. (5.1), as well as the small amount of heat liberated during the development of tension, are discussed later in this chapter, using the term *f(P,t)* as defined by Mommaerts.

LIBERATION OF INITIAL HEAT IN AN ISOTONIC CONTRACTION

During an *isotonic contraction* (i.e., when the muscle shortens while lifting a constant load) external work is performed. In addition, however, another increment of energy appears as heat. Because of the nature of the initial heat during shortening, the equations defining heat liberation during an isotonic contraction are more complex than that for the isometric contraction described above.

In 1938 Hill found that a quantity of heat (*ax*, Fig. 5.11) is liberated during shortening. This "shortening heat" is independent of the load and is determined

FIG. 5.11. Time course of initial heat liberation by a muscle allowed to shorten a constant distance while lifting a light load *(dashed line,* 1) or a heavy load *(dotted line,* 2). For reference, the time course of initial heat liberation by an isometrically contracting muscle (Fig. 5.10) is also shown. Although the rate of heat liberation subsequent to activation heat is slower when the muscle shortens while bearing a heavier load, the total amount of heat liberated during shortening (ax) is independent of load. s, time of stimulation.

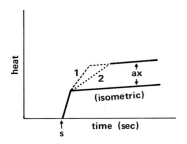

by the distance shortened. When a muscle is arranged so that it can shorten only 1 cm, heat liberation can be measured as a function of the load on the muscle as it shortens over this constant distance (Fig. 5.11). Thus when the muscle shortens against a light load (curve 1, Fig. 5.11), the total amount of heat liberated *(ax)* is the same as that which appears when the muscle shortens the same distance in the more heavily loaded contraction (curve 2, Fig. 5.11). When the distance the muscle shortens is increased, the liberation of shortening heat increases proportionately with the extent of shortening (Fig. 5.12).

In studies of the sort described in Fig. 5.11, the total *amount* of extra heat associated with a given degree of shortening is independent of load, but the *rate* at which this heat is liberated decreases as the load is increased. This is apparent when the slopes of curves 1 and 2 in Fig. 5.11 are compared.

The term *a,* which defines the amount of heat liberated for each centimeter of shortening, is a constant for any given type of muscle. The constant *a* has the dimensions of a force. If x is the distance the muscle shortens, the total amount of heat liberated during shortening is equal to $a \times x$:

$$\text{Shortening heat} = a \times x \qquad (5.3)$$

It must be remembered, however, that even though the *amount* of shortening heat is independent of load, depending only on the distance shortened, the *rate* at

FIG. 5.12. Time course of initial heat liberation by a muscle allowed to shorten to various lengths against a constant load. The shortening heat (ax) increases in proportion to the distance shortened (given as centimeters). Thus a muscle shortening 2 cm liberates twice as much shortening heat (2ax) as a muscle shortening 1 cm (ax), while the muscle shortening 3 cm liberates a shortening heat of 3ax. s, time of stimulation.

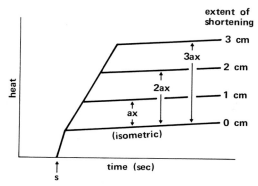

which the shortening heat appears is inversely related to the load on the muscle. As we have already seen (Fig. 5.8), the speed with which the load is lifted in an isotonic contraction is, similarly, inversely proportional to load. As a result, the rate of energy liberation, both as work and as heat, decreases at heavier loads. These important relationships are described later in this chapter.

The energy balance in an isotonic contraction was defined in 1938 by Hill as

$$\Delta E = A + W + ax \qquad (5.4)$$

where A is the activation heat [Eq. (5.1)], W is the external work done (internal work is ignored in this formulation), and ax is the shortening heat. Viewed in terms of Eq. (5.2), the right side of Eq. (5.4) can be divided into two portions; the first, corresponding to Q in Eq. (5.2), contains the heat terms A and ax. W, which corresponds to work, is equal to $P \times x$, i.e., the load P times the distance shortened x [see Eq. (5.7), below].

"TENSION-TIME" HEAT

The formulations in Eqs. (5.1) and (5.4) were revised during the mid-1960s when greater precision in the measurement of heat liberation became possible. As a result of these later studies, activation heat (A) appeared not to be constant during isometric contractions at different loads, but was found instead to be proportional to developed tension. The heat of shortening also was found to depend on load. One interpretation for these findings was offered by Mommaerts, who separated the heat of activation into two components. The first, A, is the true heat of activation, which results from processes already described. The second term, $f(P,t)$, represents heat liberation which is a function of both the tension on the muscle (P) and the length of time (t) the tension is maintained. This tension-time heat, which is related in part to internal work, can be included in Eq. (5.1) to give, for an isometric contraction

$$\Delta E = A + W_i + f(P,t) \qquad (5.5)$$

For an isotonic contraction, the term $f(P,t)$ can be included in Eq. (5.4) to give

$$\Delta E = A + W + ax + f(P,t) \qquad (5.6)$$

For simplicity in subsequent discussions we omit $f(P,t)$, the tension-time heat, from consideration. This simplification, while introducing a quantitative error in the following analyses, makes it easier to clarify the important relationships between force, velocity, the rate of extra energy liberation, and the behavior of the contractile proteins.

THE HILL EQUATION

The Hill equation, often called the "characteristic equation of muscle," defines the energetics of muscular contraction in a manner that predicts several key features of the chemistry of the contractile proteins.

The Hill equation is derived from analysis of the "extra energy" liberated during contraction as work and as heat. In a muscle that lifts the load P a distance equal to x, the extra energy liberated as work is $P \times x$. That liberated as heat is $a \times x$, i.e., the shortening heat [Eq. (5.4)]. Thus:

$$\text{Extra energy} = \underset{\text{(work)}}{P \times x} + \underset{\text{(heat)}}{a \times x} = (P + a)x \qquad (5.7)$$

Activation heat (A, Eq. 5.4) is omitted from Eq. (5.7) because it is not related to contraction, but is instead liberated before the muscle develops tension (Fig. 5.10). If for simplicity the $f(P,t)$ term is omitted, the quantity $(P + a)x$ represents the total amount of extra energy liberated by a muscle contracting under isotonic conditions.

The rate at which this extra energy is liberated is obtained by differentiating the quantity $(P + a)x$ with respect to time:

$$\text{Rate of extra energy liberation} = (P + a) \; dx/dt \qquad (5.8)$$

Because $dx/dt = $ velocity (v), the rate of extra energy liberation is $(P + a)v$.

The terms in Eq. (5.8) can be rewritten:

$$\text{Rate of extra energy liberation} = (P + a)v \qquad (5.9)$$

The meaning of this equation is apparent from the experimental finding that the rate of extra energy liberation by a contracting muscle is an inverse, linear function of load (Fig. 5.13). In an isometrically contracting muscle, where $P = P_0$, the rate of extra energy liberation is zero because there is neither shortening heat (ax) nor work (Px) due to the fact that the distance shortened (x) is zero. In an unloaded, freely shortening muscle, where $P = 0$, the rate of extra energy release is maximal (Fig. 5.13). Furthermore, a direct linear proportionality is found between the rate of extra energy liberation and the difference between the maximal load the muscle can lift (P_0) and the actual load on the muscle (P). It follows therefore that the rate of extra energy release is directly proportional to $P_0 - P$; i.e., the smaller the load (P), the greater is this rate.

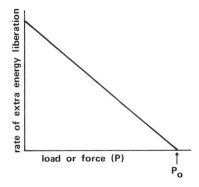

FIG. 5.13. Relationship between load (P) and the rate of extra energy liberation (as work plus heat) by contracting muscle. This inverse relationship between load and the rate of energy liberation led Hill to conclude that the active points in muscle could exist in two states. In one of these, the active points maintain tension but do not participate in energy liberation (where $P = P_0$, the latter being the maximal tension the muscle can develop). In the other state, the active points liberate energy (where $P = 0$), but as the load is zero they cannot maintain tension.

Using a constant of proportionality *(b)*, Hill was able to equate the rate of extra energy release $(P + a)v$ to load expressed as $P_0 - P$:

$$(P + a)v = b(P_0 - P) \qquad (5.10)$$

Equation (5.10) can be rearranged algebraically so as to put all of the constants (a, b, P_0) on the right. The result is the famous Hill equation.

The Hill equation is given in Eq. (5.11):

$$(P + a)(v + b) = (P_0 + a)b \qquad (5.11)$$

The beauty (and significance) of this equation lies in the fact that, because all the terms on the right are constants, Eq. (5.11) resembles the general equation for a hyperbola: $x \times y = constant$.

When Hill's data for the rate of extra energy liberation are plotted in the form of a force-velocity curve, a hyperbolic relationship is found (Fig. 5.14). This curve, which is based on measurements of heat and work, and *not* on direct measurement of muscle shortening velocity, was found by Hill to be identical to that obtained a few years earlier by Fenn and Marsh (Fig. 5.8), who measured directly the dependence of muscle shortening velocity on load.

Significance of the Hill Equation

The reader who has patiently toiled through the concepts (and algebra) described above is entitled to ask how these features of muscular contraction—energetics, heat production, velocity, etc.—contribute to an understanding of the biochemistry and biophysics of muscular contraction. This question is answered at this point in general terms, which it is hoped indicate the nature of the link between physiology and chemistry. After this topic is discussed more fully from a biochemical standpoint in Chapter 6, we return to the subject in Chapter 7 so as to define more precisely the relationship between the mechanics of muscular contraction and the chemical events that underlie this process.

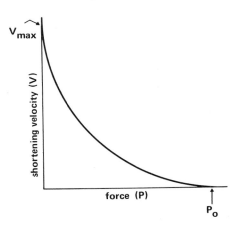

FIG. 5.14. Hyperbolic force-velocity relationship predicted from the Hill equation (Eq. 5.11). This curve is similar to that observed in studies of muscle mechanics (Fig. 5.8).

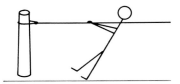

FIG. 5.15. Depiction of one of the active points of muscle in the state in which it develops tension but is not liberating energy.

It is fitting to quote directly from Hill's 1938 report in order to define the significance of Eq. (5.11). After examining this relationship, and especially data such as those in Fig. 5.13, Hill stated very eloquently how these experiments provided an insight into the chemistry of the working muscle:

> The control exercised by the tension P existing in the muscle at any moment, on the rate of its energy expenditure at that moment, may be due to some such mechanisms as the following. Imagine that the chemical transformations associated with the state of activity in muscle occur by combination at, or by the catalytic effect of, or perhaps by passage through, certain active points in the molecular machinery, the number of which is determined by the tension existing in the muscle at the moment. We can imagine that when the force in the muscle is high the affinities of more of these points are being satisfied by the attractions they exert on one another, and that fewer of them are available to take part in chemical transformation. When the tension is low the affinities of less of these points are being satisfied by mutual attraction, and more of them are exposed to chemical reaction. The rate at which chemical transformation would occur, and therefore, at which energy would be liberated, would be directly proportional to the number of exposed affinities or catalytic groups, and so would be a linear function of the force exerted by the muscle, increasing as the force diminished.

Written at a time when virtually nothing was known of the biochemistry of the contractile apparatus, and a year before myosin was discovered to have the ability to hydrolyze ATP, Hill's paragraph explains the energetics of muscular contraction by postulating two states for the interactions at hypothetical "active points" within the muscle. To explain the inverse relationship between load and the rate of energy release (Fig. 5.13), Hill postulated that, at any given time, the active points of muscle could exist in one of these states. In the *first state* the active points are attached and are developing tension, much as a man pulling against a rope (Fig. 5.15). In the *second state,* the active points are free to liberate chemical energy and thus to move, as when the same man runs freely (Fig. 5.16). To explain the type of result shown in Fig. 5.13, Hill postulated that the distribution of the active points of muscle between these two states is determined by the load on the muscle.

FIG. 5.16. Depiction of one of the active points of muscle in the state in which it is liberating energy but is not developing tension.

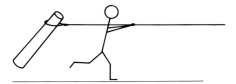

P = P$_o$, V = 0

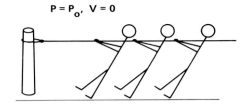

FIG. 5.17. Depiction of the active points of a muscle contracting under isometric conditions ($P = P_0$, $V = 0$). All active points are in the state in which they develop tension.

When the load P is equal to P_0 (i.e., during an isometric contraction), all active points are in the state in which they develop tension (Fig. 5.17). Under these conditions force is maximal and the rate of energy liberation zero. The latter interpretation is tenable because even though it takes energy to reach the state shown in Fig. 5.17 (the activation energy), according to the Hill equation it costs no energy to maintain tension. This is a simplification which assumes that each active point undergoes no further chemical change once tension is established. As was already pointed out, however, there is a tension-time heat. This probably reflects a slow turnover in the active points, which has been postulated to occur in an isometric contraction (much like the "little men" in Fig. 5.17 shifting their feet). The latter consideration can explain the $f(P,t)$ term in Eqs. (5.5) and (5.6).

When the load is zero and the muscle is shortening freely, all of the active points are in the second state (Fig. 5.18). As long as there is no resistance to shortening, all of the active points move at their maximal intrinsic rate. Hence the rate of energy turnover during unloaded shortening, which can be looked on as movements of knees and ankles (Figs. 5.16 and 5.18), is maximal. The rate of energy expenditure therefore is maximal when the load P is zero (Fig. 5.13).

On a theoretical basis and from examination of Fig. 5.18, the shortening velocity of unloaded muscle should be independent of the number of active points in the muscle. Thus one man capable of running at a top speed of 10 mph pulls an unloaded rope at the same speed as three (or any number) of such men linked together. For this reason, V_{max} in the force-velocity curve (Fig. 5.14) can be expected to be independent of the number of active points.

The other intercept of the force-velocity curve (P_0) represents the maximal force-generating capacity of the muscle. In terms of the analogy of the "little men" (Figs. 5.15–5.18), P_0 depends on the number of men pulling on the rope. It has been found experimentally that the maximal force that can develop in a muscle is related little if at all to its maximal shortening velocity. Thus P_0 is

P = 0, V = V$_{max}$

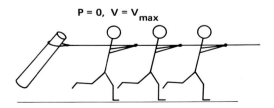

FIG. 5.18. Depiction of the active points of a muscle contracting against zero load ($P = 0$, $V = V_{max}$). All active points are in the state in which they liberate energy.

probably independent of the intrinsic maximal rate of energy expenditure; instead, it is related to the number of active points in the muscle (Chapter 7).

It is obvious, of course, that the active points in muscle are interactions between the thick and thin filaments (Chapter 1). These interactions are now at least partly understood in terms of the properties of the contractile proteins which make up these filaments. To provide an understanding of the biochemical basis for the energetic properties of muscle described in this chapter, the following chapter examines the contractile proteins and their interactions.

BIBLIOGRAPHY

Evans, C. L., and Matsuoka, Y. (1914–1915): The effect of the various mechanical conditions on the gaseous metabolism and efficiency of the mammalian heart. *J. Physiol. (Lond.)*, 49:378–405.

Fenn, W. O. (1923): The relation between the work performed and the energy liberated in muscular contraction. *J. Physiol. (Lond.)*, 58:373–395.

Fenn, W. O., and Marsh, B. S. (1935): Muscular force at different speeds of shortening. *J. Physiol. (Lond.)*, 85:277–297.

Hill, A. V. (1938): The heat of shortening and the dynamic constants of muscle. *Proc. R. Soc. (Lond.) [Biol.]*, 126:136–195.

Mommaerts, W. F. H. M. (1969): Energetics of muscular contraction. *Physiol. Rev.*, 49:427–508.

6

Contractile Proteins

To proceed from the energetics of muscular contraction to the chemistry of the contractile proteins and thus to move from a discussion of the liberation of heat and work by the living muscle to a description of protein-protein interactions and of ATP hydrolysis may seem to represent a drastic shift in topics. Yet these are but different ways of approaching a single process: the ability of muscle to function as a mechanochemical transducer.

The chemistry of the contractile proteins which effect this mechanochemical transduction is described in this chapter. In addition, the control of the interactions between the contractile proteins is examined to define the molecular basis for the transitions between rest and activity.

At the present time the molecular basis for myocardial contraction and its control can be understood in terms of the interactions between four named proteins (Table 6.1). When assembled *in vitro,* these proteins exhibit properties that reflect the three salient features of cardiac contraction: (a) They hydrolyze ATP and thus are able to liberate chemical energy; (b) they undergo changes in their physicochemical properties that, associated with ATP hydrolysis, are manifestations of the development of tension and shortening as seen in the intact muscle; and (c) their interactions are subject to control by calcium ion in a manner which appears to reflect the ability of this cation to couple excitation at the cell surface to the initiation of contraction in the living muscle. To understand the molecular basis for each of these characteristics—ATPase activity, contraction, and the mediation of excitation-contraction coupling—we first examine the structural and functional characteristics of each of these proteins.

MYOSIN

It is now established that myosin is the major protein of the thick filament of muscle in which individual myosin molecules are arranged so as to take advantage of their structural characteristics. Furthermore, a close and functionally significant relationship exists between the enzymatic characteristics of the myosin molecule and the expression of these biochemical properties in the function of muscle.

Molecular Characteristics

Myosin is a large, elongated molecule with a globular end where the important biological activities of the protein are located and a filamentous end which main-

TABLE 6.1 Contractile proteins

Protein	Location	Approximate molecular weight	Number of components	Salient biochemical properties
Myosin	Thick filament	480,000	Two heavy chains of 200,000; four light chains, two of 19,000 and two of 24,000	ATP hydrolysis; interacts with actin
Actin	Thin filament	42,000	One	Activates myosin ATPase; interacts with myosin
Tropomyosin	Thin filament	68,000	Two nonidentical chains of 34,000	Modulates actin-myosin interaction
Troponin complex	Thin filament	Three different proteins (see Table 6.2)		Ca^{2+} binding; with tropomyosin confers Ca^{2+} sensitivity to contractile proteins

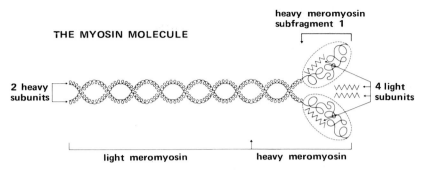

FIG. 6.1. Myosin molecule. Myosin is an elongated molecule consisting of a "tail" *(left)* and a "head" *(right)*. The tail consists of a coiled coil (composed of two α-helical chains wound around each other) that extends into the paired globular head of the molecule. The latter contains, in addition, four light subunits. Enzymatic cleavage at the point indicated by the lower arrow produces heavy and light meromyosins, while enzymatic cleavage of heavy meromyosin at the point indicated by the upper arrow yields heavy meromyosin subfragment 1.

tains the structural rigidity of the thick filament. The length of the myosin molecule is approximately 1,600 Å, and the molecular weight of both cardiac and skeletal myosin is approximately 480,000 daltons. The filamentous end of the molecule, which imparts rigidity to the thick filament, exists as a coiled coil, a nonflexible structure made up of two α-helical peptide chains wound around each other (Fig. 6.1). Each of these α-helices is derived from one of the two heavy subunits of the myosin molecule. The "head" of this molecule, which has a globular conformation, is also a paired structure. In addition to two heavy (~200,000 daltons) polypeptide chains, each derived from one of the paired myosin subunits, the myosin "head" contains two pairs of light (19,000 and 24,000 daltons) peptide chains, the function of which is discussed subsequently (Fig. 6.2).

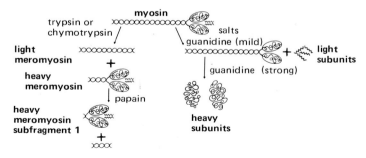

FIG. 6.2. Means of producing myosin subfragments *(left)* and subunits *(right)*. The subfragments are produced by proteolytic digestion. Mild treatment with salts releases the light subunits, while concentrated salts can dissociate and denature the two heavy subunits.

Early studies of myosin indicated that proteolytic enzymes (e.g., *trypsin* and *chymotrypsin*) are able to split the molecule into two fragments (Fig. 6.2). *Light meromyosin,* the smaller of these fragments, is derived from the "tail" of the molecule and exhibits the solubility properties which characterize myosin. The larger fragment, *heavy meromyosin,* contains the "head" of the myosin molecule to which is attached a small portion of the tail. Further digestion of heavy meromyosin with the proteolytic enzyme *papain* can remove the remainder of the tail. The remaining globular protein, *heavy meromyosin subfragment 1,* represents the head of the molecule (Fig. 6.2). In this head region, which contains the myosin light subunits, are found the important biochemical activities of the molecule.

The significance of the two points of proteolytic cleavage of myosin has only recently become apparent. In earlier studies light and heavy meromyosins were often referred to as "subunits" of the molecule. However, if one accepts the usual definition of a subunit as a discrete polypeptide chain within the parent molecule, this interpretation is in error. It now appears that the point at which myosin is cleaved into the meromyosins represents a flexible region of the tail because the susceptibility to cleavage by proteolytic enzymes is greater where the coiled-coil conformation is less rigid. Following this reasoning, it is likely that the second point of proteolytic cleavage at the base of the head, which yields a small portion of the tail and heavy meromyosin subfragment 1, represents a second region of flexibility. The significance of these two putative points of flexibility lies in the manner in which the myosin head is believed to move in the thick filament (Chapter 7).

Biological Properties

Purified myosin, as already indicated, possesses two important biological properties. The first, discovered in 1939 by Engelhardt and Ljubimova, is its ATPase activity. Myosin thus has the ability to hydrolyze the polyphosphate chain of ATP, liberating the terminal phosphate and thereby releasing chemical energy. The ability of myosin to bind actin, the second of the biological properties of myosin, represents an *in vitro* manifestation of the interaction between the thick and thin filaments of the sarcomere.

Both of these biological properties are found in heavy meromyosin and in heavy meromyosin subfragment 1, and thus can be localized to the globular head of the myosin molecule. This location is seen later to be of central importance to the contractile process.

The filamentous tail of the myosin molecule lacks enzymatic and actin-binding activities but tends to form aggregates under the ionic conditions that exist in the muscle. Its coiled-coil conformation confers structural rigidity to this portion of the molecule and thus also to aggregates of myosin tails. In this way the coiled-coil conformation of the tail of the myosin molecule reinforces the backbone of the thick filament of the sarcomere (see below).

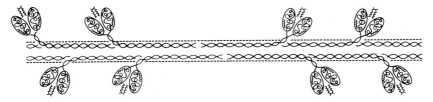

FIG. 6.3. Organization of individual myosin molecules in the thick filament. The "backbone" of the thick filament is delineated by dashed lines. Individual myosin molecules have opposite polarities in the two halves of the sarcomere (*right* and *left*). The bare area in the center of the thick filament is a region devoid of cross-bridges, which can be seen to arise from the "tail-to-tail" organization of myosin molecules unique to the center of the thick filament. The cross-bridges represent the "heads" of the individual myosin molecules, which project at right angles to the long axis of the thick filament.

Organization in the Sarcomere

Myosin is not found in a monomeric state in the myocardial cell. Instead, the protein is aggregated in a regular array as the *thick filament* (Fig. 6.3). In the thick filament the myosin tails are wound together to form a rigid backbone, from which the myosin heads project to make up the cross-bridges. The orientation of the elongated myosin molecules in the thick filament becomes reversed at the center of the filament so that the heads of the molecule (i.e., the cross-bridges) extend away from the center of the thick filament at both sides of the sarcomere (Fig. 6.3).

The cross-bridges in resting muscle are perpendicular to the long axis of the thick filament, whereas in active muscle their tips shift toward the center of the sarcomere (Fig. 6.4). The result of repeated cycles of this spatial translation is believed to be a "rowing" motion that begins when the thick filaments become attached to the thin filaments, after which the thin filaments are drawn toward the center of the sarcomere, causing the sarcomere to shorten. If the ends of the muscle are fixed so that shortening cannot take place, tension develops.

The shift in orientation of the cross-bridges clearly involves at least one flexible "joint" in the myosin molecule. The significance of a second joint arises from the finding that the strength of the interactions between thick and thin filaments

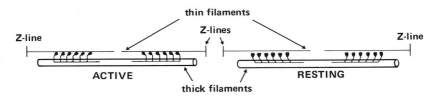

FIG. 6.4. Myosin cross-bridges in the thick filament. In resting muscle *(right)* the cross-bridges are oriented perpendicular to the longitudinal axis of the thick filament. In active muscle *(left)* the cross-bridges interact with the thin filaments, which then are "pulled" toward the center of the sarcomere.

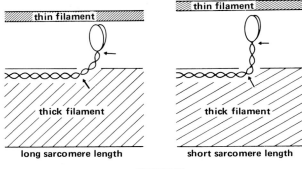

thin filament

thin filament

thick filament

thick filament

long sarcomere length   short sarcomere length

RESTING

FIG. 6.5. Relationship between cross-bridges and thin filaments in resting muscle at long and short sarcomere lengths. Two flexible points in the myosin molecule *(arrows)* allow the relationship between the tip of the cross-bridge and the thin filament to remain the same in spite of changes in the distances between thick and thin filaments.

does not necessarily diminish at shorter sarcomere lengths. In view of the fact that muscle volume remains virtually constant as the muscle shortens, the lateral distance between the thick and thin filaments must increase at shorter sarcomere lengths. Yet the intensity of the interaction between the myosin cross-bridges and the thin filaments can be relatively constant at varying sarcomere lengths. This finding can be explained if the tips of the cross-bridges are able to extend away from the backbone of the thick filament to maintain their contact with the thin filaments as sarcomere length decreases. Such a high degree of mobility was suggested by H. E. Huxley to reflect the existence of two joints in the myosin molecule (Fig. 6.5). As was already indicated, each of the putative joints in this molecule may give rise to a point of susceptibility to proteolytic enzymes.

Functional Implications

Myosins purified from muscles which serve different functions exhibit different intrinsic ATPase activities (Chapter 2). This difference is seen even when the muscles are from the same animal. In general, muscles adapted for continuous or sustained activity shorten slowly, e.g., postural muscles, leg muscles of the hare, and pectoral muscles of flying birds. Such slow muscles characteristically contain myosins that have a low ATPase activity. Conversely, muscles adapted for brief bursts of rapid acceleration (e.g., leg muscles of the rabbit) generally contract rapidly. Myosins isolated from fast muscle exhibit a high rate of ATP hydrolysis. The functional significance of these differences and the similarity to slow muscle of both the energetics of myocardial function and the low cardiac myosin ATPase activity are described in Chapter 2.

A possible relationship between the chemistry of myosin and the functional characteristics of muscle is suggested by studies of the subunit structure of myosins from different skeletal muscles. When the light subunits of slow and fast muscles are separated and examined by polyacrylamide gel electrophoresis, different electrophoretic mobilities are found. The light subunits of cardiac myosin, which is functionally a slow myosin, are similar to those of slow skeletal muscle, both differing electrophoretically from those of fast skeletal muscle myosin. These and other findings indicate that the myosins represent a class of isozymes in which the chemical reactivity of the protein and its functional role in the living muscle are determined, at least in part, by the nature of the light subunits.

> The possibility that myosin ATPase activity and muscle shortening velocity are both determined by the nature of the myosin light subunits is suggested by the finding that maximum velocity of shortening and myosin ATPase are not invariable but are subject to modification by influences arising outside the muscle. Best understood of these influences is the effect of cross innervation in mammalian skeletal muscle. In an animal in which fast and slow muscles coexist in a single limb, the muscles can be cross-innervated so that the nerve initially supplying the fast muscle goes instead to the slow muscle and vice versa. Such cross innervation causes both the biochemical and physiological characteristics of the muscles to become reversed: The maximal shortening velocity of the fast muscle becomes slower at the same time that the ATPase activity of its myosin decreases. Conversely, both shortening velocity and myosin ATPase activity increase in the muscle that was originally slow.
>
> Changes in the structure of the myosin molecule accompany these changes in ATPase activity. Most striking are alterations in the electrophoretic mobilities of the light subunits found in the head of the myosin molecule. These light subunits, which differ electrophoretically in fast and slow muscles (see above) assume the characteristics of the muscle originally innervated by the newly implanted nerve. Thus when a fast muscle is innervated surgically with a nerve that originally supplied a slow muscle, decreased muscle shortening velocity and myosin ATPase activity are accompanied by the replacement of the myosin light subunits characteristic of the fast muscle with those whose electrophoretic mobilities are characteristic of the slow muscle. Opposite changes are seen in the cross-innervated slow muscle, suggesting that changes in the nature of these light subunits are responsible, at least in part, for alterations in both myosin ATPase activity and muscle-shortening velocity.

Direct demonstration of a role for the myosin light subunits in determining the intrinsic rate of ATP hydrolysis has been difficult because of the lability of the heavy chains after the light chains are removed. Some workers have made "hybrid" myosins in which light chains derived from fast muscle myosin are combined with heavy chains isolated from slow muscle myosin and vice versa. A limited number of studies with these chimeric myosins supports the view that the light chains determine the ATPase activity of the molecule at least in part.

ACTIN

Between 1864, when myosin was first described by Kühne, and the early 1940s the asymmetrical protein isolated by salt extraction from muscle minces was assumed to consist of a single protein species. As studies of "myosin" became more searching, however, it became apparent that not all myosin preparations were the same. Thus the physicochemical properties of *myosin A,* which was isolated after brief salt extraction of minced muscle, were found to differ from those of *myosin B,* which was obtained after more prolonged extraction. These differences were explained when Straub, working in the laboratory of A. Szent-Györgyi, found that myosin B contained an additional protein not present in myosin A. This second protein, first isolated in 1942, was called *actin* because of its ability to activate myosin ATPase activity.

Molecular Characteristics

Actin is much smaller than myosin, having a molecular weight of approximately 42,000 daltons. Unlike myosin, which is highly asymmetrical, actin is a globular protein having a slightly ovoid shape with an average diameter of approximately 55 Å. When studied *in vitro,* actin can be stabilized either in a monomeric form, called G-actin (G = globular), or as a highly asymmetrical polymer, F-actin (F = fibrous). G-actin polymerizes readily if the highly charged actin monomers are allowed to approach each other, e.g., when their negative charges are screened by the addition of salts. Depolymerization of F-actin can be effected most simply by removal of salts.

Actin has a very interesting chemistry which is described here only briefly because these chemical properties are not clearly relevant to the process of muscular contraction. G-actin contains both a bound nucleotide and a bound divalent cation. The nucleotide that binds to G-actin with greatest stability is ATP, while either Ca^{2+} or Mg^{2+} can occupy the metal-binding site. Both the nucleotide and cation bound to G-actin are freely exchangeable, although removal of either reduces the stability of G-actin in that it rapidly loses its ability to polymerize. The F-actin polymer, like G-actin, contains bound nucleotide and bound cation. In the polymer, however, both are tightly bound and do not freely exchange with nucleotides and cations in the solution. Furthermore, during polymerization actin-bound ATP is converted to ADP. Thus the polymerization of actin is associated with the hydrolysis of loosely bound ATP, which in F-actin becomes tightly bound ADP according to the reaction

$$G\text{-actin} \cdots ATP \longrightarrow F\text{-actin-ADP} + P_i$$

Depolymerization of F-actin is associated with loosening of the binding of ADP to the protein. To recover a G-actin that can again polymerize, it is necessary to provide free ATP (represented as A*TP) which replaces the bound nucleotide according to the reaction:

$$F\text{-actin-ADP} + A^*TP \longrightarrow G\text{-actin} \cdots A^*TP + ADP$$

When actin is sonicated or held at higher temperatures, both reactions can alternate rapidly, thereby allowing free ATP to be hydrolyzed. Thus actin can have the properties of an ATPase enzyme. According to the usual definition of the term, however, actin is not considered to represent an ATPase because under ordinary conditions the protein does not hydrolyze free ATP.

Biological Properties

Neither actin-bound nucleotide nor metal ion appear to have a role in muscular contraction. Actin-bound nucleotide is not exchanged during muscular contraction, indicating that ATP hydrolysis by the reactions described above does not occur in the living muscle. Furthermore, when F-actins are prepared under special conditions so as to contain neither bound nucleotide nor bound metal, the actomyosins reconstituted from such nucleotide- and metal-free actins exhibit all of the features of muscular contraction when studied *in vitro* (see below). For these reasons it is now generally believed that actin-bound nucleotide and cation are only of structural significance. Possibly they act to stabilize the structure of the actin polymer.

Two other biological properties of actin appear to be involved directly in muscular contraction: (a) the ability to activate myosin ATPase activity; and (b) the ability to interact physicochemically with myosin. Both of these properties allow the "two-protein" actomyosin reconstituted from highly purified actin and myosin to liberate chemical energy from ATP and undergo physicochemical changes, two of the three salient features of the contractile process.

Organization in the Sarcomere

Like myosin, actin is not present in living muscle in its monomeric form. Instead, actin exists in the sarcomere as the F-actin polymer, which provides the "backbone" of the thin filament of the sarcomere. The basic structure of both F-actin and the thin filament is that of a double-stranded helix (Fig. 6.6). Each of the two strands of F-actin and the thin filament is made up of a chain of actin monomers so that the structure of these polymers resembles two strands of pearls wound around each other. This structure differs from the coiled-coil structure of the tail of the myosin molecule, which is made up of chains of amino acids rather than of macromolecules.

The distance between the nodes of F-actin is approximately 385 Å, so that each half-turn of the F-actin filament contains approximately seven pairs of actin monomers (Fig. 6.6). These quantitative characteristics are important to an un-

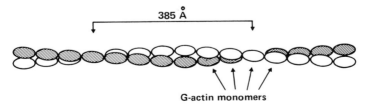

385 Å

G-actin monomers

FIG. 6.6. The F-actin polymer is composed of two strands of G-actin monomers (ovals) wound around each other. The G-actin monomers in the two strands are identical; one strand is shaded here only to illustrate the two-stranded structure of F-actin. The internodal distance is approximately 385 Å.

derstanding of the functional organization of the thin filament, as will become clear when we examine the interactions between actin and the regulatory proteins tropomyosin and the troponin complex.

TROPOMYOSIN

For almost 15 years tropomyosin was the "orphan" of the contractile proteins. Discovered in 1948 by Bailey, tropomyosin alone was found to have no biological activity—it did not hydrolyze ATP nor interact with myosin. However, its structure proved to be of considerable interest to the physical chemist, for like the tail of the myosin molecule, tropomyosin was found to be a coiled coil.

Molecular Characteristics

Like light meromyosin, tropomyosin contains two peptide chains in a coiled coil conformation. Unlike light meromyosin, the two peptide chains of tropomyosin are linked by a single disulfide bridge (Fig. 6.7). The two chains of tropomyosin are similar but probably not identical. The molecular weight of each is 34,000 daltons, giving a total molecular weight of 68,000 for tropomyosin.

Biological Properties

Tropomyosin itself has no important biological properties. In combination with actin, however, tropomyosin possesses the very important property of modulating the interactions between actin and myosin.

The action of tropomyosin to modulate the interactions between actin and myosin that cause tension and shortening is complex in that tropomyosin can both inhibit and enhance these interactions. The characteristics of these modulating functions depend on the state of the interactions between actin and myosin (Chapter 7). Most important of the regulatory effects is the ability of tropomyosin, along with troponin, to serve as the calcium-receptor mechanism of the contractile apparatus.

Organization in the Sarcomere

Among the first clues pointing to tropomyosin as a regulator of the contractile process was the discovery that tropomyosin commonly appeared in actin preparations as a contaminant. This finding led to the recognition that tropomyosin

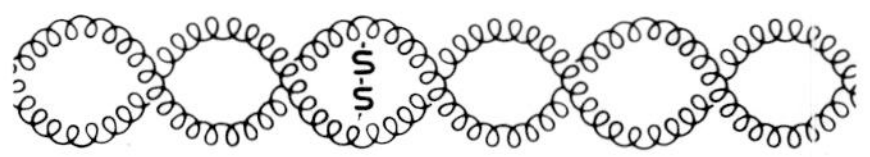

FIG. 6.7. The tropomyosin molecule is composed of two α-helical peptide chains wound around each other in a coiled coil conformation. Unlike the tail of the myosin molecule (Fig. 6.1), the two polypeptide chains are joined by a single disulfide bond (–S–S–).

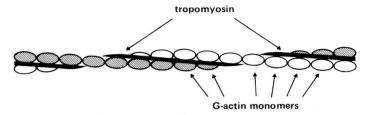

FIG. 6.8. Tropomyosin is found along with actin in the thin filament, where it is located in the "groove" between the two strands of G-actin monomers.

bound stoichiometrically to F-actin, and thus to the view that tropomyosin was present along with actin in the thin filament. More recently it has been possible to show that one molecule of tropomyosin lies in each of the two grooves that run longitudinally between the two strands of actin in the thin filament (Fig. 6.8). Thus besides its regulatory function, tropomyosin adds structural rigidity to the thin filament.

TROPONIN

The last of the four named proteins of the myofibril to be discovered, the troponin complex is now recognized to be made up of three discrete proteins. Each of the components of troponin possesses one of the salient properties of the troponin complex, which along with tropomyosin serves to regulate the interactions between actin and myosin that give rise to the contractile process.

Molecular and Biological Characteristics

The troponin complex was described in 1965 by Ebashi and was suggested initially to be a globular protein having a molecular weight of approximately 50,000 daltons. It soon became apparent, however, that these preparations of troponin were in fact made up of three proteins, each of which possesses one of the three important biological properties of the complex. *Troponin I*, like tropomyosin, has the ability to regulate the interactions between actin and myosin. The regulatory effect of primary interest is that of an interaction inhibitor—hence the designation troponin I. *Troponin T* serves primarily to bind the troponin complex to tropomyosin; and *troponin C* contains two high- and two low-affinity binding sites for Ca^{2+}.

Calcium binding to the two low-affinity binding sites of troponin C exhibits *positive cooperativity*, which indicates that there is a strong interaction between the two sites such that when the first binding site is occupied by calcium the affinity of the second calcium-binding site for Ca^{2+} is increased. In this way the binding of the first calcium ion to troponin C facilitates binding of the second calcium ion, thereby amplifying the effects of an increase in ionized calcium concentration within the cell.

TABLE 6.2 *Approximate molecular weights of the components of troponin*

	Approximate molecular weight (daltons)	
Component	Fast skeletal muscle	Cardiac muscle
Troponin T	37,000	41,000
Troponin I	21,000	28,000
Troponin C	18,000	18,000

Although cardiac and skeletal muscles each contain the full complement of three troponin components, the molecular weights of the components of cardiac and fast skeletal troponin differ (Table 6.2). From a functional standpoint as well, each of the troponin components is specific for the muscle from which it is isolated (see below).

Organization in the Sarcomere

Like tropomyosin, the troponin complex is found along with actin in the thin filament of the sarcomere where the troponin complex is distributed along the thin filament at approximately 400 Å intervals. This distribution is determined by the longitudinal separation of troponin-binding sites on the elongated tropomyosin filaments in the thin filament (Fig. 6.9).

The binding of the three components of troponin to the actin and tropomyosin of the thin filament of the sarcomere probably follows the order shown in Fig. 6.10. The binding between troponin I and actin (represented in Fig. 6.10 as a dashed line) appears to depend on whether troponin C contains bound calcium. Whether troponin I binds to actin depends on whether the calcium binding sites of troponin C are occupied by calcium. In this way the variable affinity of troponin I for actin appears to represent an essential element in the mechanism

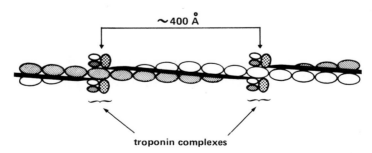

FIG. 6.9. Troponin complexes are found along with actin and tropomyosin in the thin filament. The troponin complexes are bound to tropomyosin at approximately 400-Å intervals along the thin filament.

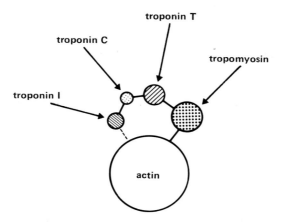

FIG. 6.10. Cross section of half of the thin filament at the level where the troponin complexes are located. This shows proposed relationships between actin, tropomyosin, and the three components of the troponin complex. The dashed line between troponin I and actin represents a bond postulated to vary in strength depending on the binding of calcium to troponin C.

by which calcium triggers the contractile process, as is described more fully in Chapter 7.

MODELS OF THE CONTRACTILE PROTEINS

Starting with the highly purified contractile proteins described above, it is possible to reconstitute an actomyosin that exhibits properties *in vitro* that are remarkably similar to those of the intact muscle. These properties, already noted at the beginning of the chapter, are: (a) ATP hydrolysis, which corresponds to energy liberation in the muscle; (b) physicochemical changes, in which the chemical energy derived from ATP hydrolysis is converted to mechanical work; and (c) regulation by calcium, which corresponds to the response of the contractile proteins to excitation-contraction coupling. The first two can be identified in the two-protein actomyosins (comprised only of actin and myosin). The third, control by calcium, requires in addition the presence of the regulatory proteins tropomyosin and troponin.

Actin Plus Myosin: The Two-Protein Actomyosin

The actomyosins reconstituted from highly purified actin and myosin are able to hydrolyze ATP and undergo physicochemical changes analogous to those which generate tension and shortening in the intact muscle. Many factors govern these interactions *in vitro*. Some are of interest only to the biochemist, but others appear to reflect the operations of control mechanisms relevant to regulation of the contractile process *in vivo*.

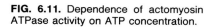

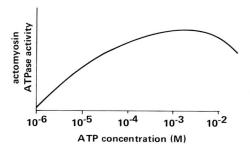

FIG. 6.11. Dependence of actomyosin
ATPase activity on ATP concentration.

    In general terms, the ATPase activity of the two-protein actomyosin is stimu-
lated by both Ca^{2+} and Mg^{2+}. The ATPase activity of myosin alone is also
stimulated by Ca^{2+} but, in contrast, is inhibited by Mg^{2+}. Conversion of the
inhibitory effect of Mg^{2+} on myosin to a stimulatory effect on actomyosin reflects
the role of this cation as a cofactor in the activating effects of actin. Concomitant
with its ability to stimulate myosin ATPase activity in the presence of actin,
Mg^{2+} also promotes the physicochemical interactions between actin and myosin
that represent an *in vitro* manifestation of muscular contraction. In this way
Mg^{2+} is essential for the contractile process in actomyosins studied *in vitro*.
    High concentrations of the alkali metal salts (e.g., Na^+ and K^+) inhibit both
actomyosin ATPase activity and the interactions between actin and myosin which
give rise to contraction. Slight differences exist between the inhibitory effects of
the different alkali metal ions. Na^+, for example, is less effective than K^+ as an
inhibitor of the interactions between actin and myosin, so that replacement of
K^+ by Na^+ slightly increases these contraction-promoting interactions. This effect
is so slight, however, that it appears not to account for a postulated effect of
Na^+-K^+ exchange in the regulation of myocardial contractility (Chapter 11).
    ATP itself has an interesting and important dual effect on actomyosin. Like
the elf in Aesop's fable who blew hot and cold with the same breath (hot to warm
his chilled hands, cold to cool his soup), ATP can cause either stimulation or
inhibition of the interactions between actin and myosin (Fig. 6.11). At low
concentrations ATP promotes these interactions and causes muscle to contract.
In contrast, high ATP concentrations (above approximately 1mM) inhibit actomyosin ATPase activity. This latter effect, which is prominent at the ATP concentrations found in resting muscle, reflects dissociation of the thick and thin
filaments and thus inhibition of the interactions between actin and myosin that
promote contraction. High ATP concentrations are therefore said to have a
"plasticizing" effect in that they decrease the interaction between the two types
of filaments. Reduction in ATP concentration can, by abolishing this plasticizing
effect, promote contraction (Chapter 7).
    Manifestation of these physicochemical interactions *in vitro* depends on the
physical state of the actomyosin. Most striking are the changes observed during
the early 1940s by A. Szent-Györgyi, who prepared actomyosin threads in which

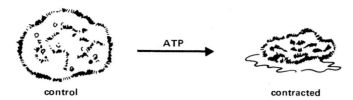

control   contracted

FIG 6.12. Contraction of a floc of an actomyosin gel *in vitro* (shown here as a sponge), which during superprecipitation (contraction) squeezes water out of itself to become smaller and denser.

the asymmetrical actin and myosin filaments were oriented parallel to each other. Addition of ATP causes such actomyosin threads to shorten, and if a load is attached to the actomyosin threads mechanical work is performed. While the mechanical properties of actomyosin threads are similar to those of muscle (e.g., hyperbolic force-velocity curves can be recorded), their tensile strength is low so that they break quite easily.

It is more convenient to study the physicochemical properties of actomyosin gels in which the orientation of the asymmetrical molecules is more or less random. Under these conditions the physicochemical changes associated with contraction cause the individual flocs of actomyosin to shrink (Fig. 6.12). This process, which resembles a sponge squeezing water out of itself, is often called *syneresis*, i.e., a drawing together of the molecules of the gel. If these gels are examined after low-speed centrifugation, the volume of the insoluble actomyosin pellet is found to have decreased (Fig. 6.13). Hence the term "superprecipitation" was coined to describe this *in vitro* manifestation of the contractile process.

Another useful way to study the "contraction" of actomyosin gels is to follow the turbidity changes initiated by addition of ATP (Fig. 6.14). Higher concentrations of ATP cause actin and myosin to dissociate, so that two distinct effects are seen. The initial effect of ATP is to cause an abrupt fall in turbidity, called "clearing" (Fig. 6.14), which results from dissociation of actin and myosin. Clearing is seen only in the presence of Mg^{2+}. As a result of the dissociation of actin and myosin, ATPase activity during clearing is low, approximating that of the ATPase of myosin alone which is inhibited by Mg^{2+} (see above). With

FIG. 6.13. Superprecipitation (contraction) of an actomyosin gel *in vitro*. Shrinkage of the individual flocs of actomyosin (Fig. 6.12) reduces the volume of the pellet that is obtained after centrifugation.

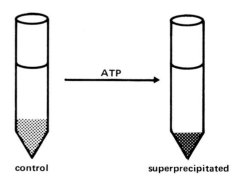

control   superprecipitated

FIG. 6.14. Turbidity changes that follow addition of ATP to an actomyosin gel *in vitro*. Following a brief "clearing" phase, during which actin and myosin are dissociated by high ATP concentration, these proteins become reassociated when ATP levels fall. Under the latter conditions ATP hydrolysis is accelerated and the actomyosin gel contracts (superprecipitation) and becomes more turbid.

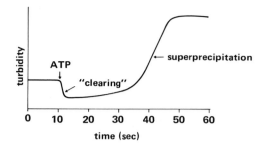

the passage of time, ATP concentration in the medium falls because of ATP hydrolysis by myosin. Eventually the plasticizing effect is lost (Fig. 6.11) at which time actin and myosin recombine in a manner that allows actin to interact with myosin so as to promote ATP hydrolysis and syneresis (Fig. 6.12). The resultant shrinkage of the actomyosin gel causes turbidity to increase (superprecipitation) (Fig. 6.14). ATPase activity becomes high during superprecipitation, reflecting the rapid conversion of the chemical energy released by ATP hydrolysis to mechanical work.

From the preceding discussion it is apparent that the state of the interactions between actin and myosin are dependent on the composition of the medium. Thus changing concentrations of the alkali metal ions, Mg^+ and ATP, either individually or together, can modify the properties of the actomyosins. For this reason it was once believed that the physiological control of the interactions between actin and myosin, and thus the reversible transitions between rest (manifest, for example, as clearing) and activity (manifest as superprecipitation, syneresis, or contraction of actomyosin threads), could be effected by changes in ATP concentration. For over a decade, however, it has been clear that the reversible control of muscular contraction is exerted not by changes in the concentration of ATP (or the other modifying reactants described above), but instead by variations in the concentration of Ca^{2+} around the myofibrils. The significance of this control is apparent if one compares the magnitude of the changes in ATP, Mg^{2+}, or alkali metal ion concentration needed to effect the contractile process with the changes in Ca^{2+} concentration. Normally both Mg^{2+} and ATP concentrations are in the *millimolar* range, whereas that of K^+ in the cell is 0.1 M. Considerable expenditure of energy therefore would be needed to alter significantly their concentration around the contractile proteins. In the case of Ca^{2+}, on the other hand, normal concentrations in the cell are between 0.1 and 10 μM. Thus much less energy is needed to effect the changes in Ca^{2+} concentration needed to bring about the reversible transitions from rest to activity.

As the role of Ca^{2+} in controlling the state of activity of the contractile proteins became apparent, it was recognized that this action of Ca^{2+} was not manifest in the two-protein actomyosins. Instead, the calcium sensitivity of the contractile proteins requires the presence, in addition to actomyosin, of the regulatory proteins tropomyosin and the troponin complex.

"Complete" Actomyosin and Its Control by Calcium Ion

Each of the proteins just discussed—myosin, actin, tropomyosin, and the three components of troponin—is now recognized to play a specific role in the interactions that enable muscle to contract and relax. These interactions can, from the standpoint of the intact muscle, be grouped into two types: (a) those responsible for the contractile process itself; and (b) those which permit this process to be controlled. Let us examine our current understanding of the molecular basis for the control of contraction.

The ability of Ca^{2+} to trigger muscle contraction has been known since the 1940s. However, the mechanism of this stimulatory action became clear only during the early 1960s, when it was recognized that the stimulatory action of Ca^{2+} arose from a direct effect on the contractile proteins. Prior to that time it had been believed that calcium promoted contraction by inactivating a "relaxing factor." As the stimulation of various actomyosin systems by Ca^{2+} became better understood, it was noted that not all actomyosins could be controlled by this cation. It was this observation that led Ebashi to identify, and eventually to isolate, the proteins that mediate this important regulatory function.

What Ebashi and others found was that actomyosins made only of actin and myosin were "Ca^{2+}-insensitive." This Ca^{2+} insensitivity was found not to involve loss of a stimulatory effect of Ca^{2+}. Instead, these two-protein actomyosins remained fully "active" even when Ca^{2+} concentrations were drastically lowered, as by the calcium chelator EGTA. In this way Ca^{2+} was recognized not to be a direct activator of actomyosin. Instead, Ca^{2+} reverses an inhibition of contraction, as shown in Table 6.3. Ca^{2+} removal has no effect in the two-protein actomyosin, whereas in the "complete" actomyosin this cation is needed to activate those interactions between actin and myosin that give rise to manifestations of contractile activity *in vitro*, e.g., superprecipitation and high ATPase activity (see preceding section).

The role of the regulatory proteins in modulating the interactions between actin and myosin can be seen by reading downward in column a of Table 6.3. When Ca^{2+} concentration is low, actomyosins that do not contain the regulatory proteins are active in that ATPase activity is high and superprecipitation takes place. Inclusion of tropomyosin and the troponin complex inactivates the system as long as Ca^{2+} concentration remains low. When Ca^{2+} concentration is high (column b, Table 6.3) the actomyosins are active, regardless of whether the regulatory

TABLE 6.3. *Actions of Ca²⁺ on the contractile activity of different actomyosins in vitro*

Actomyosin	(a) Low Ca^{2+}	(b) High Ca^{2+}
"Two-protein" (actin + myosin)	Active	Active
"Complete" (actin + myosin + tropomyosin + troponin complex)	Inhibited	Active

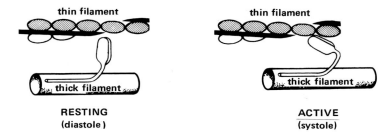

FIG. 6.15. Transition from rest (diastole) to activity (systole), showing attachment of the cross-bridges to the thin filament. A shift in the orientation of the cross-bridges is associated with longitudinal movement of the thin filament.

proteins are included. Table 6.3 thus demonstrates two essential facets of the physiological control of interactions between actin and myosin: (a) *the regulatory proteins are inhibitory in the absence of Ca^{2+}*; and (b) *the ability of Ca^{2+} to initiate contraction results from a reversal of this inhibitory effect.*

The relationships described in the preceding paragraphs are illustrated in Fig. 6.15, which is discussed again in Chapter 7. On the left are shown the contractile proteins of the resting heart, in which the myosin cross-bridge projecting from the thick filament (top) does not interact with actin in the thin filament (bottom) because of the inhibitory effects of the tropomyosin-troponin complex. This inhibition persists as long as the high-affinity Ca^{2+}-binding site on the troponin complex is devoid of calcium. Delivery of Ca^{2+} to the contractile proteins (Fig. 6.15, right) permits the cation to bind to troponin C, the Ca^{2+}-binding component of troponin. The binding of Ca^{2+} to troponin C leads to a series of conformational changes in the regulatory proteins that cause active sites on the actin of the thin filament (Fig. 6.15, right) to be exposed to the myosin cross-bridge. The availability of these active sites on actin to bind to the myosin cross-bridge sets into motion those processes which effect myocardial contraction. The nature of these processes, which involve the hydrolysis of ATP by myosin, and the mechanism of their control by Ca^{2+} are discussed in Chapter 7.

BIBLIOGRAPHY

Bárány, M. (1967): ATPase activity of myosin correlated with speed of muscle shortening. *J. Gen. Physiol.*, 50: No. 6 Pt. 2, 197–216.

Cold Spring Harbor Symposia on Quantitative Biology (1973): *The Mechanism of Muscle Contraction,* Vol. 37. Cold Spring Harbor Lab., New York.

Ebashi, S. (1974): Regulatory mechanism of muscle contraction with special reference to the Ca-troponin-tropomyosin system. In: *Essays in Biochemistry,* Vol. 10, edited by P. N. Campbell and F. Dickens, pp. 1–36. Academic Press, London.

Ebashi, S., and Endo, M. (1968): Calcium ion and muscular contraction. *Prog. Biophys. Mol. Biol.,* 18:123–183.

Huxley, H. E. (1969): The mechanism of muscular contraction. *Science,* 164:1356–1366.

Katz, A. M. (1970): Contractile proteins of the heart. *Physiol. Rev.,* 50:63–158.

Weber, A., and Murray, J. M. (1973): Molecular control mechanisms in muscle contraction. *Physiol. Rev.,* 53:612–673.

7

Mechanism and Control of the Cardiac Contractile Process

The molecular characteristics and interactions of the cardiac contractile proteins *in vitro* provide an important clue to the mechanisms of muscular contraction and their control in the intact heart. Thus actomyosins reconstituted from highly purified myosin, actin, tropomyosin, and the troponin complex exhibit the three salient properties of muscle, two of which are found in the "two-protein" actomyosins (comprised of actin and myosin). The latter are able to hydrolyze ATP and to undergo physicochemical changes analogous to contraction. The third of these properties, the ability to respond to Ca^{2+}, requires, in addition, the presence of the regulatory proteins (tropomyosin and the troponin complex). By building up contractile systems from the individually purified proteins, it has been possible to define the functional role of each of these components of the contractile machinery.

In this chapter we first examine the mechanism by which the regulatory proteins recognize the arrival of Ca^{2+} at the region of the cell which contains the contractile proteins. This mechanism permits the availability of Ca^{2+} to be translated into a signal which initiates contraction. Second, our current understanding of the interactions between actin and myosin that give rise to the contractile process is examined. Finally, these properties are re-examined in terms of the principles of muscular contraction described in Chapter 5.

RESPONSE TO CALCIUM IONS

It has already been pointed out that Ca^{2+} triggers the contractile process by reversing an inhibitory effect of the regulatory proteins. This occurs when Ca^{2+} becomes bound to troponin C, the Ca^{2+} receptor protein of the myofibril. The following scheme, based on evidence available at the time of writing, is attractive but cannot yet be accepted as proved.

The inhibitory effect of the regulatory proteins seen in the absence of Ca^{2+} requires that tropomyosin be present in the groove that runs along both sides of the double-stranded F-actin polymer which makes up the backbone of the thin filament of the sarcomere (Fig. 6.8). Seen in cross section, the backbone of the thin filament is a pair of actin molecules, one derived from each of the two strands of the F-actin polymer. Two filamentous tropomyosin molecules parallel the thin filament, lying adjacent to the paired chains of actin monomers (Fig. 7.1).

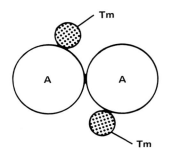

FIG. 7.1. Cross section of the thin filament at a level away from a region containing the troponin complex, showing the location of tropomyosin molecules (Tm) in the groove between adjacent strands of actin mono-mers (A).

The actin-tropomyosin complex shown in longitudinal view in Fig. 6.8 and in cross section in Fig. 7.1 cannot respond to the Ca^{2+} released during excitation-contraction coupling. This effect of Ca^{2+} to regulate the contractile process, as was already discussed, requires the presence of the troponin complex in the thin filament.

The binding of Ca^{2+} to troponin C is now believed to initiate a series of cooperative interactions among the proteins of the thin filament. These result in a shift in the position of the filamentous tropomyosin molecules as they parallel the double-stranded actin polymer. When troponin C is not bound to Ca^{2+}, tropomyosin is in a position that keeps the muscle at rest. This position of the

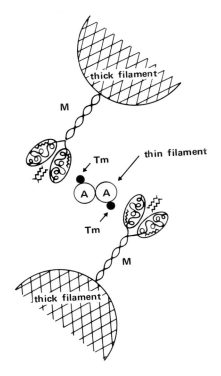

FIG. 7.2. Cross section of resting sarcomere. The tropomyosin molecules (Tm) in the thin filament are located toward the periphery of the groove between adjacent actin strands (A), thereby preventing their interaction with the myosin cross-bridges (M). (Troponin complex is not shown.)

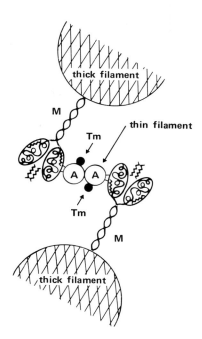

FIG. 7.3. Cross section of an active sarcomere. A shift in the position of the tropomyosin molecules (Tm) toward the center of the groove between adjacent actin strands (A) in the thin filament allows the latter to interact with the myosin crossbridges (M). (Troponin complex is not shown.)

tropomyosin filaments is believed to be toward the outside of the grooves between the two chains of actin. In this position tropomyosin inhibits the development of chemical interactions between actin and myosin. Figure 7.2 represents a cross section of one A-band in resting muscle, showing actin *(A)* and the myosin cross-bridges *(M)*. Tropomyosin *(T)* in the thin filament of resting muscle is thus oriented so as to "block" the formation of bonds between actin and the myosin cross-bridges (see also Fig. 6.15).

Contraction is initiated when Ca^{2+} binds to troponin C. Resulting cooperative interactions among the proteins of the thin filament are believed to cause tropomyosin to shift toward the center of the groove between the two strands of actin (Fig. 7.3). In other words, tropomyosin is caused to "move out of the way" so as to allow physical and chemical interactions to develop between the myosin cross-bridges of the thick filament and the active sites of actin in the thin filament (see also Fig. 6.15). The muscle returns to its relaxed state when Ca^{2+} is removed from troponin C, causing tropomyosin to return to its original inhibitory position in the thin filament (Fig. 7.2).

It must be emphasized that the full story of the cooperative interaction between actin, myosin, and the modulatory proteins is not yet known. Of greatest biological significance among the phenomena that are now understood is the ability of the regulatory proteins to inhibit the onset of the contractile process when troponin C is not bound to Ca^{2+} (Chapter 6). In addition, however, the regulatory proteins can stimulate the interactions between actin and myosin once the contractile process has begun. The stimulatory effect occurs when the interactions between actin and myosin are fully active (Fig. 7.3), so that once the muscle begins to contract the regulatory proteins appear to enhance the contractile process. Although the functional significance of this stimulatory effect is not yet clear, its importance in the control of muscular contraction is probably less than the inhibitory effects described above.

Each unit of the troponin complex is spaced approximately 400 Å from the neighboring troponin complexes along the long axis of the thin filament (Fig. 6.9). As a result, the effects of Ca^{2+} binding to any one troponin complex can exert its effect on approximately seven actin monomers. This quantitative relationship is based on the spacing of actin monomers at intervals of approximately 55 Å along the thin filament (Fig. 6.6).

The mechanism by which Ca^{2+} binding to troponin C could cause a shift in the position of tropomyosin along the thin filament is not yet fully understood.

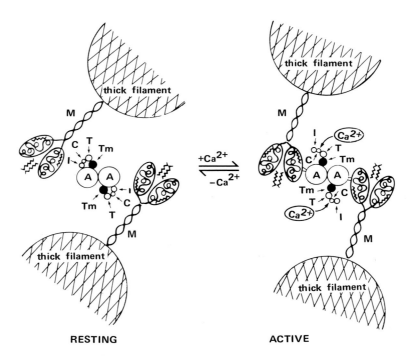

RESTING   ACTIVE

FIG. 7.4. Possible mechanism by which calcium binding to troponin initiates contraction. The basic diagrams are similar to those shown in Figs. 7.2 and 7.3. In resting muscle *(left)* the three components of the troponin complex (I, C, and T) hold tropomyosin (Tm) toward the periphery of the groove between adjacent actin strands (A), preventing their interaction with the myosin cross-bridges (M). Binding of Ca^{2+} to troponin C *(right)* sets into motion a series of cooperative interactions between the proteins of the thin filament which reduces the affinity between troponin I and actin. The resulting detachment of bonds between troponins I and actin causes tropomyosin to shift its position toward the center of the groove between the actin strands, allowing the latter to interact with the myosin cross-bridges and thereby initiate muscular activity.

It is apparent, however, that this response arises from a series of cooperative interactions between tropomyosin and the three proteins of the troponin complex. Studies of these interactions indicate that troponins I and T bind to both tropomyosin and troponin C, while tropomyosin and troponin I bind to actin (Fig. 6.10). It has been postulated that the binding of Ca^{2+} to troponin C effects a change in the affinity of troponin I for actin. The resulting changes in binding angles between these proteins could cause the elongated tropomyosin molecules to shift toward the center of the groove between the two strands of actin (Fig. 7.4). In this way a shift of tropomyosin away from the outer "edge" of the thin filament (Fig. 7.4) might allow the myosin cross-bridges to approach and interact with the active sites on actin in the thin filament, thus allowing the contractile process to be triggered by Ca^{2+}. According to this theory removal of Ca^{2+} from its binding sites on troponin C would cause troponin I to bind to actin. The resulting shift in the binding angles between the proteins of the thin filament would allow tropomyosin to return to its inhibitory position, allowing Ca^{2+} removal to cause the muscle to relax.

The three components of the cardiac and skeletal troponin complexes are functionally homologous, as was described in Chapter 6 (Table 6.2), and it is possible to make hybrids from the individual proteins of the cardiac and skeletal troponin complexes. Most of these hybrids can mediate some degree of Ca^{2+} control in the actomyosins of either muscle type. The ability of various hybrid troponin complexes to control contraction, however, is generally much less than that of the homologous troponin complexes containing troponins C, T, and I from only cardiac or only skeletal muscle. The failure to recover full calcium-sensitizing activity in hybrid troponin complexes indicates that the troponin components of an individual muscle type are functionally interdependent. In other words, the troponin complex is tissue-specific and behaves biologically as part of a highly organized and specific molecular complex.

CHEMICAL BASIS FOR CARDIAC CONTRACTION

The finding that two-protein actomyosins are able to convert the chemical energy obtained from hydrolysis of ATP into mechanical work (Chapter 6) indicates that the contractile process results from interactions between actin, myosin, ATP, ADP, and P_i, the products of ATP hydrolysis. Many aspects of the reaction mechanisms involved in muscular contraction are both poorly understood and controversial. Yet in spite of these limitations, certain aspects of the chemical basis of muscular contraction are now reasonably well understood.

Motion of the Myosin Cross-Bridge

The motion of the cross-bridge that now appears to be of central importance to the contractile process is the shift in cross-bridge orientation relative to the long axis of the thick filament that occurs when the muscle is activated (Fig. 6.4). This finding indicates the existence of at least one point of flexibility in the myosin cross-bridge.

Because muscle volume does not change significantly during contraction, its cross-sectional area must increase with shortening. When viewed in relation to the thick and thin filaments, this finding requires that the distances between the

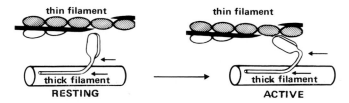

FIG. 7.5. Transition from resting *(left)* to active *(right)* muscle requires interaction between myosin cross-bridges and the thin filament, and a shift in the angle of the former relative to the longitudinal axis of the muscle. The shift in the angle of the myosin cross-bridge appears to involve two points of flexibility *(arrows)*. For simplicity, the troponin complexes on the thin filament are omitted in this and the following figures.

myosin and actin filaments increase markedly as the sarcomere length decreases (Chapter 6). Intermolecular forces generally become weaker in proportion to the square of the distance between the molecules, so that the "constant volume" properties of muscle might be expected to cause the strength of contraction to decrease markedly as the sarcomere shortens. It has been found experimentally, however, that the apparent strength of the interactions between the myosin cross-bridges and actin changes very little over a significant range of sarcomere length. This finding means either that the forces between the proteins of the thick and thin filaments are exceptional, by being virtually independent of the distance between the filaments, or else that the tips of the myosin cross-bridges move away from the axis of the thick filament as the thin filament becomes more distant at shorter sarcomere lengths. As shown in Fig. 6.5, the latter explanation is currently believed to be correct. Thus preservation of the full intensity of interactions between thick and thin filaments can result from a second point of flexibility in the myosin cross-bridge which allows the tip of the myosin molecule to extend outward from the axis of the thick filament to engage the actin of the thin filament at shorter sarcomere lengths (Fig. 7.5). These two "joints" in the molecule, as suggested in Chapter 6, may correspond to regions of susceptibility to proteolytic cleavage (Fig. 6.2).

> The existence of paired heads in each myosin cross-bridge (Chapter 6) has given rise to a number of complex theories regarding a possible interaction between myosin heads in the genesis of this and other properties of the myosin-actin interaction. It now appears, however, that "one-headed" myosin can exhibit the salient properties of contraction, although a cooperative interaction between the two components of the normal paired head remains a definite possibility.

Is ATP Essential for Contraction or Relaxation?

It has long been apparent that hydrolysis of ATP is essential for the cycle of chemical reactions which underlies the ability of muscle to function as a mechanochemical transducer. Yet the precise role of ATP in this cycle has remained obscure. Theories of muscular contraction such as the new elastic body theory (Chapter 5) suggested that ATP may be essential for establishing those cross links in the molecular machinery which give rise to the ability to shorten and to develop tension:

$$\text{Actin} + \text{myosin} \xrightarrow{\text{ATP}} \text{actomyosin} + \text{ADP} + \text{P}_i \qquad (7.1)$$
$$\text{(relaxed)} \qquad\qquad\qquad \text{(active)}$$

$$\text{Actomyosin} \longrightarrow \text{actin} + \text{myosin} \qquad (7.2)$$
$$\text{(active)} \qquad\qquad \text{(relaxed)}$$

Identification of the plasticizing effect of ATP (Chapter 6), which reflects a requirement for ATP in maintaining the contractile machinery in a relaxed state, suggested the opposite view, i.e., that the role of ATP in the contractile process is primarily to cause actomyosin systems to relax:

$$\text{Actomyosin} \xrightarrow{\text{ATP}} \text{actin} + \text{myosin—ATP} \qquad (7.3)$$
$$\text{(active)} \qquad\qquad\qquad \text{(relaxed)}$$

$$\text{Actin} + \text{myosin-ATP} \longrightarrow \text{actomyosin} + \text{ADP} + \text{P}_i \qquad (7.4)$$
$$\text{(relaxed)} \qquad\qquad\qquad\qquad \text{(active)}$$

With the growing ability to dissect the processes of muscular contraction into a series of steps—each involving different modifications of the interactions between myosin, actin, ATP, ADP, and inorganic phosphate—this question has assumed new dimensions. The number of known steps in the sequence of chemical reactions responsible for muscular contraction has grown, and it is now apparent that ATP and the products of ATP hydrolysis, ADP and P_i, can be bound to the contractile proteins at many steps in this process. For this reason attempts to distinguish between the simple alternatives set forth earlier in this paragraph have lost much of their relevance.

Reaction Mechanism

The reaction mechanism responsible for the ATPase activity of myosin alone has assumed considerable functional significance in view of the relationship between myosin ATPase activity and the speed of shortening of unloaded muscle (Chapter 6). Thus the specific step in these chemical reactions that is rate-limiting for myosin ATPase activity *in vitro* probably also accounts for the rate-limiting step in the shortening of the intact muscle.

Much controversy remains as to the reaction mechanisms which permit the contractile proteins to utilize ATP for the generation of mechanical work. Certain steps in this sequence of chemical reactions, however, are generally accepted. These are: (a) binding of ATP to myosin; (b) hydrolysis of myosin-bound ATP; (c) formation of an "active" actomyosin complex; (d) mechanochemical transduction; and (e) release of hydrolytic products. A renewed sequence is then initiated when ATP is again bound to myosin.

Binding of ATP to Myosin

The tendency for myosin to bind ATP

$$\text{Myosin} + \text{ATP} \longrightarrow \text{myosin—ATP} \qquad (7.5)$$

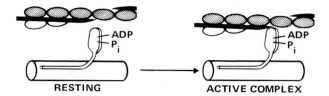

FIG. 7.6. Formation of the active complex *(right)* occurs when the myosin cross-bridge interacts with the thin filament. No changes occur in myosin-bound nucleotide and phosphate, and the cross-bridge does not alter its angle.

is sufficiently great that under resting conditions it is likely that virtually all of the myosin cross-bridges of resting muscle contain either bound ATP [Eq. (7.5)] or bound products of ATP hydrolysis [Eq. (7.6), below]. The presence of bound nucleotide is presumed to inhibit the binding of the cross-bridge to actin, thus accounting for the "plasticizing" effect of ATP (Chapter 6).

Hydrolysis of Myosin-Bound ATP

The enzymatic site of myosin has the intrinsic ability to hydrolyze ATP. The split products of ATP do not immediately dissociate, however. Instead, a complex is formed in which ADP and P_i remain attached to the myosin molecule:

$$\text{Myosin—ATP} \longrightarrow \text{myosin} \underset{P_i}{\overset{ADP}{<}} \qquad (7.6)$$

This reaction can proceed in the absence of actin, but the subsequent dissociation of ADP and P_i from myosin is slow, being manifest as the low ATPase activity of myosin alone. When actin is present, however, the latter reaction is activated.

Formation of the "Active" Actomyosin Complex

The activation of myosin ATPase by actin is accompanied by the formation of a strong interaction between these two proteins of the thick and thin filaments:

$$\text{Actin} + \text{myosin} \underset{P_i}{\overset{ADP}{<}} \longrightarrow \left(\text{actin-myosin} \underset{P_i}{\overset{ADP}{<}} \right)_{\text{(active complex)}} \qquad (7.7)$$

Initially this interaction develops by a mechanism that neither releases high-energy phosphate bond energy nor brings about a shift in the orientation of the myosin cross-bridge. As a result, the cross-bridge remains perpendicular to the thick filament (Fig. 7.6). Because the chemical energy made available by ATP hydrolysis has not yet been utilized to perform mechanical work, this complex contains considerable potential energy—hence the term "active complex." The active complex shown in Fig. 7.6 is unstable, however, and is rapidly transformed

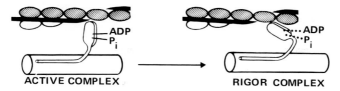

FIG. 7.7. Formation of the rigor complex involves a shift in the angle of the myosin cross-bridge. It is not known if the myosin-bound ADP, P_i, or both are released at this initial step in the formation of the rigor complex.

into a different form of actin-myosin complex in which release of phosphate bond energy is associated with a shift in position of the myosin cross-bridge.

Mechanochemical Transduction

The tendency of the active complex shown on the right side of Fig. 7.6 to break down and transform chemical energy to mechanical energy can be represented as a change in the nature of the actin-myosin complex:

$$\left(\text{Actin-myosin}\begin{smallmatrix}\text{—ADP}\\\text{—P}_i\end{smallmatrix}\right)_{\text{active complex}} \longrightarrow \left(\text{actin-myosin:}\begin{smallmatrix}\text{ADP}\\\text{P}_i\end{smallmatrix}\right)_{\text{rigor complex}} \quad (7.8)$$

The degradation of the active complex can thus be accompanied by a shift in the orientation of the myosin cross-bridge that causes the thin filament to be drawn toward the center of the sarcomere (Fig. 7.7). The resulting form of the actin-myosin complex is called the rigor complex. The mechanisms involved in this step, which represents the mechanochemical transduction of the contractile process, remain unclear. It may be that release of either or both of the products of ATP hydrolysis, ADP and P_i, accompanies this process.

The actomyosin complex depicted as the rigor complex is in a low-energy state—unlike that of the active complex which is in a high-energy state. This change in state can readily be appreciated because in the transition from the active complex to the rigor complex chemical energy must be released by the actomyosin complex in order to effect motion.

Release of Hydrolytic Products

Prior to rebinding of ATP, both ADP and P_i derived from hydrolysis of myosin-bound ATP must be released:

$$\left(\text{Actin-myosin:}\begin{smallmatrix}\text{ADP}\\\text{P}_i\end{smallmatrix}\right)_{\text{rigor complex}} \longrightarrow \left(\text{actin-myosin}\right)_{\text{rigor complex}} + \text{ADP} + P_i \quad (7.9)$$

ADP, P_i, or both may remain bound to the cross-bridge during formation of the rigor complex. Alternatively, one or both of the split products of ATP may be released while the cross-bridges remain fixed to the thin filaments as rigor complexes (Fig. 7.8). As long as the contractile proteins remain devoid of bound nucleotide, the physiocochemical state of actomyosin is that of the rigor complex.

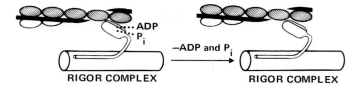

FIG. 7.8. The products of ATP hydrolysis (ADP and P_i) are eventually released by the myosin cross-bridge after it has formed a rigor complex with the thin filament.

Thus this complex is quite stable, becoming dissociated only on readdition of ATP.

The rigor complex, which accounts for muscular rigidity in *rigor mortis,* and possibly the "stone heart" (Chapter 11), dissociates when ATP is once again bound to myosin [Eq. (7.5)]. In this way the binding of ATP by myosin allows the muscle to return to its original resting state (Fig. 7.9).

The preceding description of the chemistry of the contractile process is incomplete in that a number of important details regarding these reaction mechanisms are still lacking. It is apparent, however, that the question of whether ATP is essential for contraction or relaxation is not now meaningful because this nucleotide is in fact essential for both. In general terms, one might state that ATP is essential for relaxation, and its hydrolysis is essential for contraction.

Relationship Between the Contractile Process and the Energetics of Contraction

The important findings of Hill regarding the relationship between the load on a muscle and the energetics of contraction were set forth in Chapter 5. The remarkably prescient interpretation that the load a muscle lifts determines the distribution of "active points" between two different states is now re-examined in terms of the chemical processes reviewed in this and the preceding chapter.

In his analysis of the finding that the rate of energy liberation by a contracting muscle is inversely proportional to load, Hill postulated that when the load is great, more of the active points are attached to each other and so are in a state

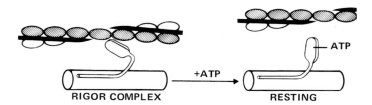

FIG. 7.9. Muscle relaxation occurs when ATP binding to the myosin cross-bridge causes the rigor complex to be dissociated. The muscle thus returns to its resting state *(right)*. It is not known if the stable resting state involves myosin bound to ATP (as shown here) or to ADP and P_i, the products of subsequent hydrolysis of myosin-bound ATP (as shown in Fig. 7.6, *left*).

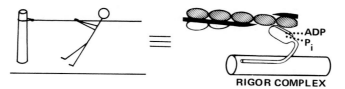

RIGOR COMPLEX

FIG. 7.10. The state of the active points in muscle when they are holding tension is identical to that of the rigor complex.

in which chemical energy is not being released. Conversely, in unloaded, freely shortening muscle, all of these active points are free to liberate chemical energy. This interpretation can be tentatively related to the reaction mechanism set out in Eqs. (7.5)–(7.9) and illustrated in Figs. 7.6–7.9.

Active Points Maintaining Tension

The decrease in the rate of energy liberation at higher loads indicates that the tension the muscle encounters during shortening influences the rate of ATP hydrolysis. Because the rate of energy liberation per unit time is slowed at higher loads, conditions where actin and myosin interact in a manner that gives rise to greater active tension, it is reasonable to relate the "little men" (in Chapter 5) holding tension to the rigor complex [Eqs. (7.8) and (7.9)]. In other words, increasing the tension on the ends of the muscle inhibits the reactions shown in Figs. 7.8 and 7.9, thereby leaving more of the rigor complexes intact at any instant (Fig. 7.10). The mechanism by which resistance to muscle shortening inhibits the breaking of the rigor complex is not known.

Active Points Liberating Chemical Energy

The rate of energy liberation per unit time is maximal in the freely shortening muscle, which by definition is contracting against zero load. Furthermore, maximal shortening velocity of a given muscle is characteristic of that individual muscle type and correlates closely with the intrinsic ATPase activity of its myosin. When myosin ATPase activity is high, maximal shortening velocity (V_{max}) is high; whereas when myosin ATPase activity is low, V_{max} is also low. A very

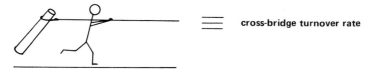

cross-bridge turnover rate

FIG. 7.11. The active points in muscle when the muscle is shortening against zero load are probably passing repeatedly through the cycle shown in Figs. 7.6–7.9 at a rate determined by the intrinsic properties of the myosin cross-bridge.

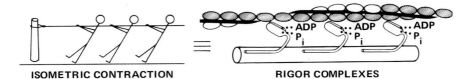

ISOMETRIC CONTRACTION   RIGOR COMPLEXES

FIG. 7.12. During an isometric contraction, where all active points are maintaining tension *(left),* the myosin cross-bridges are probably linked to the thin filament via rigor complexes *(right).*

close correlation between myosin ATPase activity and maximal shortening velocity was found by Bárány, who studied muscles in which both parameters varied over an almost 200-fold range. For this reason it appears that the same property which determines myosin ATPase activity *in vitro* also governs the maximal velocity of shortening in the unloaded muscle (see above).

In the terms set out in Eqs. (7.5)–(7.9), the rate-limiting step in the turnover cycle of the myosin cross-bridges in their interaction with the thin filament can be considered to be the same as that which is rate-limiting for the turnover of ATP by the isolated myosin. For this reason the maximal speed at which the "little men" can run corresponds to the limiting rate of the overall cycle shown in Figs. 7.6–7.9 (Fig. 7.11).

These interpretations are supported by the finding that P_0, the maximal isometric tension a muscle can generate, is independent of both the maximal velocity of shortening and the myosin ATPase activity of the muscle. Instead, P_0 appears to reflect the number of active cross-bridges (Fig. 7.12).

The existence of two independently determined parameters of muscle function suggests two mechanisms by which muscular performance can be controlled. One depends on the characteristics of the myosin molecule, and the other on the number of active cross-bridges. In view of the importance of intrinsic control of the contractile process in the regulation of myocardial function, the preceding analysis indicates the potential existence of at least two distinct biochemical control mechanisms in the regulation of myocardial contractility. We return to this analysis in Chapter 11, where the control of myocardial contractility is discussed in detail.

BIBLIOGRAPHY

Gergely, J. (1974): Some aspects of the role of the sarcoplasmic reticulum and the tropomyosin-troponin system in the control of muscle contraction by calcium ions. *Circ. Res. (Suppl. III),* 34–35: III–74–81.

Huxley, A. F. (1974); Muscular contraction. *J. Physiol. (Lond.),* 243:1–43.

Also see bibliography to Chapter 6.

8

Series Elasticity, "Active State," Length-Tension Relationship, and Cardiac Mechanics

Chapters 5 through 7 attempted to relate the mechanical properties of contracting muscle to the chemical interactions between the contractile proteins. Much of this discussion focused on information generated in studies of the well-characterized frog sartorius in which both the simple geometry of the muscle (Chapter 11) and the ability to study brief tetani greatly simplified the analyses of mechanical performance. The latter especially permits the mechanochemical transduction process to be described without the added complexity of changes in time-dependent properties of muscular contraction. These properties, however, present a greater obstacle to analysis of muscle mechanics in the myocardium, which cannot normally be tetanized. Thus cardiac mechanics must ordinarily be evaluated during the rise and fall of tension such as occurs in the skeletal muscle during a twitch, in which the time dependence of the interactions between the contractile proteins poses a number of analytical problems.

SERIES ELASTICITY

Several features of the time-dependent properties of the mechanical response during a twitch can be explained on the basis of an elasticity that is found in series between the contractile element and the ends of the muscle (Fig. 8.1). The extension of this "series elasticity" during shortening of the contractile element absorbs some of the energy generated by the latter, while at the same time the slow increase in tension within the series elasticity delays the appearance of tension at the ends of the muscle after the contractile element shortens. As a result of absorption of energy by the series elasticity, the tension developed at the ends of the muscle during a twitch (in which activation of the contractile element is very brief) is both attenuated and delayed.

Latent Period

A significant delay between the application of a stimulus to a skeletal muscle and the first appearance of tension has long been recognized. If the muscle is held under isometric conditions, as shown in Fig. 8.2, a slight fall in tension precedes the development of tension. The brief interval between stimulation and the rise of tension is called the latent period, and the fall of tension is often called latency relaxation. These phenomena cannot be attributed simply to the time needed for

FIG. 8.1. Simplified model of muscle showing contractile element in series with a
spring-like series elasticity (longitudinal direction of muscle is left to right).

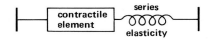

the impulse to reach the contractile elements because important changes occur
within the muscle during the latent period. In addition to the fall in tension
illustrated in Fig. 8.2, the optical properties of the muscle are altered during the
latent period so that translucency increases well before tension appears at the ends
of the muscle. The term latency relaxation is in some ways a misnomer because
the slight decrease in tension that occurs during the latent period is not an
indication that the contractile element has relaxed. Instead, an increased capacity
of the contractile element to maintain tension occurs during the latent period,
even though these changes in the contractile element are not immediately manifest as an increase in tension developed at the ends of the muscle.

That the contractile process begins during the latent period is clearly evident
when muscle stiffness is measured. Even before tension appears at the ends of
the muscle, the muscle becomes less plastic so that when the muscle is stretched
an increase in tension is apparent. This increased stiffness during the period of
latency relaxation indicates that contraction had already begun. In other words,
muscular contraction starts during the latent period, even before tension appears
at the ends of the muscle.

The delay between tension development within the contractile element and its
appearance as tension at the ends of the muscle can be attributed to an extension
of the series elasticity. Therefore the time course of activity within the contractile
element cannot be measured unless the series elasticity is first extended and its
effects eliminated (see below).

Twitch, Summation, and Tetanization

In a skeletal muscle, where the duration of the action potential is much shorter
than the mechanical response, it is possible to restimulate the muscle while

FIG. 8.2. Latency relaxation in a skeletal
muscle contracting under isometric conditions. Tension initially declines during the
first few milliseconds after stimulation (S).
This decline is the latency relaxation. (The
time scales in this and other figures in this
chapter are adapted from studies of amphibian muscle at 0°C. These events occur
much more rapidly in mammalian muscles
contracting at 37°C.)

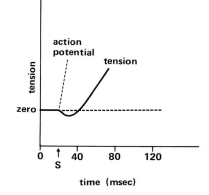

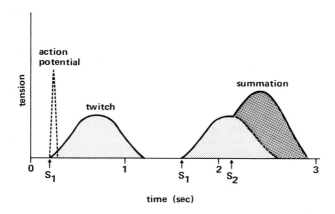

FIG. 8.3. Twitch and summation in a skeletal muscle contracting under isometric conditions. **Left:** The symmetrical contraction *(solid line)* following a single action potential *(dashed line)* produced by a single stimulus (S_1) is a twitch. **Right:** The application of a second stimulus (S_2) during the falling phase of the twitch produces a second action potential (not shown), which causes the renewed development of tension, a phenomenon called summation.

tension is still high (Fig. 8.3). The response to a single stimulus (S_1, Fig. 8.3) is the *twitch.* If a second stimulus is applied before relaxation is complete, a second contraction is added to the first contraction. Tension in the second contraction (S_2, Fig. 8.3) exceeds that developed during the twitch. Because the tension response to the second stimulus has been added to that of the first, the term *summation* has been introduced to describe this phenomenon.

If a series of stimuli is delivered so rapidly that each successive stimulus arrives before the muscle begins to relax, a new steady-state level of tension is reached in a muscle made to contract isometrically. The isometric tension in this new steady state exceeds twitch tension two- or threefold (Fig. 8.4). The higher, sustained form of contraction is called a *tetanus,* and the new level of tension is the *tetanic tension.* This isometric tension corresponds to P_0 of the force-velocity curve as discussed in the preceding chapters.

> Confusion can arise regarding the term tetanus. The distinction between the tetanus shown in Fig. 8.4 and the disease caused by the endotoxin of the bacteria *Clostridium tetani* (a condition sometimes called lockjaw) is obvious. Tetany, a pathological condition that represents sensitization of the muscles to physical and chemical stimuli, accompanies systemic alkalosis or hypocalcemia. This abnormality is quite different from the tetanus shown in Fig. 8.4, as tetany arises from a lowered threshold to nerve and muscle stimulation rather than the summation of the mechanical responses to a train of rapidly applied stimuli.

The striking increase in tetanic tension, compared to that developed in a twitch, remained unexplained for many years. It could be postulated, for example, that the level of activity by the contractile proteins is heightened by a train of stimuli. This explanation, however, is not correct. Instead, it can be shown that the

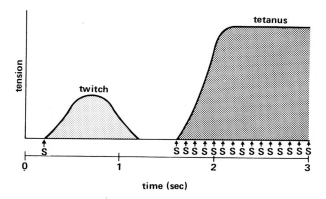

FIG. 8.4. Twitch and tetanic contractions in a skeletal muscle contracting under isometric conditions. **Left:** Twitch, as shown in Fig. 8.3. **Right:** Application of a train of stimuli (S) causes tension to rise to a higher level than that developed during the twitch. Tension remains at this high level until the train of stimuli is interrupted or the muscle fatigues.

tension which appears at the ends of the muscle during a twitch is considerably less than the maximal tension that would be developed by the contractile element were the series elasticity to be eliminated. Like the phenomenon of the latent period, the relatively low tension developed during a twitch is due to the absorption of energy as the series elasticity is lengthened.

Location of the Series Elasticity

Figure 8.1 implies that the series elasticity lies outside the contractile element. To some extent this is correct in that the tendinous ends of the muscles contribute an elasticity to experimental muscle preparations. Elasticities in such studies also may arise from nonfunctional portions of the muscle, e.g., in damaged regions of the muscle adjacent to the clamps which hold the muscle to the recording apparatus. Other artifactual elasticities, such as those due to elasticities in the recording apparatus and asynchrony of contraction in the muscle after incomplete stimulation, can usually be avoided by careful experimental design. Even when all of these elasticities are eliminated or compensated for, *a significant elasticity remains that appears to be located in the cross-bridges of the myofilaments themselves.* If muscle elasticity were located at the cross-bridges, this elasticity would behave quite differently from a passive elasticity that was separate from the contractile element. Thus an elasticity which transmits force from the cross-bridges to the ends of the muscles would not be constant but would change as the number of active cross-bridges varies with time or muscle length (see below). Muscle stiffness would therefore be expected to vary with the number of active cross-bridges, increasing, for example, as force rises at the onset of contraction. There is now considerable experimental evidence that this is the case, and that much of the series elasticity arises at the cross-bridges.

ACTIVE STATE

Because of the absorption of mechanical energy by the series elasticity, the mechanical events of the twitch do not accurately reflect the state of activity in the contractile element of the muscle. For this reason experimental techniques have been developed to allow more precise analyses of the mechanical properties of the contractile element during the twitch. These experiments use sudden changes in muscle length to circumvent the effects of the series elasticity.

Quick-Stretch Experiment

If the tension developed by the contractile elements fails to reach its maximum because of extension of the series elasticity, one way to compensate for this damping effect would be to eliminate the elasticity early in the contraction. In practical terms this can be achieved when a sudden stretch is applied to the muscle during the latent period. Such a "quick stretch," achieved by "pulling out" the series elasticity, permits the full extent of the potential for tension development by the contractile element to become apparent at the ends of the muscle. Analysis of quick-stretch experiments therefore is based on the postulate that in the stretched muscle a steady state is quickly reached in which the total tension at the ends of the muscle, the tension developed by the contractile element, and the tension on the series elasticity all become equalized at a level that approaches the maximal tension that can be generated by the contractile element.

The effects of stretches to three different lengths are shown in Fig. 8.5. When

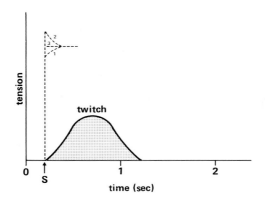

FIG. 8.5. Measurement of the active state by application of quick stretches to a skeletal muscle contracting under isometric conditions. *Solid line:* Twitch, as shown in Fig. 8.3. *Dashed lines:* 1, The muscle is quickly stretched a short distance immediately after stimulation. Tension continues to develop slowly after the stretch as the tension at the end of the quick stretch is less than that produced by the contractile element. 2, The muscle is quickly stretched a long distance immediately after stimulation. Tension declines slowly after the stretch as the tension at the end of the quick stretch exceeds that developed by the contractile element. 3, The muscle is quickly stretched immediately after stimulation to a length where the tension maintains a plateau equal to that developed by the contractile element. This tension is the "active state intensity."

FIG. 8.6. Time course of active state intensity in a skeletal muscle contracting under isometric conditions. The tension developed by the contractile element (active state intensity) greatly exceeds that which appears at the ends of the muscle during an isometric twitch because in the twitch a significant amount of energy is absorbed by the series elasticity. This energy is returned as tension during the latter period of the twitch, when twitch tension exceeds the active state intensity.

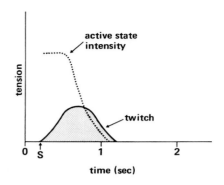

the muscle is stretched immediately after stimulation, the tension manifest at the ends of the muscle depends on the length to which the muscle is stretched. In the case of a short stretch, in which the tension on the series elasticity fails to reach the maximal tension that can be developed by the contractile element, muscle tension rises as the series elasticity is stretched further by the contractile element (curve 1, Fig. 8.5). On the other hand, if a quick stretch to a longer length causes muscle tension to exceed the maximum that can be developed by the contractile proteins, the muscle lengthens until tension falls to a level that can be maintained by the contractile element (curve 2, Fig. 8.5). When a stretch is applied that brings muscle tension to a level equal to that developed by the contractile element, the muscle neither lengthens nor shortens. Instead, tension remains at a relatively stable level during the initial phases of the contraction (curve 3, Fig. 8.5). This level of tension, measured as the force the muscle can just hold without lengthening or shortening, is called the *intensity of the active state*. This can be understood most simply as the tension that would be developed by the undamped contractile element, were it to be held at constant length.

It is apparent that the active state in skeletal muscle develops very rapidly, although its manifestation as twitch tension is both attenuated and delayed because extension of the series elasticity absorbs much of this mechanical energy during the brief period of activity in the twitch. The finding that maximum active state intensity is rapid in onset agrees with the finding that "initial" heat is

FIG. 8.7. Composite drawing showing the relation of tetanic tension (*dashed line;* see also Fig. 8.4) and the active state intensity (*dotted line;* see also Fig. 8.6). By maintaining the contractile element in a constant state of activity, the train of stimuli that produces the tetanic contraction allows the full intensity of the active state to appear at the ends of the muscle.

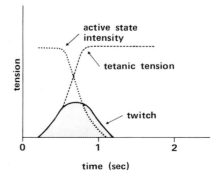

produced mainly in the early stages of the mechanical response (Chapter 5).

The time course of the intensity of the active state can be determined by applying quick stretches during the upstroke of the twitch (Fig. 8.6). As already shown, the capacity to develop maximal active state tension occurs well before the time that twitch tension reaches its peak.

The concept of the active state explains the greater tension developed during a tetanus than during a twitch (Fig. 8.7). The maximum intensity of the active state in a twitch has been shown by quick-stretch experiments to be essentially the same as that developed during a tetanus. Thus the high level of tetanic tension can be seen to reflect the true intensity of the active state when the series of stimuli that produces a tetanic contraction prevents the active state from declining from its maximum intensity.

Quick-Release Experiment

We have already seen that the contractile state of a muscle depends on at least two properties of the contractile proteins (Chapter 7). One of these properties,

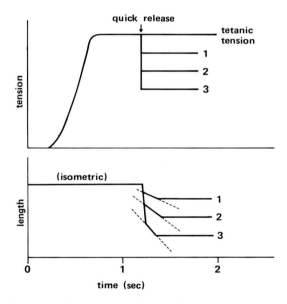

FIG. 8.8. Quick releases to shorter muscle lengths during the maintenance of tension by a skeletal muscle contracting under isometric conditions. **Top:** The tension developed during a tetanic contraction (Fig. 8.4) abruptly falls when the muscle, by quick releases, is allowed to shorten to a relatively longer length (1), a moderate length (2), or a relatively short length (3). **Bottom:** The quick releases allow the muscle to shorten to the new lengths. The initial, rapid length changes represent shortening of the series elasticity. Subsequent rates of shortening, to which tangents are drawn *(dashed lines)*, represent shortening rates of the contractile element at the levels of tension shown in the top diagram. Shortening of the contractile element is more rapid when the quick release is to a shorter length, i.e., when the contractile element shortens at a lower tension.

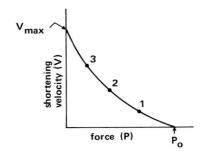

FIG. 8.9. Force-velocity curve constructed from the quick-release experiment shown in Fig. 8.8. The forces at points 1, 2, and 3 are the tensions achieved after the quick releases to different lengths (Fig. 8.8, top). Shortening velocities are the rates of the length change shown by the dashed lines in the bottom part of Fig. 8.8. This hyperbolic curve is similar to that shown in Fig. 5.14.

which is manifest as the *ability to generate tension,* can be measured by quick-stretch experiments which eliminate the absorption of tension by the series elasticity (see above). This type of experiment, however, does not provide information as to the maximal speed at which the contractile element is able to shorten. The latter property, which is an index of the *energy-turnover rate,* can be evaluated in "quick-release" experiments in which an isometrically contracting muscle is allowed to shorten suddenly against a series of light loads. When tension is abruptly reduced, the muscle shortens (Fig. 8.8). As the new load is reduced (*1, 2,* and *3,* Fig. 8.8, going from heaviest to lightest), muscle length decreases. The decrease is initially very rapid and reflects shortening of the series elasticity. Subsequently the muscle shortens at a slower rate, determined by the load to which the muscle is released (dashed lines drawn tangentially to the second phase of shortening in Fig. 8.8). This slower phase of shortening, which becomes more rapid as quick releases are made to progressively lighter loads (Fig. 8.8), is a measure of the shortening velocity of the contractile element. When the relationship between this shortening velocity and the load against which the muscle shortens after a quick release is plotted, the familiar hyperbolic force-velocity curve is obtained (Fig. 8.9; see also Fig. 5.14). Thus the quick-release experiment provides a means to evaluate both the maximal number of active force-generating sites and the maximal rate of turnover of actin-myosin interactions (Chapters 9 and 11).

LENGTH-TENSION RELATIONSHIP

The dependence of tetanic tension on muscle length, the length-tension relationship, has been recognized for over a century. In modern terms this relationship states that the intensity of the active state is maximal at a muscle length (l_0) which is approximately that of the muscle in the body, declining at both longer and shorter lengths. With the acceptance of the sliding filament hypothesis of muscular contraction (Chapter 1), it became possible to explain at least part of this relationship in skeletal muscle. These explanations, which were based on the classic studies of Gordon, A. F. Huxley, and Julian, appeared initially to provide a basis for understanding also the length-tension relationship in the heart.

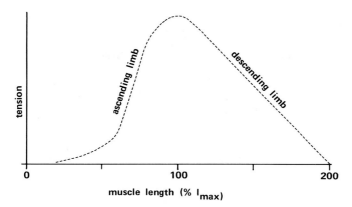

FIG. 8.10. Length-tension curve for a whole muscle, which defines the tension developed when the muscle contracts isometrically during tetanic contractions at different rest lengths. Muscle length is expressed as percent of l_{max}, which is defined as that rest length at which developed tension is maximal. Curves of this sort are conventionally scanned from left to right; thus the ascending limb is to the left, where tension rises with increasing muscle length, and the descending limb is to the right, where tension declines with increasing muscle length.

During the past few years, however, a growing body of evidence has come to demonstrate that this "classic mechanism" fails to explain a large number of important observations in cardiac muscle. The classic mechanism for the length-tension relationship is described in the following pages. This mechanism is then utilized as a starting point for a description of recent findings that provide a more accurate view of the molecular basis of the length-tension curve in cardiac muscle.

Classic Mechanism

As originally shown in whole skeletal muscles, the curve relating active tension developed in a tetanic contraction to muscle length was relatively broad (Fig. 8.10). With the development of techniques that permit the length-tension relationship to be recorded at the level of a small group of sarcomeres, it became apparent that the developed tension relationship reflected, at least in part, length-dependent changes in the positions of the thick and thin filaments of the sarcomere. The resulting sarcomere length-tension curve was narrower along the length axis than was the curve for the whole muscle (Fig. 8.11). The relatively narrower sarcomere length-tension curve reflects the elimination of inhomogeneities that in the whole muscle produce significant variations in sarcomere length at long and short muscle lengths.

At the longer muscle lengths, where not all sarcomeres of a whole muscle are equally stretched, the decline in tension due to increased sarcomere length becomes masked by the greater tension developed by the relatively shorter sarcomeres (Fig. 8.11, right). A similar deviation between the sarcomere length-tension curve and that for the whole muscle is seen also at shorter lengths (Fig.

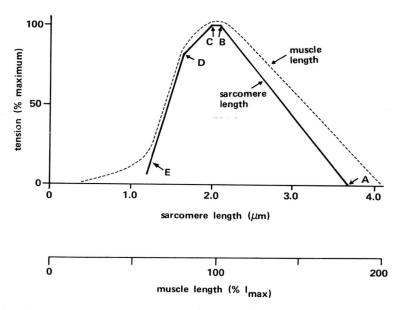

FIG. 8.11. Length-tension curve for a small group of sarcomeres *(solid line)* compared with that for the whole muscle shown in Fig. 8.10 *(dashed line)*. Sarcomere length is shown as the upper abscissa. At a sarcomere length of 3.65 μm, no tension is developed (A). Tension becomes maximal as the sarcomere shortens to a length of approximately 2.2 μm (B). As the sarcomere length decreases below approximately 2.0 μm (C), tension begins to decline with further shortening. At lengths below approximately 1.65 μm (D), tension declines more rapidly with extreme sarcomere shortening (E).

8.11, left). Here inhomogeneities in sarcomere length allow some sarcomeres in the muscle to remain less shortened and so better able to develop tension.

The classic mechanism for the sarcomere length-tension curve is best understood by beginning at the point at the right of the "descending limb" of the sarcomere length-tension curve (i.e., *B* to *A*, Fig. 8.11), where developed tension is zero. Examination of sarcomere structure at this point (*A*, Fig. 8.11), which in the frog semitendinous muscle corresponds to a sarcomere length of 3.65 μm, shows that at this length there is no overlap between the thick filaments

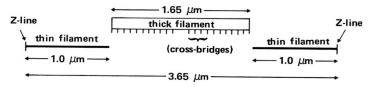

FIG. 8.12. Portion of a single sarcomere at a length of 3.65 μm (A, Fig. 8.11). At this sarcomere length there is no overlap between the thick filament *(above)* and the thin filaments *(below)*, so that no interactions are possible between the myosin cross-bridges and actin.

FIG. 8.13. Portion of a sarcomere at a length of 2.2 μm (*B*, Fig. 8.11). All myosin cross-bridges are adjacent to the thin filaments, so the number of potential interactions between the contractile proteins is maximal.

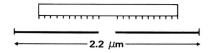

2.2 μm

(length = 1.65 μm) and the two thin filaments of the sarcomere (length = 2 × 1.0 μm) (Fig. 8.12). Note from Fig. 8.12 that the absence of overlap between the thick and thin filaments at these long sarcomere lengths allows no potential for interaction between the myosin cross-bridges and actin, and therefore no tension can be developed.

As sarcomere length is reduced (moving from *A* to *B* in Fig. 8.11), tension increases, reaching a maximum at a sarcomere length of approximately 2.2 μm (*B*, Fig. 8.11). At this sarcomere length, l_{max}, all of the myosin cross-bridges are adjacent to one of the two thin filaments of the sarcomere (Fig. 8.13). A small gap remains between the ends of the thin filaments, but this space of approximately 0.20 μm corresponds to a "bare" area in the center of the thick filament that is devoid of cross-bridges (see also Fig. 6.3).

Reduction in sarcomere length from 2.2 μm to approximately 2.0 μm (*B* to *C*, Fig. 8.11) is associated with no change in active tension. This plateau in the sarcomere length-tension curve probably occurs because as the thin filaments lose their apposition to cross-bridges in the region at the center of the sarcomere, where the thick filament lacks cross-bridges, the peripheral portions of the thin filaments become able to interact with cross-bridges at the ends of the thick filament (Fig. 8.14). For this reason sarcomere shortening from 2.2 to 2.0 μm is associated with neither an increase nor a decrease in the number of potential interactions between thick and thin filaments.

The decline in tension that occurs as the sarcomere shortens at lengths less than 1.9–2.0 μm (*C*, Fig. 8.11) cannot be fully explained ultrastructurally. It was initially postulated that at short sarcomere lengths the thin filament from the opposite half of the sarcomere, by passing beside a region of the thick filament in which the polarity of the cross-bridges did not allow interactions with the thin filament, might interfere with the ability to develop tension (Fig. 8.15).

Recently, however, it has been postulated that the degree of activation of the contractile proteins is reduced at short sarcomere lengths. This explanation is based on a number of findings, among which is evidence that at short rest lengths the core of each muscle fiber is not fully activated. The mechanism responsible for this phenomenon can be understood if it is remembered that at short sarcomere lengths muscle diameter increases because muscle volume remains essentially constant. As a result, muscle shortening causes the distance from the cell

FIG. 8.14. Portion of a sarcomere at a length of 2.0 μm (*C*, Fig. 8.11). All myosin cross-bridges remain in a position to interact with the thin filaments.

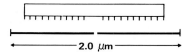

2.0 μm

FIG. 8.15. Portion of a sarcomere at a length of 1.7 μm (segment *D–C*, Fig. 8.11). The central ends of the thin filaments have crossed in the middle of the sarcomere ("double overlap"), but a direct causal relationship between this position of the myofilaments and the loss of tension at shorter sarcomere lengths has not convincingly explained the ascending limb of the length-tension curve.

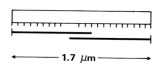

surface to the core of each muscle fiber to increase. The way in which these changes alter the effectiveness of the activation process is discussed later in this chapter.

The abrupt decline in tension seen when sarcomere length becomes extremely short, below 1.65 μm, is probably due to both reduced activation of the contractile proteins and deformations of the myofilaments. The length of the thick filament is approximately 1.65 μm, so that sarcomere lengths less than 1.65 μm can be reached only when the thick filament "crumples" (Fig. 8.16). Such deformations are apparent microscopically as "contraction bands," which appear at the ends of the thick filaments when there is extreme sarcomere shortening.

Physiologically, most skeletal muscles probably operate on the ascending limb of their length-tension curves (*D* to *C,* Fig. 8.11). This follows from the fact that at rest most muscles are at a length that corresponds to the peak of their length-tension curve (l_0, Fig. 8.10), so that shortening brings sarcomere length into the range when tension decreases as the muscle shortens. This response, in which muscle tension increases as the preload on the muscle becomes greater (e.g., *D* to *C,* Fig. 8.11), is of special significance in the heart (Chapter 13).

Length-Tension Relationship in Cardiac Muscle

A number of observations were made during the past decade that make it extremely unlikely that the classic mechanism for the length-tension relationship can explain many important features of this relationship. This is especially true in the heart, in which sarcomere lengths are normally in the shorter range where the length dependence of tension is least well understood. Furthermore, under

FIG. 8.16. Portion of a sarcomere at a length of 1.6 μm (segment *D–E,* Fig. 8.11). At this sarcomere length the Z-lines (vertical lines at the peripheral ends of the thin filaments) encroach on the ends of thick filaments. This causes the latter to "crumple," giving rise to contraction bands at the periphery of the A-band. These deformations contribute to the precipitous fall of tension as the sarcomere shortens further on this unphysiological portion of the sarcomere length-tension curve.

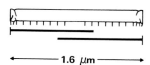

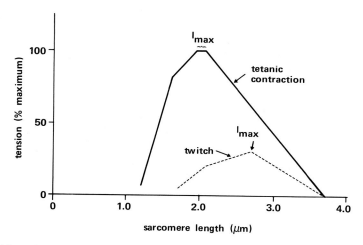

FIG. 8.17. Length-tension curve for a small number of sarcomeres measured during an isometric tetanic contraction *(solid line)* and an isometric twitch *(dashed line).* Not only is tension less during the twitch, but the maximum of the length-tension curve (l_{max}) of the twitch is shifted to a longer sarcomere length.

these conditions (i.e., at shorter sarcomere lengths) time-dependent variations in the degree of activator release and removal introduce a further mechanism for variation in tension. These time-dependent factors are of much greater importance in the twitch-like contractions of the heart than in tetanized skeletal muscle. The difficulties in understanding the basis for the length-tension curve of cardiac muscle thus arise partly from the time-dependent variations in activation in cardiac muscle and the fact that the myocardium functions on the ascending limb of the sarcomere length-tension curve. Furthermore, the degree of activation of the contractile proteins of the heart is normally less than that which would cause maximum tension to be generated and is variable.

The importance of time-dependent variations in the degree of activation is readily appreciated in skeletal muscle when the length-tension diagrams of twitches are compared to those of tetanic contractions. It has been known for more than 50 years that the length of a skeletal muscle at which tension is maximal (l_{max}) is greater during a twitch than during a tetanic contraction. This phenomenon, which reflects both length- and time-dependent factors governing the availability of Ca^{2+} for binding to troponin, was recently carefully studied by Close, who defined one way by which variations in the duration of activation release can alter the shape of the length-tension relationship. As shown in Fig. 8.17, the shapes of these curves are quite different in the twitch than in a sustained tetanus, and l_{max} is greater in the twitch.

The different length-tension relationships shown in Fig. 8.17 can be explained in terms of time-dependent variations in the degree of activation of the contractile proteins. Alterations in muscle geometry probably influence the extent to which the contractile proteins are activated in that the ability of the sarcoplasmic reticulum to deliver enough activator Ca^{2+} for binding to all of the Ca^{2+}-binding sites on troponin (Chapter 9) is reduced at shorter sarcomere lengths. Altered balances between activator release and removal are seen even during a sustained tetanus where the active state is prolonged. When the duration of the active state is shortened in addition, as in a twitch, time-dependent factors that limit Ca^{2+} release become significant. Thus the decline in twitch tension at short sarcomere lengths (Fig. 8.17) may be explained if the brief duration of activation in the twitch reduces the ability of the sarcoplasmic reticulum to release enough Ca^{2+} to saturate the Ca^{2+}-binding sites of troponin, due possibly to the increased cross section that occurs at short sarcomere lengths. An interplay between the classic and time-dependent mechanisms for the length-tension relationship can explain the rightward shift of l_{max} that is seen when the twitch is compared to the tetanus (Fig. 8.17). As the muscle shortens, its cross-sectional area increases, so the distance through which the activation processes must be transmitted increases. This increase in cross-sectional diameter seems to impair the ability of the action potential to initiate Ca^{2+} release to the contractile proteins, especially in the core of the fiber. As a result, the ability of the sarcomeres in the center of a muscle fiber to develop tension becomes disproportionately reduced at short sarcomere lengths when the twitch is compared to a tetanic contraction.

Additional explanations for the impediment to activation in the muscle operating at short sarcomere lengths are possible. For example, as the muscle fibers become shorter and thicker, the T-tubules may narrow, elongate, or both, thereby interfering with "communication" between the cell surface and its core. Other possible explanations for the loss of activation at shorter sarcomere lengths include a change in the Ca^{2+} sensitivity of the contractile proteins caused by altered muscle length and an influence of muscle geometry on the ability of the sarcoplasmic reticulum to maintain a high intracellular Ca^{2+} concentration during activity. While there is still no clear explanation for the apparent length dependence of the activation process and time dependence of the length-tension relationship, it is now obvious that the classic mechanism for the length-tension relationship in skeletal muscle is inadequate to account for these phenomena as they occur in twitch-like contractions which take place at short sarcomere lengths in the heart.

CARDIAC MECHANICS

The relatively straightforward nature of the time- and length-dependent features of skeletal muscle mechanics are in marked contrast to the situation in the heart. In keeping with the general rule that all aspects of the contractile process are more complex in cardiac than in skeletal muscle, the field of cardiac mechanics remains in a state of confusion and contradiction. In the evaluation of skeletal muscle mechanics, it is possible to analyze the contractile characteristics of muscles in which the fibers parallel each other and where the active state is extremely rapid in onset. More importantly, it is possible to tetanize these skeletal muscles so that force-velocity, heat, and length measurements can be made in the presence of a constant level of the active state. In the myocardium, as was already indicated, the active state appears to be slow in onset and the muscle cannot ordinarily be tetanized, so that analyses of mechanical properties must be attempted in the face of time-dependent changes in contractile conditions. In addition, the elasticity and nonparallel arrangement of the fibers in cardiac muscle preclude the attainment of true isometric conditions, so mechanical studies of the myocardium are also complicated by length-dependent changes in contractile conditions. Finally, the fact that the length-dependent basis for changes in tension remain poorly understood virtually rules out the precise evaluation of the forces and velocities that are generated by the contractile elements of the myocardium.

The fundamental differences between the mechanical properties of cardiac and skeletal muscle can be clearly seen in an analysis by Brady, who studied the effects of quick stretch. As shown in Fig. 8.5, sudden stretching of a skeletal muscle reveals the rapid onset of the active state in the contractile element, which manifests as a plateau of tension early in the course of the twitch. In cardiac muscle, where the contractile event lasts several hundred milliseconds as opposed to the much shorter twitch of a skeletal muscle, no such plateau is seen after a quick stretch (Fig. 8.18). Thus an early quick stretch (*A*, Fig. 8.18) that initially exceeds the ability of the muscle to hold tension (as evidenced by the fall in tension immediately after the stretch) is not followed by a plateau of tension. Instead, tension slowly rises, this increase closely following the time course of the contraction in the unstretched muscle. A quick stretch to a greater length

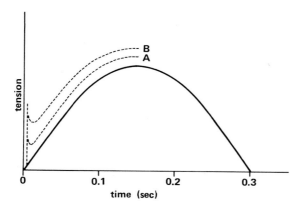

FIG. 8.18. Results of a quick-stretch experiment in cardiac muscle (cf. Fig. 8.5). *Solid line,* normal isometric contraction. *Dashed lines,* tension developed after quick stretches to two different lengths (B is stretched to a longer length than A). Even though the quick stretches cause the muscle initially to reach a length that causes total tension to exceed that developed by the contractile element—as evidenced by a transient fall in tension—total tension resumes its rise later. No plateau of tension is seen.

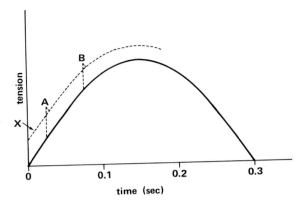

FIG. 8.19. Results of a quick-stretch experiment in cardiac muscle where a quick stretch is applied at two times after stimulation (A and B). Although the tension developed in each stretch initially exceeds that developed by the contractile element—as evidenced by a transient fall in tension—total tension resumes its rise so that both curves become superimposed by the time tension reaches its peak. This increment in tension is the same when the muscle is stretched to the same increased length prior to stimulation (X).

(*B*, Fig. 8.18) is followed by an even greater initial drop in tension before its subsequent slow rise.

The time course of tension development in cardiac muscle subsequent to a quick stretch is essentially independent of the time at which stretch is applied (Fig. 8.19). Thus the curves following two stretches to the same length (*A* and *B*, Fig. 8.19) are virtually superimposable. In fact, the increased tension following these quick stretches is not due primarily to the elimination of a damping effect of the series elasticity, as can be shown when the muscle is stretched to the same final length *before* stimulation (X, Fig. 8.19). That the increased tension following the quick stretches (*A* and *B*, Fig. 8.19) is the same as that observed when muscle length is increased by the same amount prior to stimulation means that the added tension following the stretches (dotted lines, Figs. 8.18 and 8.19) is due mainly to the expression of the length-tension relationship.

That the slow development of tension in cardiac contraction is largely independent of damping effects of the series elasticity indicates that in the myocardium, unlike skeletal muscle, the active state is slow in onset and thus is *time-dependent*. This interpretation is supported by the finding that heat liberation at the start of contraction in cardiac muscle is slower than in skeletal muscle.

That the onset of the active state is slower in cardiac than in skeletal muscle is probably due to the slow arrival of Ca^{2+} at the region of the cell occupied by the myofilaments. This in turn reflects a more limited amount of Ca^{2+} available for cardiac excitation-contraction coupling, which contrasts with the saturating amounts of calcium normally released during this process in skeletal muscle, as well as a more complex mechanism of excitation-contraction coupling in the myocardium. The complexity and variability of this Ca^{2+}-release mechanism provides the basis of one mechanism for the regulation of myocardial contractility (as becomes apparent in subsequent chapters).

Another distinguishing feature of cardiac muscle that complicates the analysis of cardiac mechanics is the much higher resting tension of heart muscle. In contrast to skeletal muscle, in which resting tension is practically zero at muscle lengths below l_0, cardiac muscle has a high resting tension at all lengths along the resting length-tension curve (Fig. 8.20). Although the relationships between sarcomere length and developed tension are similar in cardiac and skeletal muscle, the curve relating muscle length to developed tension in the myocardium is superimposed on high levels of resting tension. Stated another way, the heart has a very steep resting length-tension curve owing to the fact that it has a much lower resting compliance than skeletal muscle. While the basis for this resting stiffness is not known, it is of considerable functional significance since at normal levels of resting tension the myocardium always functions on the ascending limb of its active length-tension relationship. In other words, it is not possible to pull the myocardial cell onto the descending limb of its sarcomere length-tension curve unless resting tension becomes abnormally high (Chapter 13).

One of the very promising findings in some of the early studies of cardiac mechanics was that V_{max} appeared to be independent of initial fiber length. This early finding indicated that accurate measurements of V_{max} could provide an index of the length-independent contractile properties of cardiac muscle. These length-independent properties of the contractile process reflect the intrinsic ability of

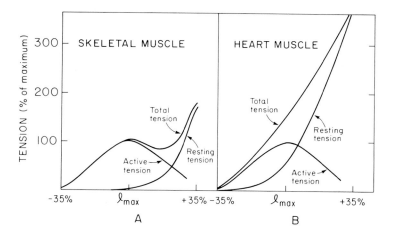

FIG. 8.20. Comparison of total and active length-tension curves in skeletal (A) and cardiac (B) muscle allowed to contract under isometric conditions. Active tension, which is the tension developed during contraction, equals total tension after stimulation minus the tension recorded in the resting muscle prior to stimulation. Although the active length-tension curves are similar for the two muscle types, the resting tension in cardiac muscle is much higher and, unlike skeletal muscle, is significant at lengths below l_{max}. (Modified from Jewell: *The Physiological Basis of Starling's Law of the Heart,* 1974. Ciba Foundation Symposium, 24. Elsevier, Amsterdam.)

the heart to perform mechanical work at any given initial muscle length, the so-called level of "myocardial contractility" (Chapters 10–13). Unfortunately the promise of the early studies of cardiac mechanics has not been fulfilled in that recent investigations show significant length-dependence of V_{max}, which decreases with decreasing initial length.

The complexities of interpreting the mechanical expression of the properties of the interactions between the cardiac contractile proteins, many of which were described above, reduce our ability to utilize studies of cardiac mechanics to obtain precise measurements of changes in myocardial contractility. This is especially unfortunate in light of the fact that myocardial contractility is controlled largely by changes in the biochemical mechanisms within the cardiac muscle cell that are responsible for contraction.

BIBLIOGRAPHY

Brady, A. J. (1965): Time and displacement dependence of cardiac contractility: Problems in defining the active state and force-velocity relations. *Fed. Proc.,* 24:1410–1420.

Davson, H. (1964): *A Textbook of General Physiology,* Chap. XXI. Little, Brown, Boston.

Gordon, A. M., Huxley, A. F., and Julian, F. G. (1966): The variation in isometric tension with sarcomere length in vertebrate muscle fibers. *J. Physiol. (Lond.),* 184:170–192.

Hill, A. V. (1949): The abrupt transition from rest to activity in muscle. *Proc. R. Soc. (Lond.)* [*Biol.*], 136:399–420.

Porter, R., and Fitzsimons, D. W., editors (1974): *The Physiological Basis of Starling's Law of the Heart.* Ciba Foundation Symposium. Associated Scientific Publishers, Amsterdam/New York.

Sonnenblick, E. H. (1965): Determinants of active state in heart muscle: Force, velocity, instantaneous muscle length, time. *Fed. Proc.,* 24:1396–1409.

9

Excitation-Contraction Coupling

Cardiac systole, like contraction in skeletal muscle, is set into motion by a series of steps that begins when the action potential depolarizes the sarcolemma. The final step in this series is the delivery of Ca^{2+} to bind to troponin C, the Ca^{2+} receptor of the cardiac contractile proteins (Chapter 6). Knowledge of this complex process, called excitation-contraction coupling, remains spotty. Much like the early explorers' maps of the Western Hemisphere, some areas of our present knowledge of excitation-contraction coupling can be clearly and accurately outlined. Other regions, however, are only poorly defined, in many cases being understood only from limited and incomplete data. Yet a broad outline of the structure-function relations of this process can now be drawn (Table 9.1) and related to knowledge of the ultrastructure of the myocardial cell (Fig. 9.1).

The complex reactions described in this chapter may at first sight seem to represent an unreasonably elaborate means for delivery of Ca^{2+} to troponin. Thus the level of ionized calcium in the extracellular fluid is in the range of 1 mM whereas the level of Ca^{2+} needed to saturate troponin is much less (approximately 10 μM). In view of this high concentration gradient for Ca^{2+} across the sarcolemma, it is reasonable to ask why it is necessary to have such a complex system for Ca^{2+} delivery. The answer to this question lies primarily in the relative slowness of diffusion, the simplest mechanism by which Ca^{2+} entering the cell would ultimately reach the contractile proteins. The limitations of diffusion are especially true in mammalian skeletal muscle. Here the large fiber size and great rapidity of tension development preclude a significant role for diffusion of calcium to the interior of the fiber in activating the contractile proteins.

In order to explain the rapid onset of contraction in large, rapidly contracting skeletal muscles, it is necessary to postulate the existence of an intracellular store from which activator Ca^{2+} can reach its binding site on troponin C by a short diffusion path. In cardiac muscle, where the cells are smaller and the onset of contraction is slower, this requirement for internal stores of activator Ca^{2+} is less absolute. Indeed the sarcoplasmic reticulum is very poorly developed in some fetal hearts and in the hearts of many amphibians. Adult mammalian cardiac muscle generally contains an extensive sarcoplasmic reticulum, although in the human myocardium this membrane system is less well developed than in skeletal muscle. For this reason it is theoretically possible for the Ca^{2+} which enters the myocardium from the extracellular fluid to participate in activating the contractile proteins of the heart. However, most of the Ca^{2+} that enters the cell during systole probably enters an intracellular store rather than becoming immediately available for binding to troponin C (Chapter 11).

TABLE 9.1. *Structural and functional basis for cardiac excitation-contraction coupling*

Structure	Function
Sarcolemma	Propagation of action potential; control of Ca^{2+} fluxes across the sarcolemma
Transverse tubular system	Transmission of action potential to interior of cell; control of Ca^{2+} fluxes
Sarcoplasmic reticulum	Release of Ca^{2+} to, and removal of Ca^{2+} from, troponin C; storage of Ca^{2+}
Subsarcolemmal cisternae	? Activation site at which Ca^{2+} release is initiated at the start of systole
Sarcotubular network	? Relaxation site at which Ca^{2+} is accumulated to terminate systole
Troponin C	Ca^{2+} receptor of the contractile proteins (Chapter 6)

The changing mechanical response of the heart to a variety of drugs and hormones, and the decline in tension developed by the myocardium when it is stimulated at very high rates of contraction, provides further evidence for the existence of an internal store of Ca^{2+}. Such changes in myocardial contractility,

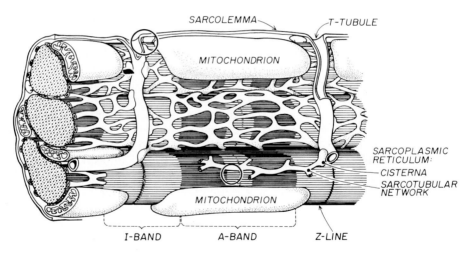

FIG. 9.1. Ultrastructure of the working myocardial cell. Contractile proteins are arranged in a regular array of thick and thin filaments (seen in cross section at the left). The A-band represents the region of the sarcomere occupied by the thick filaments into which thin filaments extend from either side. The I-band is the region of the sarcomere occupied only by thin filaments; these extend toward the center of the sarcomere from the Z-lines, which bisect each I-band. The sarcoplasmic reticulum, a membrane network that surrounds the contractile proteins, consists of the sarcotubular network at the center of the sarcomere and the cisternae, which abut on the t-tubules and the sarcolemma. The transverse tubular system (t-tubule) is lined by a membrane that extends from the sarcolemma and carries the extracellular space into the myocardial cell. Mitochondria are shown in the central sarcomere and in cross section at the left side of the figure. (From Katz: *N. Engl. J. Med.*, 293:1184, 1975.)

which are detailed in Chapter 11, are best understood by postulating a variable store of activator calcium within the myocardium. The filling of this calcium store from the extracellular fluid and its emptying to deliver Ca^{2+} to the contractile proteins are modulated by a complex interacting series of mechanisms that begins with excitation of the sarcolemma and ends when Ca^{2+} is released for binding to troponin. The variable mechanical behavior of cardiac muscle therefore arises through the operation of a control system which acts by way of this complex mechanism of excitation-contraction coupling.

SARCOLEMMA

It is well established that the cardiac contraction is initiated when an action potential depolarizes the sarcolemma. The exact nature of the mechanism by which this depolarization triggers contraction, however, remains unknown. A complex series of changes in ionic currents accompanies the cardiac action potential (Chapter 14), any of which could represent the stimulus that initiates the succeeding steps in the process of excitation-contraction. These ionic currents are determined largely by the permeability properties of the cardiac sarcolemma.

During diastole the sarcolemma is highly permeable to potassium but is impermeable to both sodium and calcium. The upstroke of the action potential (i.e., the initial phase of rapid depolarization) is caused by a fast inward current carried by sodium ions. At this time potassium permeability decreases sharply. The upstroke of the action potential ends when the membrane again becomes impermeable to sodium. The cardiac action potential now exhibits a slow inward current that is due mainly to the influx of calcium. Toward the end of the cardiac action potential, the sarcolemma once again becomes impermeable to calcium whereas potassium permeability rises to its high diastolic level. These complex ionic changes during the cardiac action potential, which are discussed more fully in Chapter 14, include a number of possible ionic mechanisms that could lead eventually to the release of Ca^{2+} in the subsequent steps of excitation-contraction coupling.

Sodium Pump

In addition to its role in controlling the ion fluxes which generate the action potential, the sarcolemma contains a number of ion transport systems which maintain cellular composition. One of these is the sodium pump.

A small amount of sodium enters the cell during depolarization, and to restore resting membrane potential a small amount of potassium is lost from the cell at the end of systole (Chapter 14). Although the amounts of this net exchange of sodium for potassium are small, some mechanism must exist for restoring cell composition at the end of each systole. This task is accomplished by the sodium pump, in which the exchange of sodium for potassium is accomplished by an

ATP-dependent enzyme. Energy is needed because both sodium and potassium are moved against a concentration gradient.

There is considerable evidence that the sites of this pump which are activated by sodium face the inside of the cell whereas those which require potassium are at the outer surface of the sarcolemma. In this way the "polarity" of this pump is such that sodium is carried from the inside of the cell to the extracellular fluid in exchange for potassium, which is brought into the cell.

It now appears that this pump is electrogenic in that three sodium ions are transported out of the cell in exchange for only two potassium ions:

$$3Na^+_i \longrightarrow 3Na^+_o \qquad\qquad (9.1)$$

$$\boxed{\text{pump}}$$

$$2K^+_i \longleftarrow 2K^+_o \qquad\qquad (9.2)$$

Thus the sodium pump generates an electrical potential by carrying a net positive charge out of the cell. The potential so generated is probably less than 10 mV (Chapter 14). The electrogenic nature of the sodium pump, which tends to make the interior of the cell more negative, thus contributes to the normal resting potential, in which the inside of the cell is negatively charged relative to the extracellular space (Chapter 14).

The identification of a membrane-bound ATPase that is activated when sodium and potassium are present together and which has the characteristics of the sodium pump led to the now generally accepted view that this Na-K-ATPase is in fact derived from the sodium pump. The reaction mechanism by which the Na-K-ATPase interacts with sodium and potassium is complex, and involves the formation of a phosphorylated intermediate that is in some ways reminiscent of that formed by the myosin cross-bridge. In the case of the Na-K-ATPase, where the physiological expression of the liberation of chemical energy from ATP is ion transport rather than motion, the specific steps in this reaction sequence reflect the formation and translocation of complexes between the enzyme and the cations it transports.

The initial step in the reactions of the Na-K-ATPase is the formation of an ATP-enzyme complex:

$$E + ATP \longrightarrow E \cdots ATP \qquad\qquad (9.3)$$

This step is then followed by conversion of the $E \cdots ATP$ complex to a phosphorylated enzyme, a reaction which requires Na^+ and Mg^{2+}:

$$E \cdots ATP \xrightarrow[Mg^{2+}]{Na^+} E_1 \sim P + ADP \qquad\qquad (9.4)$$

The breakdown of the phosphorylated enzyme, which takes place only in the presence of Mg^{2+}, has been suggested to require the conversion of the $E_1 \sim P$ complex to a lower energy state:

$$E_1 \sim P \xrightarrow[Mg^{2+}]{} E_2 - P \qquad\qquad (9.5)$$

This step, like that involving the conversion of the phosphorylated myosin complex from the "active complex" to the "rigor complex" [Eq. (7.8)], may be responsible for energy transduction, in this case translocation of Na^+. The eventual breakdown of the phosphorylated enzyme requires potassium:

$$E_2\text{-P} \xrightarrow{K^+} E + P_i \qquad (9.6)$$

The overall reaction requires both sodium and potassium ions—hence the designation Na-K-ATPase:

$$ATP \xrightarrow[Mg^{2+}]{Na^+ \text{ and } K^+} ADP + P_i \qquad (9.7)$$

Cardiac glycosides (e.g., digitalis) have a specific and highly important action to inhibit the Na-K-ATPase (Chapters 11 and 14). This effect is associated with inhibition of the potassium-dependent breakdown of the phosphorylated enzyme [Eq. (9.6)], so that the amount of E_2-P is increased in the digitalis-poisoned Na-K-ATPase. The finding that this inhibitory action can be partially reversed by increasing extracellular potassium concentration explains the pharmacologically significant effect of high serum potassium levels to overcome the toxic effects of the cardiac glycosides (Chapter 19). As both potassium and digitalis act only when presented to the outside of the cell, the inhibitory effects of the cardiac glycosides have been interpreted to reflect an inhibition of potassium loading by the sodium pump at the extracellular side of the sarcolemma.

TRANSVERSE TUBULAR SYSTEM

The transverse tubular system of the mammalian myocardium consists of narrow tubules that enter the cell at right angles to the axis of the cell. The lumens of these tubules open freely into the extracellular space. The content of the fluid within the transverse tubules cannot now be analyzed directly, but it is probable that, like the extracellular fluid, these structures contain a solution that is high in sodium and low in potassium.

In the heart the t-tubules differ from those of most mammalian skeletal muscles in several important respects. Unlike the corresponding structures in skeletal muscle, which penetrate the sarcomere at the level of the edges of the A-band (the junctions between A- and I-bands), the transverse tubular system of the mammalian myocardium runs alongside the Z-bands. In addition, these tubules can run longitudinally from one sarcomere to the next in the myocardium, thereby "connecting" adjacent sarcomeres.

A further difference between these muscle types lies in the larger diameter of the cardiac transverse tubular system. Like the sarcolemma, this system appears to participate in the transmission of a regenerative action potential. Propagation of the action potential into the t-tubules can thus facilitate the rapid activation of structures deep within the muscle cell. Because conduction of a regenerative action potential is much more rapid than the diffusion of an activator substance, the action potential passing down the t-tubules can accelerate activation of the cell interior.

One of the classic experiments in muscle physiology was the demonstration by A. F. Huxley and R. Taylor that localized (nonpropagated) depolarization of a skeletal muscle fiber at the point where the mouth of the transverse tubular system opens through the sarcolemma causes contraction only of the two half sarcomeres adjacent to the point of stimulation. This finding strongly suggests that the t-tubules transmit the signal of excitation-contraction coupling into the cell interior. Attempts to demonstrate similar localized responses to stimulation of cardiac muscle at the point of opening of the transverse tubular system through the sarcolemma, however, have failed. This finding probably reflects the longitudinal extensions of the transverse tubular system in the heart, which permits activation to spread into adjacent sarcomeres.

If the connections between the t-tubules and the surface of the cell are disrupted in a skeletal muscle (e.g., by increasing and then suddenly decreasing osmolarity), excitation-contraction coupling is significantly impaired. Changes in membrane capacitance that accompany such disruptive treatment have been interpreted to mean that this osmotic treatment disconnects the transverse tubular system from the cell surface, indicating that at least part of the propagated action potential is transmitted to the cell interior along the t-tubules.

SARCOPLASMIC RETICULUM

The sarcoplasmic reticulum, a system of tubules oriented in a longitudinal direction within the muscle cell (hence the now obsolete term longitudinal tubular system), can be divided into two regions: the subsarcolemmal cisternae and the sarcotubular network (Fig. 9.1). Subsarcolemmal cisternae are found both beneath the sarcolemma and alongside the transverse tubular system, while the sarcotubular network surrounds the contractile proteins in the center of the sarcomere. Largely on the basis of their anatomical characteristics and comparisons with analogous structures in mammalian and amphibian skeletal muscle, different functions are tentatively ascribed to these two portions of the sarcoplasmic reticulum.

Subsarcolemmal Cisternae

Where the sarcoplasmic reticulum comes in contact with the sarcolemma and the transverse tubular system, the sarcoplasmic reticulum often becomes a flattened saccular structure in which the membranes of the sarcoplasmic reticulum and transverse tubular system approach and parallel each other. These structures, which are formed by elements of each of these two membrane structures, are called *dyads* (Fig. 1.16). To some extent the term subsarcolemmal cisternae is a misnomer unless one considers the transverse tubular system to represent an extension of the sarcolemma.

The subsarcolemmal cisternae of cardiac muscle are similar to the *terminal cisternae* of skeletal muscle in several ways. The latter are large extensions of the sarcoplasmic reticulum that run along both sides of the transverse tubular system to make up the *triads* of skeletal muscle (two terminal cisternae from adjoining sarcomeres plus the transverse tubule). In the case of skeletal muscle, there is fairly convincing evidence that the terminal cisternae represent an excitation site at which calcium release for binding to troponin is initiated. This calcium is released in response to a signal originating from the action potential. In view of the overall similarity (although by no means absolute identity) between the triads of skeletal muscle and the dyads of the myocardium, it seems reasonable to postulate that the subsarcolemmal cisternae of cardiac muscle also represent a site at which calcium release begins.

Sarcotubular Network

In skeletal muscle there is evidence that the structure responsible for the removal of calcium from troponin, which thereby causes the muscle to relax, is the sarcotubular network—that portion of the sarcoplasmic reticulum which surrounds the sarcomere. These membranes must therefore have the ability to remove calcium from high-affinity Ca^{2+}-binding sites on troponin C, the capacity to retain a quantity of calcium which approximates that bound to the contractile proteins at the height of systole, and a calcium transport rate sufficiently rapid to account for the observed rates of relaxation in the intact muscle. These requirements can be met when membrane fractions enriched in fragmented sarcoplasmic reticulum are studied *in vitro*. In such preparations one can satisfy the three major requirements for a system which mediates excitation-contraction coupling: (a) the ability to retain a *quantity* of calcium sufficient to activate the troponin in cardiac muscle; (b) the ability to transport this calcium at a *rate* rapid enough to account for the observed rate of relaxation in the intact myocardium; and (c) sufficiently high *affinity* for Ca^{2+} to allow the sarcoplasmic reticulum to remove Ca^{2+} from its tight binding to troponin C. In addition to these requirements, it is also possible to identify mechanisms which may account for changes in the contractile properties of the heart that occur in response to physiological, pharmacological, and pathological influences (see below and Chapter 11).

MITOCHONDRIA

The well-known ability of mitochondria to take up large amounts of calcium has led some investigators to postulate a role for mitochondrial calcium transport and release in both cardiac excitation-contraction coupling and the regulation of myocardial contractility. There is little doubt, however, that the mitochondria are not *essential* for excitation-contraction coupling as this process is even more rapid in fast muscles that are almost devoid of mitochondria. Furthermore, the Ca^{2+} affinity of the mitochondrial calcium pump is low and the rate of calcium transport of physiological levels of intracellular Ca^{2+} very slow. It thus seems unlikely that these structures, whose primary function in the cardiac muscle cell is ATP regeneration, play an important role in regulating the calcium fluxes that are involved in excitation-contraction coupling. Mitochondrial calcium transport may, however, help to relax the myocardium when intracellular Ca^{2+} concentrations become extremely high. It is also possible that the ability of the mito-chondria to take up and store calcium can play an important role in certain pathological states, e.g., myocardial ischemia. It must be emphasized that many important questions regarding the role of the mitochondria in regulating the contractile function of the myocardium remain to be conclusively answered.

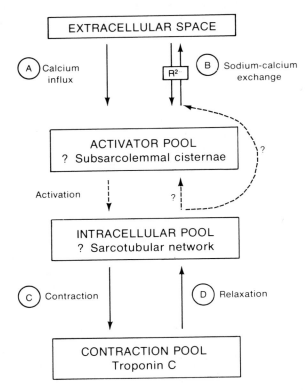

FIG. 9.2. Calcium fluxes that participate in cardiac excitation-contraction coupling represent calcium movements between the extracellular space, an activator pool that may be related to the subsarcolemmal cisternae, an intracellular pool that is probably within the sarcoplasmic reticulum, and a contraction pool that represents calcium bound to troponin. Calcium influx (A) is a "downhill" flux across the sarcolemma that occurs largely as the electrogenic slow inward current. A sodium-calcium exchange (B) can transport calcium in either direction across the sarcolemma but is involved mainly in the "uphill" transport of calcium out of the cell in a nonelectrogenic exchange for sodium, which moves down a concentration gradient into the cell. The intracellular pool that supplies calcium to the sodium-calcium exchange is not known but may be related to the sarcoplasmic reticulum. A relatively small calcium flux from the activator pool may trigger the release of a larger amount of calcium from the intracellular pool ("calcium-triggered calcium release") as shown by the arrow labeled "activation." Contraction (C) occurs when a large amount of calcium is released from the intracellular pool, most likely when an increase in the calcium permeability of the sarcoplasmic reticulum allows this ion to become available for binding to calcium-binding sites on troponin. Relaxation (D) occurs when the ATP-dependent calcium pump of the sarcoplasmic reticulum pumps calcium back into this intracellular membrane system. The resulting fall in cytosolic Ca^{2+} concentration causes calcium to become dissociated from its binding site on troponin.

CALCIUM FLUXES DURING EXCITATION-CONTRACTION COUPLING

A number of studies indicate that in both cardiac and skeletal muscle the site from which calcium is released to initiate contraction is not the same as that to which this cation is transported in the processes responsible for relaxation. In the heart, for example, contractility decreases at high rates of stimulation (the negative staircase; Chapter 11). This finding has been interpreted to indicate that calcium can be retained at a "relaxing site" (possibly the sarcotubular network) because of a relatively slow transfer of calcium to the "excitation site" (possibly the subsarcolemmal cisternae) from which it can be released to initiate further contractions. Additional evidence for this interpretation emerged from studies of the movement of labeled calcium in skeletal muscle. These studies indicate that immediately after the contraction ends calcium is found in that part of the sarcomere occupied by the sarcotubular network, whereas calcium subsequently migrates to the region of the sarcomere occupied by the terminal cisternae. On this basis it is proposed, although tentatively, that at least three pools of calcium are found within the myocardium (Fig. 9.2). One of these, the sarcotubular network, represents a relaxation site which terminates systole by removing Ca^{2+} from troponin C. This is accomplished by an ATP-dependent calcium pump, which has an affinity for Ca^{2+} sufficiently high to allow it to pump calcium into the interior of the sarcotubular network and thereby lower the cytosolic Ca^{2+} concentration to levels that cause Ca^{2+} to become dissociated from troponin C. The second calcium pool, the subsarcolemmal cisternae (which are analogous to the terminal cisternae of skeletal muscle), may represent an activator pool that initiates calcium release from the sarcotubular network, possibly in response to either a change in electrical potential across the sarcoplasmic reticulum or a calcium trigger. The third intracellular calcium pool, which contains calcium only during systole, is the Ca^{2+}-binding component of troponin. In view of the anatomical proximity between the subsarcolemmal cisternae and the extracellular space, it is proposed further that the calcium which enters the cell with the slow inward current (Chapter 14) is retained in or near the subsarcolemmal cisternae. This latter interpretation is somewhat speculative, however, and does not account for all features of the calcium exchanges that take place across the sarcolemma.

At least four calcium fluxes can participate in the control of myocardial contractility (Fig. 9.2; Table 9.2). Two of these take place across the sarcolemma, and the other two probably represent the movement of the calcium ion between intracellular pools.

Calcium Influx Across the Sarcolemma: Slow Inward Current

The small but significant quantity of calcium that enters the myocardial cell from the extracellular fluid gives rise to a "slow inward current" that occurs during cardiac systole, where it contributes to the plateau phase of the action

TABLE 9.2. *Calcium fluxes that can modulate myocardial contractility*

Calcium flux		Probably mediated by	Mechanism
From	To		
Extracellular space	Intracellular space	Sarcolemma	Slow inward current; electrogenic
Intracellular space	Extracellular space	Sarcolemma	Sodium-calcium exchange; nonelectrogenic
Intracellular pool	Troponin C	Sarcoplasmic reticulum	Passive diffusion
Troponin C	Intracellular pool	Sarcoplasmic reticulum	ATP-dependent calcium pump

potential (Chapter 14). In the mammalian myocardium this calcium is not immediately available for binding to the contractile proteins. Instead, the calcium that enters the myocardial cell during the slow inward current is first retained in an intracellular store. Only during subsequent contractions does this calcium become available to augment systolic force. Several lines of evidence suggest that the "pool" into which this calcium flows during the action potential corresponds to a space immediately beneath the sarcolemma, possibly related to the subsarcolemmal cisternae of the sarcoplasmic reticulum (the excitation site).

The finding that calcium enters the myocardium during systole raises the possibility that this calcium initiates the contractile process by binding to troponin. The amount of calcium which enters the mammalian heart during normal systole, however, is too small to activate more than a small fraction of the potential interactions between actin and myosin. Thus the number of troponin binding sites for calcium is approximately 60–90 μmoles/kg of myocardium, whereas the net influx of calcium during each action potential is on the order of 1–5 μmoles/kg. Under special conditions and in the amphibian heart, however, it appears that this calcium influx may directly activate a significant fraction of the contractile proteins.

Evidence against a direct role in the initiation of systole of the calcium influx, which manifests as the slow inward current, has been obtained in studies of the tension response of the myocardium to a series of stimuli administered after a quiescent period. During the first beat following a prolonged diastole, the slow inward current is large but little tension is generated. During subsequent contractions tension increases (the positive staircase; Chapter 11), although the slow inward current becomes smaller. These and other observations (see below) suggest that calcium influx during the slow inward current does not itself trigger contraction. Instead, this calcium appears to fill an intracellular store from which calcium can be released during subsequent contractions to initiate the contractile process.

Activation of contractile tension development takes place over the same range of membrane depolarization as does an increase in membrane permeability to calcium. Thus both the slow inward current and tension appear when the membrane is depolarized to potentials of approximately -40 mV, and both become maximal at 0 to $+10$ mV, declining as the depolarization step extends into the more positive range of membrane potential. A further similarity between the control by membrane voltage of the slow inward current and developed tension is seen in studies of the recovery of the ability to contract after depolarization. In order to obtain a mechanical response after a full depolarization, membrane potential must be returned toward its repolarized (resting) level. The extent of recovery of the ability to develop tension depends on both the duration of this period of repolarization and the potential to which the membrane is returned. Greater degrees of repolarization (i.e., return to membrane potentials closer to resting potential) and longer periods of repolarization produce greater tensions in subsequent contractions. The time dependence and voltage dependence of the recovery of this ability to respond mechanically to subsequent depolarizations are similar to the time and voltage dependence of the recovery of the slow inward calcium current, which is also inactivated by prior membrane depolarization. These similarities between the properties of the slow inward current and the contractile response are consistent with other evidence (Chapter 11) that the slow inward calcium current is an integral part of the system which regulates contractile amplitude.

Calcium Efflux Across the Sarcolemma: Sodium-Calcium Exchange

The finding that calcium enters the myocardium during each action potential indicates that some mechanism must exist to pump calcium out of the cell. This calcium efflux takes place against both a concentration and an electrical gradient as $[Ca^{2+}]_o$ is considerably greater than $[Ca^{2+}]_i$, and the outside of the cell during diastole is positively charged relative to the cell interior. For this reason movement of calcium out of the myocardium requires an expenditure of energy.

One might anticipate that calcium efflux, like that of sodium, is mediated by an ATP-dependent pump. Such a calcium pump has been described in the sarcoplasmic reticulum, in which a 90,000- to 100,000-dalton "pump" protein binds calcium and forms a phosphorylated intermediate with the terminal phosphate group of ATP, which is hydrolyzed. A Ca^{2+}-activated ATPase has not been clearly identified in the cardiac sarcolemma, and evidence on this important question remains incomplete. There are, however, a number of reasons to believe that even if such a calcium pump does exist in the sarcolemma, its activity cannot alone explain a number of peculiarities in the transport of calcium out of the myocardial cell. For example, the Q_{10} of calcium efflux is only approximately 1.35, a value much lower than that expected from an ATP-dependent ion pump. Furthermore, calcium efflux involves a highly specialized interaction with sodium that appears to be quite different from that of the Na-K-ATPase.

The significance of sodium in the metabolism of calcium by the heart has long been recognized, and a direct relationship between myocardial contractility and the ratio $[Ca^{2+}]_o/[Na^+]^2_o$ is well established. Studies of calcium efflux demonstrate that more than 80% of calcium efflux requires that either sodium or calcium be present outside the cell, and that normally most of the calcium efflux represents exchange of internal calcium for external sodium. From a quantitative standpoint this sodium-calcium exchange involves the competition of two sodium ions for one calcium ion both inside and outside of the membrane. This behavior can be explained if calcium transport involves a divalent anionic carrier (R^{2-}) that can bind either one calcium or two sodium ions.

The possibility that calcium transport across the sarcolemma involves a Na-Ca-ATPase analogous to the Na-K-ATPase is unlikely because the membrane systems responsible for sodium-calcium exchange "see" these two ions in the same way, whether they are inside or outside the membrane. In contrast, the cation-binding sites of the sodium pump are polarized in that sodium binding occurs preferentially at the inside of the myocardial cell, whereas potassium is bound preferentially at the outer surface of the membrane. In the case of the sodium-calcium exchange, however, sodium and calcium appear to bind equally well at both sides of the membrane. Furthermore, the transport of calcium by the sodium-calcium exchange mechanism, unlike that effected by the Na-K-ATPase, is insensitive to cardiac glycosides.

> Another line of evidence which makes it unlikely that calcium efflux requires an ATP-dependent pump is based on studies of metabolic inhibitors and agents that release calcium from intracellular stores. Metabolic inhibitors (e.g., cyanide and 2,4-dinitrophenol) *increase* calcium efflux. If the effects of these inhibitors of ATP production were mediated solely by the decrease in cellular ATP levels, the response of an ATP-dependent calcium pump should be a decrease in calcium efflux. The finding that, instead, calcium efflux increases in the poisoned myocardial fiber can be explained if the primary effect of the metabolic inhibitors is to increase the calcium concentration at the inner surface of the sarcolemma and so promote an ATP-independent exchange with extracellular sodium. The primary factor increasing calcium efflux would thus be the increased intracellular Ca^{2+} concentration caused by the effect of ATP depletion to slow ATP-dependent calcium pumps in other membranes, e.g., in the sarcoplasmic reticulum. This explanation is supported by the effects on calcium efflux of another agent, caffeine, which is known to release calcium from the sarcoplasmic reticulum by a mechanism that does not depend on changes in ATP levels. Like the metabolic inhibitors, caffeine also increases calcium efflux. Furthermore, calcium efflux initiated by metabolic inhibitors and that which results from administration of caffeine depend on extracellular sodium; both are abolished in a sodium-free medium.

The interpretation that the increased calcium efflux brought about by metabolic poisons and caffeine reflects increased calcium availability at the inside of the sarcolemma is supported by the finding that contracture occurs when the efflux of calcium is prevented by removing the extracellular sodium. That added extracellular sodium can relax these contractures is in accord with the role of sodium to allow calcium efflux to proceed by the exchange mechanism described above.

One scheme which can explain these complex effects is shown in Fig. 9.3. This mechanism involves a divalent negatively charged carrier (R^{2-}), which can bind either Na^+ or Ca^{2+} inside or outside the sarcolemma. Assuming that only CaR and Na_2R move freely across the membrane, the driving force for calcium efflux

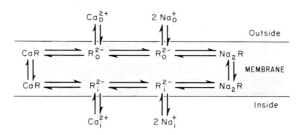

FIG. 9.3. Sodium-calcium exchange mechanism of the cardiac sarcolemma. Na^+ and Ca^{2+} binding occur competitively at both the inside and outside of the sarcolemma. The amount of each cation moving into the cell in this exchange is determined by the ratio $[Na^+]^2/[Ca^{2+}]$ at the outside of the cell; that moving outward is determined by this ratio at the inner surface of the membrane. o, extracellular. i, intracellular. R, carrier. (From Katz: *N. Engl. J. Med.,* 293:1184, 1975.)

is the concentration gradient for sodium across the sarcolemma. As a result of this sodium gradient, which is established by the Na-K-ATPase, the ratio $[Na^+]_i/[Na^+]_o$ is less than unity. This sodium gradient causes the carrier system shown in Fig. 9.3 to establish a gradient for calcium according to the equation

$$\frac{[Ca^{2+}]_i}{[Ca^{2+}]_o} = \frac{[Na^+]_i^2}{[Na^+]_o^2} \tag{9.8}$$

if the affinities of R^{2-} for sodium and calcium are the same at both sides of the membrane.

Equation (9.8) is derived from the equilibrium between Ca^{2+}_o and Ca^{2+}_i with R^{2-}:

$$Ca^{2+}_o + R^{2-}_o \rightleftharpoons CaR \rightleftharpoons Ca^{2+}_i + R^{2-}_i$$

and that between Na^+_o and Na^+_i with R^{2-}:

$$2Na^+_o + R^{2-}_o \rightleftharpoons Na_2R \rightleftharpoons 2Na^+_i + R^{2-}_i$$

which hold as long as the affinities of R^{2-} for both cations are the same on both sides of the membrane. In this case:

$$[Ca^{2+}]_o \times [R^{2-}]_o = [Ca^{2+}]_i \times [R^{2-}]_i$$

and

$$[Na^+]^2_o \times [R^{2-}]_o = [Na^+]^2_i \times [R^{2-}]_i$$

The ratio between these latter equations is:

$$\frac{[Ca^{2+}]_o}{[Na^+]^2_o} = \frac{[Ca^{2+}]_i}{[Na^+]^2_i}$$

Equation 9.8 is obtained when both sides are multiplied by $[Na^+]^2_i$ and divided by $[Ca^{2+}]_o$.

Reduction of extracellular sodium causes the equilibrium described in Eq. (9.8) to shift so that the ratio $[Ca^{2+}]_i/[Ca^{2+}]_o$ increases. When $[Ca^{2+}]_o$ is held constant, therefore, a decrease in $[Na^+]_o$ causes an increase in $[Ca^{2+}]_i$ [Eq. (9.8)]. In the model shown in Fig. 9.3 the initial effect of a reduction in $[Na^+]_o$ is a decrease in the inward movement of sodium and a corresponding increase in calcium influx. The increase in calcium influx causes $[Ca^{2+}]_i$ to rise until the relative rates of sodium and calcium efflux match the newly established relationship between sodium and calcium influx. This new equilibrium is reached, therefore, by an increase in intracellular calcium.

If both $[Na^+]_o$ and $[Ca^{2+}]_o$ are reduced so that the ratio $[Ca^{2+}]_o/[Na^+]_o^2$ remains constant, there is no change in the relative rates of sodium and calcium influx, and thus no change in the relative rates of sodium and calcium efflux. This follows from Eq. (9.8), in which a proportionate reduction in the numerators of both sides of the equation has no effect on the denominators.

The effects of inhibition of the Na-K-ATPase can also be understood in terms of Eq. (9.8). Drugs like the cardiac glycosides, which impair sodium efflux and thus increase $[Na^+]_i$, cause an increase in the $[Na^+]_i^2/[Na^+]_o^2$ ratio. According to Eq. (9.8), the $[Ca^{2+}]_i/[Ca^{2+}]_o$ ratio also increases, so that at a constant level of extracellular calcium the sodium pump inhibition can cause a net gain in intracellular calcium and thus enhancement of contractility (Chapter 11).

The findings predicted by Eq. (9.8) that were discussed in the preceding paragraphs are well documented qualitatively. From a quantitative standpoint, however, the relationship of the carrier system pictured in Fig. 9.3 to the actual situation in the mammalian heart is less clear. There is thus evidence that the $[Na^+]_i/[Na^+]_o$ ratio is between 1:10 and 1:20, so that Eq. (9.8) predicts a ratio for $[Ca^{2+}]_i/[Ca^{2+}]_o$ of between 1:100 and 1:400. As the extracellular concentration of ionized calcium is approximately 10^{-3} M, the predicted value for $[Ca^{2+}]_i$ is between 2.5×10^{-6} M and 1×10^{-5} M. However, these ionized calcium concentrations are well above those which would permit the myocardium to be in a relaxed state because of the high affinity of cardiac troponin for calcium. This discrepancy can be explained if an additional calcium efflux mechanism (e.g., one which involves an ATP-dependent calcium pump in the sarcolemma) also participates in calcium efflux. It is also possible that a "compartment" for calcium exists just beneath the sarcolemma in which ionized calcium concentration is higher than that in the cytosol surrounding the contractile proteins. A possible site for this calcium compartment is the subsarcolemmal cisternae, in which Ca^{2+} concentration can be maintained at a relatively high level by the calcium pump of the sarcoplasmic reticulum. Thus the subsarcolemmal cisternae may represent an intracellular pool for calcium which is maintained in equilibrium with extracellular calcium by the carrier system in Fig. 9.3. If this explanation is correct, calcium efflux from the myoplasm involves a two-step system. The first step is calcium transport into the sarcoplasmic reticulum by a calcium pump which utilizes stoichiometric amounts of ATP for the uphill transport of calcium (see below). The second step of uphill calcium transport, which would carry calcium from the sarcoplasmic reticulum out of the cell, utilizes the sodium gradient across the sarcolemma. While this second step would not use ATP directly, it must be remembered that the energy derived from this sodium gradient is generated by the Na-K-ATPase.

Calcium Release

The significance of an internal release of activator for muscular contraction was mentioned at the outset of this chapter. It is generally accepted that in skeletal muscle activator calcium is released from intracellular stores in the sarcoplasmic reticulum. In the mammalian myocardium, however, there remains some disagreement as to whether activator calcium is derived from a pool just beneath the sarcolemma, the sarcoplasmic reticulum, or both. It is assumed here that the major source of calcium for binding to troponin C in the myocardial cell is the intracellular calcium pool within the sarcoplasmic reticulum (Fig. 9.2).

Two different theories as to the mechanism responsible for calcium release to troponin C in the myocardium have now been proposed. The first, which can be looked on as an "electrical trigger," is now believed to be responsible for calcium release to the contractile proteins in skeletal muscle. The second, a "calcium-triggered calcium release" is less likely to be of significance in skeletal muscle but may play an important role in the myocardium, in which variations in this calcium release are of major physiological importance.

Electrically triggered release of calcium by the sarcoplasmic reticulum is suggested by the finding that anions which readily cross the sarcoplasmic reticulum when added to solutions so as to replace anions that are poorly able to cross the membrane of the sarcoplasmic reticulum can cause calcium release. Adding salts of permeant anions (e.g., chloride) produces transient contractions in "skinned" cardiac muscle fibers, i.e., fibers in which the sarcolemma has been removed, which were previously in solutions containing only nonpermeant anions (e.g., proprionate). These transient contractions are due to the release of calcium from stores within the sarcoplasmic reticulum. It is proposed that this effect of anion exchange arises from transient depolarization of the sarcoplasmic reticulum caused by the rapid entry of the negatively charged chloride ions.

There is also evidence that calcium ions can serve as a trigger which causes the sarcoplasmic reticulum to release calcium to the contractile proteins. Much like the primer charge in an old flintlock musket—which when caused to explode by the flint striking the primer pan leads to the discharge of the larger charge of powder within the barrel of the musket—the influx of a small amount of calcium from an activator pool (Fig. 9.2) has been proposed to cause the release of a larger quantity of calcium from the sarcoplasmic reticulum. This second release of calcium from a large intracellular pool (Fig. 9.2) can provide enough activator calcium to bind to troponin and lead to contraction. When a "skinned" muscle fiber is soaked in calcium, after which this cation is removed, some membrane stores remain filled with calcium. Adding to such fibers quantities of calcium that are themselves too small to evoke a mechanical response causes a brief contraction. These contractions can be shown to be initiated by the transient release of a larger quantity of calcium from stores within the sarcoplasmic reticulum. In this way calcium induces enhanced calcium release. The mechanism by which this trigger acts to release calcium is probably an increased calcium permeability of the sarcoplasmic reticulum. The significance of these findings in terms of the initiation of the physiological cardiac contraction remains in dispute.

Whether the trigger that initiates calcium release from the sarcoplasmic reticulum is electrical in nature or is related to a transient increase in Ca^{2+} concentration mediated by calcium flux from an activator pool immediately outside the sarcoplasmic reticulum, it is apparent that calcium efflux from the sarcoplasmic reticulum is a "downhill" process. Thus movement of calcium from the sarcoplasmic reticulum to the cytosol, where it becomes bound to troponin C, does not require the expenditure of energy, as by an ATP-dependent calcium pump. Instead, this excitatory calcium flux appears to be controlled by changes in the calcium permeability of the membranes of the sarcoplasmic reticulum.

Calcium Removal by Sarcoplasmic Reticulum

The characteristics of myocardial contractile function are determined not only by the release of calcium to initiate cardiac systole but also by the rate of calcium removal from the cytosol. As already described, this calcium transport is effected by the sarcoplasmic reticulum. Calcium transport by the sarcoplasmic reticulum *in vitro* was discovered independently during the early 1960s by Hasselbach and Makinose, and by Ebashi and Lipmann. These investigators described an ATP-dependent transport of calcium ion into membrane vesicles isolated in cardiac microsomal preparations enriched in sarcoplasmic reticulum vesicles.

The mechanism by which these membranes pump calcium involves at least three reactions:

$$2Ca^{2+}_o + ATP + E_o \rightleftharpoons Ca_2E_o{\sim}P + ADP \qquad (9.9)$$

$$Ca_2E_o{\sim}P \longrightarrow Ca_2E_i + P_i \qquad (9.10)$$

$$Ca_2E_i \longrightarrow 2Ca^{2+}_i + E_o \qquad (9.11)$$

where E_o and E_i are, respectively, the concentrations of the calcium carrier at the outside and inside of the membrane vesicles; $Ca_2E_o{\sim}P$ and Ca_2E_i are, respectively, the concentrations of the calcium-carrier complex at the outside and inside of the membrane; and Ca^{2+}_o and Ca^{2+}_i are, respectively, the ionized calcium concentrations outside and inside the membrane vesicles.

Equation (9.9) describes the reversible binding of calcium to a carrier (E_o) at the outside of the membrane. This binding step requires the participation of ATP, which is hydrolyzed by the carrier, so that the calcium carrier appears to be identical with the Ca^{2+}-activated ATPase. The products of ATP hydrolysis are not immediately released. Instead, the terminal phosphate of ATP becomes att'.ched to the carrier, forming an acyl phosphoprotein (see below).

Equation (9.10) describes the translocation of the calcium-carrier complex from the outside to the inside of the membrane. This transport step involves the "uphill" transport of calcium against concentration gradients greater than 3,000:1. Thus energy is required for the reaction described in Eq. (9.10), the energy probably being provided by hydrolysis of the phosphorylated ATPase intermediate.

The reaction described in Eq. (9.11) allows calcium to be released within the sarcoplasmic reticulum, while at the same time the carrier returns in an "unloaded" form to the outside of the membrane where it can again participate in calcium transport.

It is now clear that the membranes of both skeletal and cardiac sarcoplasmic reticulum contain an ATPase protein. This protein has a molecular weight of approximately 90,000–100,000 and in the presence of ATP and calcium forms an acyl phosphoprotein that is an intermediate of the ATPase reaction. This ATPase protein binds 2 moles of calcium for each mole of bound ATP or phosphate [Eqs. (9.10) and (9.11)] and thus has the characteristics expected of the calcium carrier, which transports calcium with a stoichiometry of 2 moles of calcium transport per mole of ATP hydrolyzed.

In preparations of cardiac microsomes the content of the acyl phosphoprotein is approximately 1–2 nmoles/mg protein, so that the binding of calcium to the ATPase protein can account for the association of 2–4 nmoles of calcium per milligram of membrane protein in cardiac microsomes. Yet calcium storage by cardiac microsomes reaches a level of more than 40 nmoles/mg. The mechanism responsible for the transport and retention of most of the rest of the approximately 40 nmoles of calcium per milligram of protein by cardiac microsomes is not fully understood. A portion of this calcium is probably present in a pool of freely exchangeable calcium within the microsomes, where it contributes to a high concentration gradient for calcium across the microsomal membrane. This interpretation is supported by the finding that a variety of physical and chemical means (e.g., sonication and phospholipase treatment, or addition of calcium ionophores) cause calcium to be released from microsomes that have transported calcium in the absence of calcium-precipitating anions. On the other hand, calcium release from intact microsomes is extremely slow when extramicrosomal Ca^{2+} concentration is abruptly lowered, indicating that the membranes of the sarcoplasmic reticulum are, under these conditions, impermeable to calcium. The mechanism whereby calcium permeability is increased remains unknown, but may reflect an effect of elevated Ca^{2+}_o, as was discussed earlier in reference to the calcium-triggered calcium release.

A portion of the calcium taken up by the sarcoplasmic reticulum may be bound to one or more of the acid proteins that have been identified in preparations of skeletal muscle sarcoplasmic reticulum. It has been suggested that these proteins may serve a calcium-trapping function analogous to that seen when calcium-precipitating anions are included in studies of muscle microsomes *in vitro* (see below). This proposed role for these acid proteins, however, is controversial.

The extent of calcium transport by fragmented sarcoplasmic reticulum is markedly increased when reactions are carried out in the presence of calcium-precipitating anions such as oxalate and phosphate. This anion-dependent calcium transport (usually called calcium uptake) is made possible by the ability of these anions to precipitate calcium when the internal Ca^{2+} concentration rises to moderately high levels. During oxalate-facilitated calcium uptake, for example, a calcium-oxalate precipitate forms with the calcium pumped into the microsomal vesicles, so that the calcium pump is able to continue to transport calcium until large amounts of calcium are present within the vesicles. In contrast, the calcium transport seen in the absence of calcium-precipitating anions is quickly inhibited by an inhibitory effect of the high Ca^{2+} concentration within the vesicles.

A number of studies indicate that the total *amount* of calcium rapidly transported by cardiac microsomes in the absence of calcium-precipitating anions can account for relaxation in the intact heart, and that both the *rate* of transport and the apparent *affinity* of the pump for calcium are sufficiently high to allow this pump to cause calcium to dissociate from cardiac troponin at a rate commensurate with that of relaxation in the intact heart.

Acceleration of Relaxation by the Cyclic AMP-Protein Kinase System

Agents which lead to the production of *cyclic AMP* (e.g., the β-adrenergic agonists and glucagon) characteristically accelerate relaxation in the heart. These agents are well known to enhance myocardial contractility by increasing calcium influx across the sarcolemma (Chapter 11); the accompanying acceleration of relaxation can be explained by an effect to stimulate the calcium pump of the sarcoplasmic reticulum. This action is especially important in the case of the catecholamines, which exert a dramatic effect to increase heart rate as well as to increase myocardial contractility.

The significance of the acceleration of relaxation by catecholamines stems from the ability of these agents to increase heart rate (Chapter 19). If systole was not shortened during interventions such as exercise, where heart rate can increase threefold, the heart would not relax long enough to receive the increased venous return. Thus to allow for diastolic filling, the cardiac response to agents like norepinephrine, which plays a major role in the cardiac response to exercise, includes not only enhanced contractility and tachycardia but also abbreviated systole.

The ability of these agents to enhance myocardial contractility is probably mediated in part by increased calcium influx across the sarcolemma (Chapter 11), but acceleration of relaxation can be explained by stimulation of calcium transport by the sarcoplasmic reticulum. The mechanism of this stimulatory action is of general biological interest because it illustrates one means by which cyclic AMP can effect its role as a "second messenger" through a change in an ion-transport system.

The role of cyclic AMP as a second messenger reflects its ability to translate the initial message generated by the arrival at the cell surface of a hormone (e.g., the catecholamine *epinephrine*) into a second message that can be recognized within the cell. This second message is carried by cyclic AMP, which is produced from ATP by an enzyme called *adenylate cyclase*. In the case of the heart, as in other tissues, adenylate cyclase is present in the sarcolemma and possibly in other cell membranes as well. This enzyme is activated when the catecholamine hormones interact with β-receptors located on the cardiac sarcolemma. The binding of cyclic AMP to the β-receptor initiates a complex change in this system which activates adenylate cyclase, thereby promoting the conversion of ATP to cyclic AMP.

Adenylate cyclases are now believed to consist of two types of active subunit: *regulatory subunits,* which serve as hormone-specific receptors, and *catalytic subunits,* which contain the active site responsible for cyclic AMP production. The mechanism by which hormone binding to the regulatory subunit increases the activity of the catalytic subunits is poorly understood. It has been found that nucleotides, notably GTP, participate in this activation process by both modifying hormone-binding to the receptor subunit and acting in concert with the hormones on the catalytic subunit to promote cyclic AMP production. Very recent evidence indicates that this activation process may also be sensitive to a stimulatory action that occurs when cellular ATP levels decline.

The stimulation of cyclic AMP production brought about by activation of adenylate cyclase can be written as the first half of a reaction mechanism that also describes the degradation of cyclic AMP:

$$\text{ATP} \xrightarrow[\text{cyclase}]{\text{adenylate}} \text{cyclic AMP} \xrightarrow[\text{diesterase}]{\text{phospho-}} \text{AMP} + \text{PP}_i \qquad (9.12)$$

The second half of this reaction, which leads to the inactivation of cyclic AMP by its conversion to AMP, is catalyzed by *phosphodiesterase.* In this way cyclic AMP levels can be regulated by alterations in both its synthesis by adenylate cyclase and its degradation by phosphodiesterase. Thus phosphodiesterase inhibitors such as theophylline can exert an epinephrine-like action on the heart.

The interaction of calcium with the reaction mechanism shown in Eq. (9.12) illustrates a very interesting negative feedback system in the heart. It is well established that agents which increase cyclic AMP levels in the heart increase the flow of calcium into the cell (Chapter 11). This increased cellular Ca^{2+} concentration in turn decreases cyclic AMP levels by inhibiting adenylate cyclase and activating phosphodiesterase (Fig. 9.4). In this way the actions of cyclic AMP to increase cellular Ca^{2+} can lead eventually to a decline in cyclic AMP levels.

We already noted that the effector systems of the mammalian cell cannot recognize directly the arrival of hormone such as epinephrine at the cell surface—

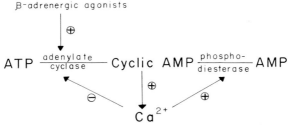

FIG. 9.4. Interrelationships between Ca^{2+} and cyclic AMP within the myocardium. β-Adrenergic agonists activate adenylate cyclase, thereby causing cyclic AMP levels to rise. This in turn increases intracellular Ca^{2+}, which tends to reverse these effects by promoting a reduction in cyclic AMP levels through the ability of Ca^{2+} to inhibit adenylate cyclase and to activate phosphodiesterase. (From Tada et al.: *Circ. Res.,* 36:8, 1976, by permission of the American Heart Association, Inc.)

that the interposition of cyclic **AMP**, which serves as a second messenger, is required. Recently it has become apparent that the processes of translation within the cell may involve "messengers" in addition to cyclic AMP. Stated in another way, effector systems within the mammalian cell are not only unable to recognize epinephrine as a signal to initiate altered function, they also appear incapable of recognizing directly the message carried by cyclic AMP. Instead, altered cell function requires the interposition of a class of enzymes which acts as still another messenger, *the cyclic AMP-dependent protein kinases.* The messenger function of the cyclic AMP-dependent protein kinases, like that of cyclic AMP, is manifested by their ability to translate one type of afferent signal into a chemically different message.

Protein kinases are enzymes which catalyze the formation of phosphoproteins. They accomplish this by transferring the terminal phosphate group of ATP to form phosphoesters with serine or threonine residues of proteins by the reaction:

$$\text{Protein} + \text{ATP} \xrightarrow{\text{protein kinase}} \text{phosphoester phosphoprotein} + \text{ADP} \quad (9.13)$$

The overall reaction scheme that mediates the effects of adenylate cyclase activators on calcium transport by the sarcoplasmic reticulum can be written as in Fig. 9.5.

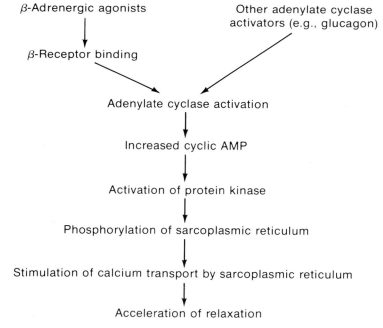

FIG. 9.5. Cascade of reactions by which agents that increase cyclic AMP levels can accelerate relaxation in the heart.

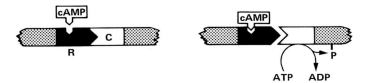

FIG. 9.6. Mechanism by which cyclic AMP (cAMP) activates a cyclic AMP-dependent protein kinase. In its basal state *(left)* the catalytic site of the enzyme (C) is inhibited by the regulatory component (R) to which it is bound. Binding of cyclic AMP to the regulatory component (sometimes also called the cyclic AMP-binding component) reverses this inhibition by causing it to be dissociated from the catalytic component *(right)*. Freed of this inhibitory effect, the latter catalyzes transfer of the terminal phosphate of ATP to various proteins (protein phosphorylation). The reaction shown here depicts a membrane-bound protein kinase which phosphorylates an adjacent membrane site. Soluble protein kinases also are found, and these can phosphorylate both soluble and membrane-bound proteins.

The activation of protein kinase occurs by the reversal of an inhibitory effect of a regulatory component. This involves the binding of cyclic AMP to the regulatory component, which also serves as a cyclic AMP-binding component (Fig. 9.6). When the regulatory (cyclic AMP-binding) component of protein kinase no longer inhibits the catalytic component, this enzyme becomes able to catalyze the phosphorylation of a number of proteins. Like the adenylate cyclases, protein kinases may be membrane-bound and so may phosphorylate the membrane structures in which they lie (Fig. 9.6). In view of the general lack of substrate specificity of the protein kinases, their orientation in membranes may confer some selectivity to the structures which are phosphorylated. Soluble protein kinases exist, however, so that the mechanism of substrate selectivity remains incompletely understood.

For the sequence of reactions shown in Fig. 9.6 to exert a physiological action in the myocardial cell, some mechanism to reverse this effect is required. In other words, if phosphorylation of the sarcoplasmic reticulum plays a role in the control of cellular function, then a system to dephosphorylate the sarcoplasmic reticulum also must exist. This effect is now attributable to another class of enzymes, the *phosphoprotein phosphatases,* which hydrolyze the phosphate ester bonds formed by the protein kinases:

$$\text{Protein} + \text{ATP} \xrightarrow[\text{kinase}]{\text{protein}} \underset{\underset{\text{ADP}}{+}}{\text{protein-P}} \xrightarrow[\text{phosphatase}]{\text{phosphoprotein}} \text{protein} + P_i \quad (9.14)$$

The significance of the dephosphorylation reaction in the regulation of cell function remains to be evaluated. It may be, for example, that the specificity of some of the regulatory phosphorylation reactions results from variations in the sensitivity of different phosphoproteins to dephosphorylation by the phosphoester phosphatases. This important question cannot yet be answered.

The relationships described in the preceding paragraphs are shown in Fig. 9.7, in which the receptor protein for protein kinase-catalyzed phosphorylation has been designated phospholamban. Phosphorylation of phospholamban can be

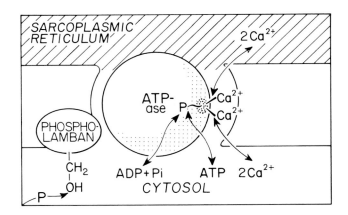

FIG. 9.7. Stimulation of the calcium pump of cardiac sarcoplasmic reticulum after phosphorylation of phospholamban. Transfer of the terminal phosphate of ATP to the hydroxyl group of a
serine residue on phospholamban to form a phosphoester bond stimulates the calcium pump
(ATPase). This enhances the ability of the latter to effect the ATP-dependent transport of
calcium into the sarcoplasmic reticulum. Also shown is the operation of the calcium pump in
which the terminal phosphate of ATP is transferred to a carboxyl group (P~) to form a high-
energy acyl phosphate bond. This allows two calcium ions to bind to and then be transported
into the sarcoplasmic reticulum by a reaction that leads to the release of ADP and P_i. Double
arrows are drawn for this reaction because the reaction is reversible; viz., the energy made
available when Ca^{2+} flows down the Ca^{2+} concentration gradient out of the sarcoplasmic reticulum can be utilized by the calcium pump to synthesize ATP from ADP and P_i.

shown to be associated with stimulation of calcium transport by the sarcoplasmic
reticulum *in vitro*. A functional role for these reactions in accelerating relaxation
in response to agents that promote cyclic AMP production in the heart is suggested by the absence of this response in skeletal muscles that do not respond
to β-adrenergic agonists with an increased rate of relaxation.

A role of sarcolemmal phosphorylation in mediating the actions of β-adrener-
gic agonists to promote calcium entry across the sarcolemma is suggested by the
ability of phosphorylated phospholamban to stimulate calcium efflux from the
sarcoplasmic reticulum. While it is possible that an analogous mechanism alters
calcium transport across the sarcolemma in response to activation of adenylate
cyclase, available evidence remains inconclusive.

We have now seen how the control of excitation-contraction coupling can be
explained as the interplay between at least four calcium fluxes. Two of these are
between the extracellular space and the cell interior. Calcium influx and efflux
therefore represent calcium movements across the sarcolemma. The other two
calcium fluxes, which take place within the cell, are controlled by the sarcoplasmic reticulum and possibly by a membrane that delimits an activator pool (Fig.
9.2).

In view of the likelihood that the phasic control of myocardial contractility
is mediated by changes in the amount of calcium made available for binding to
troponin C, the functional significance of the interplay between the calcium

movements shown in Fig. 9.2 in determining the contractile state of the myocardium can be readily appreciated. We return to this formulation in Chapter 11, where the physiological, pharmacological, and pathological mechanisms that effect the phasic control of myocardial contractility are described.

BIBLIOGRAPHY

Ebashi, S. (1976): Excitation-contraction coupling. *Annu. Rev. Physiol.,* 38:293–313.

Huxley, A. F. (1959): Local activation of muscle. *Ann. NY Acad. Sci.,* 81:446–452.

Katz, A. M., and Repke, D. I. (1973): Calcium-membrane interactions in the myocardium: Effects of ouabain, epinephrine, and 3′, 5′-cyclic adenosine monophosphate. *Am. J. Cardiol.,* 31:193–201.

Katz, A. M., Tada, M., and Kirchberger, M. A. (1975): Control of calcium transport in the myocardium by the cyclic AMP-protein kinase system. *Adv. Cyclic Nucleotide Res.,* 5:453–472.

Reuter, H. (1974): Exchange of calcium ions in the mammalian myocardium: Mechanisms and physiological significance. *Circ. Res.,* 34:599–605.

Schwartz, A., Lindenmayer, G. E., and Allen, J. C. (1975): The sodium-potassium adenosine triphosphatase: Pharmacological, physiological and biochemical aspects. *Pharmacol. Rev.,* 27:3–134.

Tada, M., Kirchberger, M. A., Iorio, J. M., and Katz, A. M. (1975): Control of cardiac sarcolemmal adenylate cyclase and sodium, potassium-activated adenosinetriphosphatase activities. *Circ. Res.,* 36:8–17.

10

Myocardial Contractility: Force, Velocity, Length, and Time

Recognition of the importance of changes in myocardial contractility in response to altered circulatory demands of the body is a relatively recent event in the history of cardiovascular research. The significance of changes in the intrinsic contractile properties of the heart was largely overlooked until the mid-1950s largely owing to earlier emphasis on length-dependent changes in myocardial performance (Frank-Starling relationship; Chapter 13). A number of observations made prior to that time indicated that cardiac muscle was able to alter its intrinsic contractile properties, but the importance of these early observations did not become apparent until a symposium on this subject was organized in 1955. This symposium, in which Sarnoff presented the concept of a "family of Starling curves," clearly integrated knowledge of the length-dependent changes in contractile performance described a half-century before by Frank and Starling with scattered bits of evidence pointing to a significant role for alterations in myocardial contractility. The impact of this symposium was immediate in that cardiovascular physiologists began to examine the contractile properties of cardiac muscle in an effort to define the mechanisms by which the heart responded to a wide variety of physiological, pharmacological, and pathological factors.

The application of the principles of muscle mechanics to the analysis of cardiac performance began in 1959 with the studies of Abbott and Mommaerts, and later those of Brady and Sonnenblick. The potential importance of muscle mechanics (Chapter 5) as an aid to understanding the regulation of cardiac performance arises from the fact that control of the pumping action of the heart is effected by mechanisms intrinsic to the myocardial cell. The significance of this intrinsic control of cardiac contractility becomes apparent after examining Table 10.1, in which four mechanisms with the potential to regulate cardiac and skeletal muscle performance are compared.

SUMMATION OF CONTRACTIONS

The tension developed by a skeletal muscle can be augmented when high stimulation frequencies cause summation (Fig. 8.3) or a tetanic contraction (Fig. 8.4). In this way tension output can be regulated by variations in the frequency at which a motoneuron is discharged. Most skeletal muscle contractions, however, are brief tetani or summated contractions. Whereas some movements of the extraocular muscle may be twitches, the twitch generally represents a functionally

TABLE 10.1. *Mechanisms regulating muscular performance*

Mechanism	Functional role in skeletal muscle	Functional role in cardiac muscle
Ability to summate individual contractile events (partial and complete tetanus)	Minor	None
Ability to vary number of active motor units	Major	None
Ability to undergo length-dependent changes in contractile properties (length-tension or Frank-Starling relationship)	Usually minor	Major in beat-to-beat regulation; minor in sustained circulatory changes
Ability to change intrinsic contractile properties (contractility)	Minor	Major in sustained circulatory changes; minor in beat-to-beat regulation

useless type of contraction, e.g., the knee jerk. Thus variations in the extent of summation of individual contractile events probably play no more than a minor role in the regulation of skeletal muscle performance.

In contrast to skeletal muscle, the cardiac action potential lasts until the end of the active state. Because the membrane of the cardiac muscle cell does not become responsive to physiological stimuli until the muscle has relaxed, summation and tetanization are not possible. This potential regulatory mechanism thus cannot operate in the heart.

VARIATIONS IN THE NUMBER OF ACTIVE MOTOR UNITS

Each skeletal muscle is composed of a number of *motor units,* which are groups of muscle cells innervated by a single motoneuron. Because each motoneuron can function independently of other motoneurons in the nerve supplying a skeletal muscle, the tension generated by the muscle can be modulated by the recruitment of a greater or lesser number of active motor units. To lift a light load only a few percent of the motor units are activated in the muscles used, whereas if the same muscles are used to lift a heavy load a much larger proportion of the motor units in the muscles involved are activated via their motoneurons. This control system, which is integrated in the central nervous system, recruits a greater or lesser number of motoneurons, and does not involve changes intrinsic to the individual muscle fibers each of which contributes a stereotyped contractile response.

This type of control is not possible in the heart, which is functionally a syncytium. Because the specialized cell-cell junction in the heart (the intercalated disc) is a pathway of low electrical resistance, impulses entering any region of the ventricular myocardium eventually are conducted to all regions of the ventricles. As a result, fractional activation of the ventricles (or atria) is not normally possible.

CHANGES IN SARCOMERE LENGTH

The dependence of muscle tension on rest-length in striated muscle is considered in some detail in Chapter 8. This length-tension relationship represents a potential control mechanism by which the level of preload can influence the tension the muscle generates. Control of muscle performance by this mechanism is probably of little importance in controlling the work output of skeletal muscles inasmuch as muscle length is determined by the angles at the joints rather than by the functional demands on the muscle. To a large extent, therefore, the position one assumes in the performance of muscular work, and especially of isometric work, is determined more by the need to achieve optimal leverage than by attempts to set sarcomere lengths to the apices of their length-tension curves.

In the heart, which is a hollow viscus whose leverage is determined by the radius of curvature of its muscular walls (Chapter 12), the length-tension relationship plays a much more important role in regulating the force generated by the walls of the atria and ventricles. In the ventricles, for example, sarcomere length is determined partly by the preload, which in turn is influenced by the volume of blood returning during diastole plus that remaining in the ventricle after the preceding systole. For this reason the length-tension relationship provides a means by which increasing preload can increase the ability of the heart to eject more blood.

It is likely that the length-tension relationship in the heart is of major importance in the mediation of beat-to-beat changes in cardiac performance. Operation of the length-tension relationship in the heart, which is manifest as the Frank-Starling relationship (Chapter 12), probably has a primary role in "fine tuning" of the heartbeat, such as occurs in the following two dynamic situations.

Response to Minor Changes in Venous Return and Resistance to Ejection

Elevating the legs causes the forces of gravity to increase blood flow into the right atrium. The resulting elevation in right atrial pressure is transmitted to the right ventricle as an increase in end-diastolic volume (dilatation) and hence in preload. Operation of the length-tension relationship thus allows dilation of the right ventricle to increase the ability of this chamber to eject blood as long as the ventricle remains on the ascending limb of the length-tension curve (Figs. 8.20 and 12.9). In this way a positive feedback is established in which increased demands for cardiac work provide for an adjustment in cardiac performance that meets the increased demands.

A similar positive feedback by the length-tension relationship can be described when the resistance to ejection of blood from one of the ventricles is increased. If, for example, the left ventricle is faced with an abrupt increase in aortic pressure, less blood is ejected. The result of this reduced emptying is retention of a larger volume of blood in the ventricle at the end of the systole, so that the return of blood to the ventricle during the next diastole causes ventricular volume to be increased beyond that seen before aortic pressure was elevated. The resulting ventricular dilatation, as long as the ventricle is operating on the ascending limb of its length-tension relationship, allows more force to be developed and so permits the left ventricle to eject a normal volume of blood in the face of an increased aortic pressure.

Note that for the length-tension relationship to mediate the cardiac response to increases in loading it is necessary for the myocardium to be operating on the ascending limb of the sarcomere length-tension curve. The functional consequences of overstretching of the sarcomeres of the heart onto the descending limb are quite serious (Chapter 12). The likelihood of such an untoward event, however, is minimized by the high resting stiffness of the myocardium and by the pericardium (Fig. 8.20 and Chapter 12).

Matching the Outputs of the Right and Left Sides of the Heart

The other regulatory function probably served largely by operation of the length-tension relationship is matching of the outputs of both sides of the heart. In view of the relative independence of contractile strength by the right and left ventricles, the two major pumping chambers of the heart, some mechanism must exist to match their outputs. Without such a control system it would be possible, for example, for the output of the right ventricle to exceed that of the left ventricle, a situation that would prove lethal by literally drowning the individual as blood accumulates in the lungs.

The positive feedback which results from the operation of the ventricles on the ascending limbs of their length-tension relationships allows the outputs of the ventricles to be kept in balance. For example, if right ventricular output is increased (e.g., by leg raising; see above), the increased flow of blood through the lungs would, by dilating the left ventricle, serve as a stimulus to the left ventricle to increase its output. Conversely, reduced ejection of blood by the left ventricle would increase left ventricular volume and thus increase left atrial pressure. The latter in turn would increase the resistance to ejection by the right ventricle, thereby leading to a rise in right ventricular diastolic pressure. The resulting increase in resistance to filling of the right ventricle, by impeding the return of blood by way of the great veins, would decrease right ventricular output. In this way the output of the right side of the heart would decrease, thereby coming into balance with that of the left side.

Although the length-tension relationship probably plays a major role in the beat-to-beat adjustments of the work of the heart, changes in developed tension arising from changing muscle fiber length appear not to be critical to most long-term circulatory changes. During exercise, for example, where cardiac work is increased greatly, the heart may become smaller; whereas in heart failure, where cardiac work decreases, the heart becomes enlarged. For this reason other regulatory systems must also operate to allow the heart to adjust its performance to major long-term changes in circulatory dynamics.

CHANGES IN CONTRACTILITY

Variations in muscle tension that arise from summation and tetanization, recruitment of a greater or lesser number of motor units, and changes in muscle length represent responses to control mechanisms that arise outside the muscle cell. Changes in contractility, on the other hand, reflect the operation of control mechanisms intrinsic to the muscle cells. In this way the muscle, by changing biochemical and biophysical aspects of the contractile process within the cell, is able to vary its response with either a stronger or a weaker contraction. Unlike the "fine tuning" effected by the Frank-Starling relationship, changing contractility represents a "coarse gain control" in the regulation of cardiac function.

Changes in the intrinsic contractile properties of the skeletal muscle cell are of little functional significance. Although slight changes in skeletal muscle contractile performance can be shown to occur in the intact animal under special circumstances, the role of these changes in altering the functional capacity of the muscle is much less important than the extrinsic control systems already discussed. For all practical purposes, therefore, one can look on a skeletal muscle as responding in a stereotyped manner. In the case of a tetanic contraction this response is of a maximal nature, as if the contractile proteins of a skeletal muscle deliver their "all" in response to any form of physiological stimulation.

The situation in the heart is quite different from that just described for a skeletal muscle. Under basal conditions the normal heart makes available only approximately two-thirds of its maximal contractile potential for the pumping of blood. Furthermore, the intensity of this response is highly variable, being subject to a large number of influences. This variability in response does not mean that the heart does not respond in an all-or-none fashion; instead, it is as if the amount of the "all" is variable (Chapter 11).

The term *inotropic* is commonly used in discussing changes in myocardial contractility. A *positive inotropic* intervention is one that causes contractility to increase, whereas a *negative inotropic* intervention reduces contractility. Inotropic changes probably mediate most important changes in the physiological function of the heart and are involved in the response of the heart to a number of drugs and disease states.

WHAT IS MYOCARDIAL CONTRACTILITY?

The concept of *myocardial contractility* is extremely difficult if not impossible to define, although a *change in myocardial contractility* is relatively easy to identify. Any change in the work performed during a single heartbeat that does not result from a change in initial fiber length can be considered to be the result of a change in contractility. In an isolated strip of cardiac muscle, for example, if a drug increases the ability of the muscle to shorten, develop tension, or both during each contraction at a fixed muscle length, contractility has been increased (Fig. 10.1). Conversely, a drug that reduces the ability of the strip of muscle to

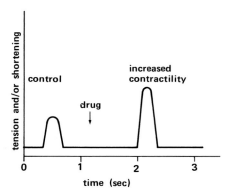

FIG. 10.1. An increase in myocardial contractility enhances the amount of tension developed, the rate of shortening, or both without an increase in rest length.

do work during each beat at constant rest length can be said to have decreased contractility (Fig. 10.2).

Changing contractility can be identified in the intact heart by measuring an increase or decrease in the work performed per beat at constant end-diastolic volume. These effects and their interplay with concurrent changes in rest length that are often seen in the living animal and man are discussed in Chapters 12 and 13.

If we accept the definition of a change in myocardial contractility set forth in the preceding paragraph, we are still left with the very difficult but important problem of defining what it is that has in fact been changed. It is at this point that virtually all definitions of contractility fall short of their goal, for myocardial contractility is really the net effect of *all* mechanisms by which the activity of the contractile proteins becomes manifest as the ability of the cardiac muscle to do work. For this reason any definition of myocardial contractility must take into account the ability of the muscle to develop tension and to shorten, which can vary independently of each other, as well as the rates of onset and decay, and the overall duration of both of these properties. Factors outside the contractile

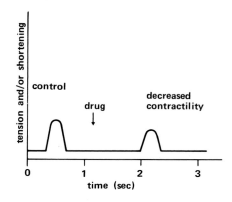

FIG. 10.2. A decrease in myocardial contractility reduces the amount of tension developed, the rate of shortening, or both without a decrease in rest length.

proteins (e.g., muscle elasticity) also may influence the ability of the muscle to do work. Because the nature of the elasticity is poorly understood, it is not possible to provide a complete and accurate description of the capacity of the contractile proteins of the cardiac muscle to shorten and develop tension.

Two partial definitions of myocardial contractility are provided here; one is based on extrapolations from the analyses of skeletal muscle mechanics provided in Chapter 5, and the other on what is known of the biochemistry of the contractile proteins as set forth in Chapters 6 and 7. The reader can thus obtain at least an approach to the understanding of myocardial contractility, since it is difficult at this time to provide an accurate and complete definition of this important parameter.

CONTRACTILITY DEFINED IN TERMS OF MUSCLE MECHANICS

Hill postulated that two states could exist in the "active points" of muscle (Chapter 5). In the first state all of the active points hold tension, and in the second state they participate in chemical reactions. The distribution of active points between these two states is determined by the load on the muscle. This situation therefore is one in which a potential to do work is established which can be "tapped" in different ways. When the muscle is presented with heavy loads, this potential to do work appears as tension so that large loads are slowly moved short distances. At lower loads the muscle performs work in a different manner. Here the lighter load is moved more rapidly over a greater distance. Thus as the load is varied, both the total work performed (Fig. 5.2) and the velocity of muscle shortening (Fig. 5.14) also vary. It is important to recognize that these load-dependent changes do *not* represent variations in contractility but are different ways in which a given state of contractility can be expressed.

A change in contractility, viewed in the context of this discussion, can represent any change in the potential of the muscle to do work. This description can be expanded by examining the force-velocity relation, which defines the mechanical properties of muscular contraction as they manifest at different loads.

In terms of Hill's formation of two states in active muscle, it is theoretically possible for each state to vary independently of the other. For example, the number of active points in muscle could increase without there being any change in their rate of turnover. This is analogous to an increase in the number of "little men" pulling on the rope shown in Fig. 5.17. Similarly, the maximum rate of energy liberation by these active points could increase, so that the "little men" in Fig. 5.18 move more quickly without there being a change in their number. As discussed in Chapter 7, therefore, it is possible to vary contractility by one or both of two independent mechanisms. Variations in the number of active points would, in theory, alter P_0, the intercept of the force-velocity curve where force is maximal. Variations in the rate of turnover of active points, on the other hand, would cause a shift in V_{max}, the intercept of the force-velocity curve at zero load, where velocity is maximal. In considering an increase in contractility, therefore,

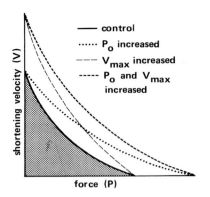

FIG. 10.3. An increase in myocardial contractility causes an upward shift in the force-velocity curve that can be brought about by an increased V_{max}, an increased P_0, or both. The force-velocity curve prior to the increase in contractility is designated the control.

an upward shift in the force-velocity could arise from increased V_{max}, P_0, or both (Fig. 10.3).

Figure 10.3 demonstrates that *all of these shifts in the force-velocity curve at constant muscle length represent an increase in contractility because the ability to do work at intermediate loads is increased.* These three theoretical mechanisms can be differentiated, however, only if the intercepts of the force-velocity curve can be measured and compared. At intermediate loads no distinction between these mechanisms is possible, as is apparent from Fig. 10.3.

In terms of the preceding discussion, it is apparent that the concept of myocardial contractility represents an expression of at least two theoretically independent properties of the contractile proteins: maximal force-generating capacity and maximal shortening velocity. Each of these parameters, however, may change at a different rate during the slow evolution of cardiac systole. As a result, alterations in the time-dependent properties of P_0, V_{max}, or both can influence myocardial contractility. Prolongation of the time that P_0 is maintained or acceleration of the development of full V_{max}, etc. can, for example, increase the ability of the heart to do work during each contraction. These time-dependent properties therefore increase the complexity of our definition of myocardial contractility because, for example, the longer the duration of the active state, the greater is the potential to do work, even if the intensity of the active state remains constant.

In cardiac muscle the active state is both slow in onset and of finite duration (Chapter 8), so at least two time-dependent properties must be included in the list of parameters that define myocardial contractility. The first is the rate of onset of the capacity to generate tension and to shorten; the second is the duration of each. Viewed in terms of the time dependence of the force-velocity curve, therefore, it is possible to imagine that this relationship undergoes a series of changes that evolve throughout each contraction. We return to these time-dependent properties later in the chapter, after first re-examining the concepts of force and velocity in terms of our current understanding of their relationship to the known interaction between the contractile proteins.

CONTRACTILITY DEFINED IN TERMS OF INTERACTIONS
BETWEEN CONTRACTILE PROTEINS

The relationship between the biochemistry of the interaction between the contractile proteins and the energetics of muscular contraction was discussed at the end of Chapter 7. Here it was postulated that Hill's first state of the active points in muscle—that in which tension was generated—occurs when the actin-myosin interactions are in a state represented by the rigor complex (Fig. 7.10), i.e., where tension is generated but no energy is being liberated. The second state, in which the active points liberate chemical energy at their maximal intrinsic rate, corresponds to the rapid cycling of actin-myosin-ATP interactions which cause muscle shortening but in which no tension is being generated (Fig. 7.11). From this formulation it can be postulated that the two intercepts of the force-velocity curve, and thus myocardial contractility, can reflect entirely different aspects of the chemistry of the contractile proteins.

Myocardial contractility can be understood in terms of the preceding discussion to represent an expression of both the number and tension-generating capacity of the rigor complexes, and the maximal rate of energy liberation in the cyclic interactions between the contractile proteins and ATP. Changes in myocardial contractility therefore can arise from alterations in either or both of these properties. The complexity of these mechanisms is readily appreciated when one considers, for example, the many reactions involved in the interactions between the cross-bridges and the thin filament [Eq. (7.5)–(7.9)].

Changes in the number of rigor complexes are most readily explained as being due to gradations in the amount of calcium delivered to the contractile proteins for binding to troponin. Because each of the troponin complexes appears to determine the ability of seven actin monomers to participate in the contractile process (Chapter 6), variations in the amount of calcium released during excitation-contraction coupling (Chapter 9) are amplified approximately sevenfold in regulating the number of potential rigor complexes. Because the number of rigor complexes determines force under isometric conditions, where force is maximal and shortening velocity is zero, changes in P_0 can be most easily explained as being due to variations in the availability of Ca^{2+} for binding to troponin C during systole.

Mechanisms by which the tension-generating capacity of the rigor complex can be varied are theoretically possible but have not yet been identified experimentally. The recent discovery of a role for a Ca^{2+}-myosin interaction in mediating the activation of primitive muscles suggests that calcium may have a second role in the control of the contractile processes in mammalian muscle. This hypothesis stems from the finding that in certain invertebrate muscles the Ca^{2+}-receptor protein of the contractile apparatus is not troponin C (which is absent) but one of the myosin light subunits. It is thus possible that a second role exists for Ca^{2+} which is mediated by its binding to one of the light subunits of cardiac myosin. This hypothesis, which could explain the suggested ability of calcium

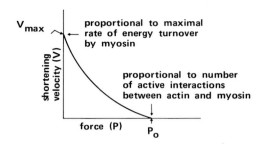

FIG. 10.4. The two intercepts of the force-velocity curve can be related to specific aspects of the interactions between the contractile proteins. As a first approximation, V_{max} is proportional to the rate of energy turnover by myosin while P_0 is proportional to the number of active interactions between actin and myosin.

to influence the intensity of the actin-myosin interaction, has not yet been critically tested. This possible mechanism for regulating myocardial contractility therefore represents both a major gap and a promising challenge in our present understanding of the interactions between the cardiac contractile proteins.

The maximal rate of energy liberation by the contractile proteins represents the other major parameter that determines the level of myocardial contractility. This property, which is correlated directly with maximal shortening velocity in a muscle at zero load, determines V_{max}, the other intercept of the force-velocity curve. Changes in this parameter can be most readily explained as being due to altered properties of the myosin molecule, possibly in the light subunits, because of the observed relationship between the structure of the myosin molecule and the absolute rates of both ATPase activity and maximal shortening velocity in the intact muscle (Chapter 6).

Two mechanisms that determine myocardial contractility were discussed in the preceding paragraphs. These can be related to the intercepts of the force-velocity curve shown in Fig. 10.4. In addition to the changes in these two properties of the contractile proteins (number of active points and their rate of interaction), alterations in the rate of activation and inactivation of the contractile process also can influence myocardial contractility.

Time-Dependent Effects

Each contraction in cardiac muscle, like each twitch in a skeletal muscle, has a characteristic rate of onset and termination. In the case of the heart, however, the slow onset of tension results primarily from the slow rate of activation, rather than a damping effect of the series elasticity. For this reason changes in the time

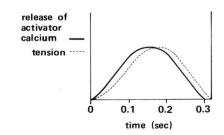

FIG. 10.5. The slow release of activator calcium *(solid line)* is partly responsible for the slow onset of tension *(dashed line)* in cardiac muscle.

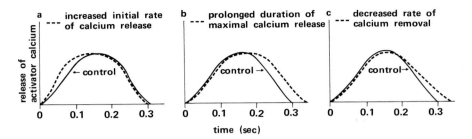

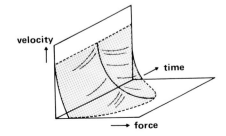

FIG. 10.6. Three ways in which time-dependent changes in the release of activator calcium can increase contractility in the absence of an increase in the maximal amount of activator calcium released. In each case the control curve represents the time course of calcium release during a control contraction (tension is not shown). More work can be performed in a contraction if: **(a)** the rate of activator calcium release is increased; **(b)** the duration of maximal activator calcium release is prolonged; or **(c)** the rate of activator calcium removal is reduced.

course of delivery of activator calcium and its removal can modify the ability of cardiac muscle to do work and thus change myocardial contractility (Fig. 10.5). One can imagine, for example, three types of change during this time course, any one or more of which would increase the work-generating capacity of the heart, even if the maximum number of active points (P_0) and the intrinsic rate of turnover of the active points (V_{max}) remained constant. These are: (a) an increased rate of delivery of activator calcium; (b) a prolonged duration of maximal activator calcium release; and (c) a reduced rate of activator calcium removal (Fig. 10.6). Conversely, a decline in myocardial contractility would occur if the rate of activator calcium delivery was decreased, the duration of its maximal release shortened, or the rate of its removal increased. It must be emphasized that these are only theoretical considerations, as evidence to define the time course of activator calcium release is not available. These potential changes in the time-dependent properties of activator calcium release must be considered, however, in any attempt to define the absolute level of myocardial contractility.

Force-Velocity-Time Relationships

Perhaps the easiest way to visualize the concept of the dependence of myocardial contractility on the number of active interactions between actin and myosin

FIG. 10.7. Three-dimensional graph showing the dependence on time (axis moving away from the reader) of a series of force-velocity curves in which V_{max} is constant *(dashed line on vertical axis)* while P_0 *(dashed line on horizontal axis)* rises and then falls during a single contraction. This graph shows the effect of the time-dependent changes in the amount of activator release during a single contraction in cardiac muscle.

(P_0), the rate of energy turnover at these active points (V_{max}), and their time dependence is as a three-dimensional graph (Fig. 10.7).

This graph was constructed with a constant V_{max} in view of the theoretical evidence that the velocity of shortening becomes maximal as soon as activator calcium reaches the contractile proteins (Chapter 7). According to Fig. 10.7, myocardial contractility would be described by the surface of the solid figure that defines the evolution of the force-velocity curve during each cardiac cycle. This area, which defines the time-dependent rise and fall of the force-velocity curve as well as its maximum, represents the total potential of the heart muscle to do work.

> Even the complex formulation of myocardial contractility shown in Fig. 10.7 is an oversimplification of our current understanding of myocardial contractility. At least two additional factors must be considered in this definition. The first is the length dependence of the active state, which causes a fall in both P_0 and V_{max} as contraction proceeds in the heart. Changes in sarcomere length occur even under isometric conditions where the ends of the muscle are fixed. These changes occur when muscle length is held constant because the elasticity of the cardiac muscle allows for some sarcomere shortening as the elastic elements are stretched. Because the heart normally functions at the apex or on the "ascending limb" of its sarcomere length-tension curve (Chapter 8), these length-dependent phenomena cause a decrease in P_0. In light of evidence that V_{max} declines when sarcomere length decreases in this region of the sarcomere length-tension curve, the length changes may also cause a progressive time-dependent fall in V_{max} (Fig. 10.8).
>
> A second complication to the analysis of myocardial contractility presented in Fig. 10.7 is the potential existence of internal resistance to shortening. Although the nature and extent of the resistance is now disputed, any such internal resistance would reduce the apparent shortening velocity, especially when the amount of activator release (and thus the number of active actin-myosin interactions) is small. Taking these length- and load-dependent changes in shortening velocity into consideration, a more accurate representation of myocardial contractility might be that shown in Fig. 10.9, in which both maximal force and maximal velocity are shown to vary with time. At this point our analysis of myocardial contractility has become so complex and involves so many unanswered questions it is of little practical use.

It should be apparent that a valid, and especially a practical, definition of myocardial contractility must now be regarded as being beyond our capabilities.

FIG. 10.8. Three-dimensional graph (constructed as in Fig. 10.7) showing a progressive decrease in V_{max} in addition to the time-dependent changes in P_0 shown in Fig. 10.7. The former is related to sarcomere shortening that occurs during each contraction in heart muscle.

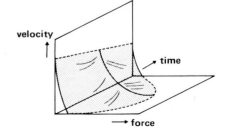

FIG. 10.9. Three-dimensional graph (constructed as in Figs. 10.7 and 10.8) showing a time-dependent initial increase in V_{max} in addition to the time-dependent changes in activator release and a decline in V_{max} later during the contraction. The former is due to the ability of the higher tension associated with greater activator release to overcome internal resistances to shortening. The surface of the solid figure represents the potential of the muscle to do work and so approximates the concept of myocardial contractility.

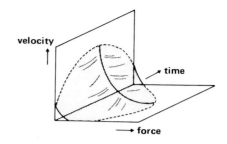

What should be remembered, however, is that the potential for the cardiac muscle to do work depends on at least four properties of the contractile element: *force, velocity, time,* and *length.* Lest the reader at this point despair of the utility of the concept of myocardial contractility, it is again emphasized that *changes* in myocardial contractility can be detected, and rather simply, as changes in the work capacity of cardiac muscle that are independent of muscle length. Furthermore, as becomes apparent in Chapters 12 and 13, approaches to such measurements are possible even in the heart of the intact animal or man. For this reason the material covered in this chapter should be held "in reserve" pending the development of more precise means to evaluate under physiological conditions the relationships between the biochemical and biophysical properties of the contractile machinery and their expression in the working heart *in situ.*

BIBLIOGRAPHY

Abbott, B. C., and Mommaerts, W. F. H. M. (1959): A study of ionotropic mechanisms in the papillary muscle preparation. *J. Gen. Physiol.,* 42:533–541.

Brady, A. J. (1974): Mechanics of the myocardium. In: *The Mammalian Myocardium,* edited by G. A. Langer and A. J. Brady, pp. 163–192. Wiley, New York.

Julian, F. J., and Moss, R. L. (1976): The concept of active state in striated muscle. *Circ. Res.,* 38:53–59.

Katz, L. N., chairman (1955): Symposium on the regulation of the performance of the heart. *Physiol. Rev.,* 35:89–168.

Parmley, W. W., Chuck, L., and Sonnenblick, E. H. (1972): Relation of V_{max} to different models of cardiac work. *Circ. Res.,* 30:34–43.

Pollack, G. H., and Krueger, J. W. (1976): Sarcomere dynamics in intact cardiac muscle. *Eur. J. Cardiol.,* 4(Suppl.):53–65.

11

Regulation of Myocardial Contractility

The central importance of changes in myocardial contractility in the physiological, pharmacological, and pathological responses of the heart has been indicated in a number of places in this book. This reliance of the heart on control mechanisms that are intrinsic to the myocardial cell provided the stimulus for a large body of research into the biochemistry of cardiac muscle and is largely responsible for the writing of this text. Much of the material already presented can be looked on as introductory to the present chapter, in which threads from the many topics already discussed are gathered in order to present a simplified and personal view of these important control mechanisms.

Two types of change in the biochemistry of cardiac muscle function have been postulated to participate in the regulation of myocardial contractility. Each corresponds theoretically to a shift in one of the intercepts of the force-velocity curve. A change in V_{max} would be expected to result from an alteration in the myosin molecule that would also be seen as a change in myosin ATPase activity *in vitro*. On the other hand, alterations in the amount of calcium released during excitation-contraction coupling would theoretically cause a change in the number of active interactions between the thick and thin filaments, and thus lead to an altered P_0. It is unfortunate that the early promise of cardiac muscle mechanics has not been realized, so that this hypothetical view of the biochemical basis for the control of cardiac contraction cannot be put to direct experimental test.

The concept that two types of mechanism participate in the control of myocardial contractility has significance beyond their potential role in shifting the force-velocity curve. Changes in myosin ATPase activity appear to represent a *tonic* form of control, in which changes in myocardial function evolve over a period measured in hours, days, or even longer, whereas changes in calcium delivery can occur from one beat to the next and so can represent a *phasic* control mechanism.

ALTERATIONS IN THE CARDIAC MYOSIN MOLECULE: A TONIC CONTROL MECHANISM

According to the theories described in the earlier chapters of this book, the maximal shortening velocity of the unloaded contractile element at any given fiber length is determined by the biochemical characteristics of the myosin molecule. Thus the rate-limiting step that determines the V_{max} of a muscle appears to be the same as that which is rate-limiting in the hydrolysis of ATP by the myosin isolated from that muscle. There is much circumstantial and some direct evidence that both of these rates are determined by the nature of the myosin molecule. For example, we have already seen how cross innervation of "fast" and "slow" skeletal muscles causes parallel changes in maximal shortening velocity, myosin ATPase activity, and the nature of the light subunits associated with the myosin molecule. These findings suggest that changes of the sort seen in the cross-innervated skeletal muscle arise from the synthesis of an altered myosin, i.e., a change in the expression of the genetic information in the cell. If this concept is correct, then changes of the sort described here require replacement of one population of myosin molecules with another. Because the turnover of cardiac myosin is slow, being measured in days, changes in myocardial contractility brought about by this means must evolve slowly. For this reason changes in myocardial function that arise from changes in the characteristics of the cardiac myosin molecule can be considered to reflect the operation of a *tonic* control mechanism.

A role for such a tonic mechanism in the regulation of cardiac function remains controversial, although changes analogous to those seen in cross-innervated skeletal muscles may occur in the myocardium in three general settings. The first is a change in endocrine balance. After hypophysectomy or in chronic hypothyroidism, where myocardial function is depressed, cardiac myosin ATPase activity has been found to be low; whereas in experimental hyperthyroidism myosin ATPase activity is high and myocardial contractility increased. A second condition in which this tonic control mechanism comes into play is in the aging heart, where a decrease in myosin ATPase has been reported to parallel depressed cardiac function. Thirdly, alterations in cardiac myosin ATPase activity have been described in hearts subjected to chronic hemodynamic overloading, where myocardial contractility is reduced (Chapter 21).

A decline in myocardial contractility caused by decreased myosin ATPase activity would reduce shortening velocity, especially at lighter loads. In addition to this deleterious hemodynamic effect, which in the intact heart would decrease the rate of ejection of blood, reduced myosin ATPase activity can increase mechanical efficiency, especially when the heart is contracting with high wall tension. This latter interpretation is based on comparisons between "fast" and "slow" skeletal muscles in which the latter have been found to use less ATP than fast muscles when shortening against heavy loads. (In contrast, fast muscles perform more efficiently when they contract at very light loads.) These differences probably represent an ontogenetic adaptation in which individual muscles contract more efficiently under the mechanical conditions they normally encounter: fast muscles during sprinting, slow muscles during sustained work. Slowing of cardiac contraction therefore may represent an adaptation either to an abnormally high, sustained demand for tension output or to an impairment of energy supply.

The mechanism by which altered enzymatic properties of myosin can influence the contractile properties of the intact muscle was discussed in Chapter 7, where the relationship between the rate-limiting step in cross-bridge movement and that of ATP hydrolysis was described. The apparent "energy-sparing" effect of slowing of this rate-limiting step may reflect a reduction in the rate at which the cross-bridge hydrolyzes ATP during the maintenance of tension. This interpretation can be understood in terms of the slow but significant turnover of cross-bridges during isometric contraction, an energy-consuming reaction that probably accounts for the "tension-time" heat: the $f(P,t)$ term in the energetic equations of Chapter 5 [e.g., Eqs. (5.5) and (5.6)]. As energy expenditure at high tensions appears to be proportional to the intrinsic rate of energy turnover by myosin, the appearance in muscle of a myosin with a low intrinsic rate of energy liberation would improve mechanical efficiency by decreasing the turnover rate of myosin cross-bridges and thus the tension-time heat generated during a sustained contraction. This energy-sparing effect, however, is accomplished at the expense of a reduction in myocardial contractility when the myocardium contracts against a light load. Conversely, when myocardial contractility is enhanced by the replacement of normal cardiac myosin with a high-ATPase myosin, the rapidity with which the heart can eject blood is increased. This effect, which results in enhanced myocardial contractility, also tends to increase energy wastage at high loads by increasing the tension-time heat.

The settings in which these tonic control mechanisms appear to operate illustrate the way in which cardiac muscle function is adapted to the needs of the body. In the hearts of the elderly, the appearance of a low-ATPase myosin has an energy-sparing effect in the face of the low demands for cardiac output usually seen in older persons. Similarly, in the chronically overloaded heart, where energy demands are increased, the synthesis of a low-ATPase myosin can improve the efficiency of the heart that must meet a high requirement for developed tension (Chapter 21). In the hyperthyroid state, on the other hand, replacement of the normal myosin with a high-ATPase myosin may represent a part of the adaptation to the increased heart rate and cardiac output that accompany hyperthyroidism. In this endocrinopathy, in contrast to most types of heart failure, the burden on the heart is an abnormally high ejection rate resulting from both a chronically increased heart rate and an increased cardiac output that is necessary to meet the abnormally high requirement for oxygen delivery to the body of the hyperthyroid individual.

There is now considerable evidence that changes in the myosin molecule can effect a tonic control of myocardial contractility by the mechanisms described above. Recent studies of developing fetal muscle point to the existence of changes in other proteins that, were they to occur in the myocardium, could contribute to this type of control mechanism. Such changes, which are seen in the troponin complex and in the calcium pump of the sarcoplasmic reticulum during development, have not yet been carefully sought in the abnormal heart, so that this represents a promising area of research into the mechanism of the tonic control of myocardial contractility.

ALTERATIONS IN CALCIUM DELIVERY TO THE CARDIAC CONTRACTILE PROTEINS: A PHASIC CONTROL MECHANISM

Changes in the amount of calcium made available for binding to the cardiac contractile proteins, unlike variations in the molecular characteristics of the contractile proteins, have the potential to modulate myocardial contractility on a beat-to-beat basis. For this reason phasic adjustments of the cardiac response to rapidly changing hemodynamic conditions can be effected at the cellular level by modulation of excitation-contraction coupling. These mechanisms, which can involve any of the processes that link excitation of the sarcolemma to the delivery of calcium for binding to troponin C, can effect abrupt increases or decreases in the pumping action of the heart (Chapters 12 and 13).

Variations in the proportion of troponin complexes in the myocardium which receive a calcium ion during excitation-contraction coupling would be expected to modify the number of active interactions between actin and myosin (Chapter 6). Such changes would cause variations in the number of force-generating sites that participate in systole and thus should cause a shift in maximum isometric tension (Chapter 7). At least on theoretical grounds, therefore, this phasic mechanism has the potential to shift P_0 of the force-velocity curve. Thus the predicted physiological expression of this phasic mechanism for the control of myocardial contractility differs strikingly from that of the tonic control mechanism described above.

Phasic changes in the intensity of the interactions between the contractile proteins can be brought about by: (a) alterations in the ability of calcium to bind to the troponin complex; (b) changes in the intracellular environment that affect the intensity of the interactions between the contractile proteins; and (c) variations in the amount of calcium released during excitation-contraction coupling.

Changes in Calcium Binding by the Troponin Complex

Alterations in the ability of troponin to bind calcium were recently suggested to participate in the increased myocardial contractility that is effected by agents which increase cyclic AMP production in the heart. This change in the calcium affinity of the calcium receptor of the contractile apparatus has been found in some studies to occur when the cyclic AMP-dependent protein kinase system is activated so as to phosphorylate the regulatory proteins of the myofibril. The proposed cascade of reactions (Chapters 3 and 9) that leads to altered calcium-binding properties of cardiac troponin is set into motion when catecholamines (e.g., epinephrine) interact with the β-receptor at the cell surface in a manner that stimulates sarcolemmal adenylate cyclase. The resulting increased cellular levels of cyclic AMP activate cyclic AMP-dependent protein kinases (as shown in Fig. 9.5), thereby leading to formation of phosphoester bonds in which the terminal phosphate group of ATP becomes attached to troponin I, one of the components of the troponin complex. A resulting decrease in the calcium affinity of the cardiac troponin complex appears to reduce the ability of the calcium released during excitation-contraction coupling to bind to troponin and thus to activate the contractile machinery of the heart. The physiological significance of this mechanism in the positive inotropic response of the heart to catecholamines remains unclear, although it does illustrate the way in which altered calcium binding by cardiac troponin is able to influence myocardial contractility.

Changes in the Intracellular Environment

For a number of years changes in the intracellular environment (besides those involving modulation of calcium release for binding to troponin, discussed later in this chapter) were thought to play a major role in the regulation of myocardial contractility. As evidence regarding these possible mechanisms accumulates, however, it has become apparent that control of contractility by such factors as varying intracellular potassium is of only minor physiological importance. Under certain pathological conditions changes in the intracellular concentrations of hydrogen ion (and under extreme conditions, ATP) may influence myocardial contractility.

Hydrogen Ion

The negative inotropic actions of acidosis have been recognized since the work of Gaskell in 1880. Studies of the effects of pH on the calcium sensitivity of actomyosin carried out during the late 1960s indicated that the curve defining the Ca^{2+} dependence of actomyosin ATPase and of the tension generated by certain actomyosin preparations *in vitro* was shifted to the right as pH was lowered in the physiological range. These data suggested that H^+ (by competing with Ca^{2+} for binding sites on troponin which lead to activation of the contractile process) can modulate tension development in the heart. Recently these experimental findings were challenged by the finding that only extremely high H^+ concentrations can displace Ca^{2+} from its binding to purified troponin C. However, there remain several lines of evidence to suggest that hydrogen and calcium ions compete for a physiological regulatory site on troponin C when it is present within the troponin complex. Thus the negative inotropic effect of acidosis now appears, at least in part, to reflect a direct effect of H^+ on the ability of the troponin complex to bind Ca^{2+}.

Potassium Ion

It is a well established fact that increased extracellular potassium ion concentration can reduce myocardial contractility. This effect, however, does not appear to be due to a direct effect of K^+ on the contractile process (see below). Instead, high extracellular K^+ probably exerts its negative inotropic effect by an effect to accelerate repolarization of the cardiac action potential, thereby shortening the duration of both the active state and the plateau of the action potential during which calcium is able to enter the cell (Chapter 14). Either or both of these consequences of high $[K^+]_0$ can explain the negative inotropic response to increased extracellular potassium concentration.

> The pioneering work of Albert Szent-Györgyi over a quarter of a century ago showed that high potassium ion concentration depressed the activity of contractile proteins studied *in vitro*. These observations, which reflect an action of increasing ionic strength to attenuate the interactions between actin and myosin (Chapter 6) were later correlated with changes in potassium fluxes that occur when cardiac muscle is subjected to various inotropic interventions. Although there is often a positive correlation between potassium loss and enhanced myocardial contractility, a number of recent studies indicate that this relationship is indirect. Furthermore, the total potassium loss is quite small and represents mainly exchange of intracellular potassium for sodium derived from the extracellular fluid, so that the ionic strength within the myocardium changes very little, if at all. The interactions of the contractile proteins, however, are only slightly sensitive to exchange of K^+ for Na^+, so that the observed changes in intracellular potassium ion concentration have little influence on the contractile proteins of the intact heart and probably are not directly involved in the modulation of myocardial contractility.

ATP

Recognition of the role of ATP in providing chemical energy for the contractile process suggests that ATP lack might directly impair myocardial performance in the overloaded heart. It remains probable that many changes in myocardial contractility, especially those which occur in response to situations resulting from an imbalance between energy production and energy utilization in the heart, are caused by lack of chemical energy (Chapter 22). However, ATP depletion itself lacks the ability to act directly on the contractile proteins in a manner that would depress myocardial contractility. This conclusion is based on many reports that high-energy phosphate contents, especially ATP, are not significantly lowered in the energy-depleted heart at a time when contractility is reduced (Chapter 22). Furthermore, besides its role to supply energy for contraction, ATP has a "plasticizing" effect on the contractile proteins, which requires even higher levels of the nucleotide than are needed to fuel contraction (Chapter 6). This "plasticizing" effect is essential for muscle relaxation, so that the initial effect of ATP depletion on the contractile proteins is to cause the heart to develop *rigor*. For example, rigor mortis in a skeletal muscle can be attributed to loss of the plasticizing effect of ATP. In view of the irreversible nature of rigor in the heart (Chapter 22), ATP lack is unlikely to be directly responsible for a decline in myocardial contractility in any but the most extreme situations. This conclusion, it must be stressed, does not mean that a relative deficiency in ATP supply is not responsible for other changes in regulatory function when the demand for chemical energy exceeds the ability of the myocardium to regenerate ATP.

Variations in the Amount of Calcium Released During Excitation-Contraction Coupling

Modulation of the processes of excitation-contraction coupling provides the basis for most of the important regulatory mechanisms that control myocardial contractility. These processes, which modulate calcium fluxes within the myocardial cell, have come to occupy a central position in our understanding of the important physiological, pharmacological, and pathological mechanisms which regulate the contractile performance of the heart. For this reason the material discussed in Chapter 9 is reconsidered at this point in an attempt to relate specific aspects of the processes of cardiac excitation to mechanisms by which varied delivery of calcium to the cardiac contractile proteins can control myocardial contractility.

Calcium derived from at least three pools can participate in modulating the intensity of excitation-contraction coupling (Fig. 11.1). The calcium pool of the *extracellular space* provides a source for calcium that can enter the cell to fill

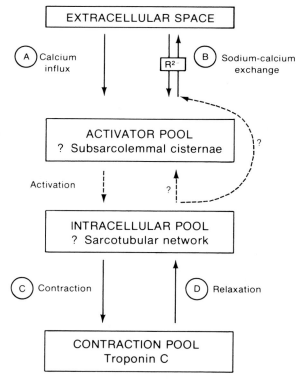

FIG. 11.1. Calcium fluxes that participate in cardiac excitation-contraction coupling (see legend to Fig. 9.2). Alterations in these calcium fluxes can modulate myocardial contractility in response to a variety of physiological, pharmacological, and pathological stimuli.

intracellular stores more immediately involved in activation of the contractile proteins. As already indicated, however, most of the calcium that enters the cell from the extracellular space does not participate directly in the initiation of contraction. Instead, this calcium plays a modulatory role in that it is involved in determining the amount of calcium made available for binding to troponin C. Thus the calcium which enters the cell from the extracellular space appears to contribute to the filling of an *intracellular pool* of activator calcium, probably located within the sarcoplasmic reticulum, possibly the sarcotubular network (Fig. 9.1). This intracellular pool serves as the direct source of the calcium that is made available for binding to troponin C, and thus for the initiation of cardiac systole. There is some evidence for a third pool of calcium which controls calcium release from the intracellular pool. This *activator pool* may be related to the subsarcolemmal cisternae of the sarcoplasmic reticulum (Fig. 9.1). The possibility that additional calcium pools exist within the myocardial cell is indicated by a number of isolated findings, but evidence for their existence remains incomplete. Because of the tenuous and controversial nature of these additional calcium pools, as well as for simplicity, the following discussion focuses only on three pools of calcium highlighted above.

The existence of three pools through which calcium can move to be delivered to, and removed from, the high-affinity calcium-binding sites on troponin C indicates that several calcium fluxes participate in the regulation of myocardial contractility. These calcium fluxes are outlined in Fig. 11.1.

In an attempt to provide a systematic, although in some places speculative, review of the relationship between these putative calcium fluxes and several important physiological, pharmacological, and pathological changes in myocardial contractility, two general mechanisms are considered: (a) altered calcium fluxes across the sarcolemma; and (b) alterations in the rates of calcium movement between intracellular pools.

Alterations in Calcium Fluxes Across the Sarcolemma

Changes in calcium fluxes across the sarcolemma (arrows *A* and *B,* Fig. 11.1) which would cause either a net gain or net loss of intracellular calcium have been implicated in a number of inotropic mechanisms. Most important of these are the positive staircase, postextrasystolic potentiation, the action of catecholamines, Na^+-Ca^{2+} competition, and the effects of cardiac glycosides.

Positive Staircase.

The positive staircase—also called treppe, Bowditch staircase, or the positive inotropic effect of activation (PIEA)—is named after Bowditch, who during the last quarter of the nineteenth century described these rate-dependent variations in the intensity of the contractile response of cardiac muscle.

It is fitting that Bowditch also described the "all-or-none" law, which states that as the intensity of stimulation is varied, an excitable tissue either does or does not respond to the stimulus, and that the intensity of the response is not determined by that of the stimulus. It is essential to recognize that even though changes in myocardial contractility represent variability in the mechanical response of the myocardium, they do not violate this fundamental property of excitable tissue because it is the intrinsic state of the myocardium and not the intensity of stimulation that is responsible for rate-dependent and other changes in myocardial contractility. In other words, changes in myocardial contractility do not violate the "all-or-none" law. Instead, they reflect variations in the amount of the "all."

While myocardial contractility is independent of the *intensity* of the stimulus, it is dependent on the *frequency* of stimulation. Thus Bowditch found that for any given frequency of stimulation a characteristic tension was developed (Fig. 11.2). At moderate to low heart rates, an increase in frequency causes tension to rise with each succeeding beat until a new plateau of tension is reached. This new and higher tension builds by a series of small steps (Fig. 11.2)—hence the designation staircase, or its German translation *treppe*. Conversely, a decrease in the frequency of stimulation causes the developed tension to decrease, so that each stimulation frequency is associated with a characteristic tension. Bowditch interpreted the greater tension seen when contractions came rapidly one after another to mean that each contraction leaves behind it a condition or substance that increases tension in the subsequent beat. At sustained high frequencies of stimulation this positive inotropic condition is assumed to build up to a new steady state, whereas when the frequency of stimulation is reduced this condition declines to a lower steady state.

For many years the positive staircase was believed to reflect a positive inotropic effect associated with the loss of potassium that occurred when the frequency of action potentials was increased at higher rates of stimulation. Although there is general agreement that increasing frequency of contraction causes a slight loss of potassium due to the greater number of action potentials per unit of time (Chapter 14), the correlation between loss of cellular potassium and the gain in contractility now appears to be indirect and not the manifestation of a causal relationship (see above). Instead, the positive staircase is probably caused by increased filling of intracellular calcium pools, most likely the result of an increase

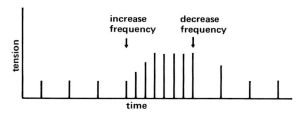

FIG. 11.2. The positive (Bowditch) staircase (Treppe). The tension developed by a strip of cardiac muscle during a series of isometric contractions (represented as vertical lines here and in Figs. 11.3, 11.9, and 11.10) increases in a stepwise manner after the frequency of stimulation is increased, and decreases when stimulation frequency is reduced.

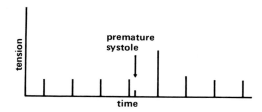

FIG. 11.3. Postextrasystolic potentiation. The tension developed during the first contraction following a premature systole ("extrasystole") is markedly potentiated. The positive inotropic state left behind by the premature systole decays slowly; it also potentiates slightly the tension developed during the second contraction after its occurrence in this example.

in the number of action potentials, each of which allows calcium to enter the myocardial cell. This explanation is based on evidence that calcium enters the cell with each systole (Chapter 14) and is pumped out during diastole. Because the relative amount of time spent during diastole decreases at higher contraction rates at the same time that the number of systoles is increasing, there is no difficulty in identifying a mechanism by which a net gain of intracellular calcium can account for the positive staircase.

Postextrasystolic Potentiation.

A special manifestation of the inotropic mechanism responsible for the positive staircase, postextrasystolic potentiation was once believed to hold considerable promise as an adjunct in the therapy of heart failure. The inotropic response during the beat following a premature systole (Fig. 11.3) is among the most intense seen in cardiac muscle. Even though this inotropic mechanism can be sustained by interposing a premature systole after every beat, for practical purposes the electrical stimulation needed to effect such "paired pulse stimulation" carries with it sufficient arrhythmogenic potential as to make this an exceedingly dangerous form of therapy (Chapter 17). Yet this inotropic mechanism has proved to be extremely useful in providing an understanding of the phasic control of myocardial contractility.

The tension developed by the contraction following a premature systole is markedly augmented (Fig. 11.3). The extent to which the following contraction is potentiated does not depend on the tension response in the premature systole; indeed, the positive inotropic effect of the premature systole is greater when its prematurity is such that it develops little or no tension. Marked potentiation of the tension response during the beat which follows the premature systole can be seen even when the latter comes so early as merely to delay relaxation of the preceding normal beat. This positive inotropic effect, like that seen in the positive staircase, is thus related to a change in the chemical properties of the myocardium that occur when two contractions follow each other in close succession.

The nature of the mechanism responsible for postextrasystolic potentiation was shown in a study carried out during the late 1960s by Wood, Hepner, and

Weidmann. Using intracellular electrodes, these investigators applied small currents across the cell membrane during systole (Fig. 11.4). These currents caused either slight depolarization or hyperpolarization at a time when the potential changes were unable to induce a regenerative action potential (the absolute refractory period; Chapter 14). Depolarizing currents (*1*, Fig. 11.4) caused membrane potential to become more positive (Chapter 14) but did not affect the tension during the systole when the currents were applied. The systole that followed the beat during which the depolarizing current was applied was markedly potentiated, however. Conversely, a hyperpolarizing current that tended to return membrane potential toward its resting level (*2*, Fig. 11.4) caused marked inhibition of tension during the subsequent beat, while having no effect on the contraction during which this current was applied. These findings are in accord with evidence that increased depolarization of the sarcolemma during or shortly after the end of the plateau of the cardiac action potential tends to promote calcium entry by way of the slow channel (Chapter 14). Conversely, lowering the membrane potential toward its resting level during the plateau phase of the cardiac action potential tends to reduce this calcium influx. These and other types of experiments also show that the calcium fluxes across the sarcolemma during systole have little influence on the tension developed by the contraction during which the currents flow, but do have marked effects on *subsequent* contractions. These experiments thus indicate that the calcium fluxes across the sarcolemma during systole contribute to a pool of calcium which becomes available for binding to troponin only during the subsequent contractions. Most of the calcium carried by the slow inward current therefore does not go directly to the contractile proteins. Instead, the calcium that enters the cell during systole contributes to

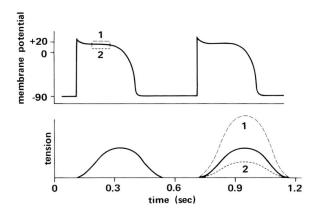

FIG. 11.4. Effects of altered membrane potential **(top)** on mechanical performance **(bottom)**. A depolarizing (1) or hyperpolarizing (2) electrical current which alters membrane potential only during the plateau of the cardiac action potential has no effect on tension developed during the contraction in which the current is applied. Tension developed in the subsequent contraction, however, is markedly increased following the depolarizing current (1) and markedly decreased following the hyperpolarizing current (2).

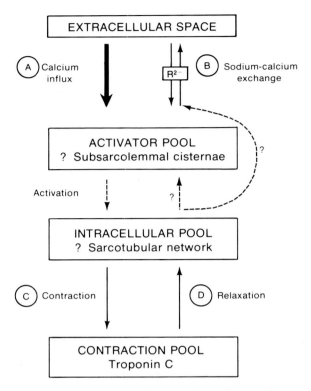

FIG. 11.5. Enhancement of myocardial contractility by an intervention that increases calcium influx via the slow inward current. The increased influx of calcium (A) probably augments tension during the subsequent contraction by increasing the calcium content of the activator pool and possibly by increasing the filling of the intracellular calcium pool which provides calcium for release to the contractile proteins.

an intracellular pool from which it is released only during subsequent contractions. In the context of the calcium movements shown in Fig. 11.1, the inotropic effects of depolarizing currents can be postulated to reflect an increase in calcium influx (Fig. 11.5). It is likely that a similar increase in calcium influx is brought about by premature systoles (postextrasystolic potentiation) and by an increased frequency of contraction (the positive staircase).

Catecholamines.

   Catecholamines and other agents that increase cyclic AMP levels in the cell probably act by modifying the gating mechanism which controls calcium entry during the slow inward current. Like the rate-dependent inotropic effects described above, the effect of these agents is to increase calcium influx across the sarcolemma (Fig. 11.5), possibly by increasing the number of calcium channels that open during the plateau of the action potential. The mechanism responsible for this effect remains poorly understood but may result from the phosphorylation of the sarcolemma by a cyclic AMP-dependent protein kinase (Chapter 9).

> There is evidence that the cardiac sarcolemma may be phosphorylated by cyclic AMP-dependent protein kinases, and that sarcolemmal phosphorylation is associated with a change in calcium binding by these membranes. These studies remain difficult to interpret, however, because of the low density of calcium transport sites in the sarcolemma, and because of the absence of measurable biochemical reactions that can be clearly attributed to the operation of the gating mechanism which controls the slow inward current.

Altered Extracellular Calcium and Sodium.

Altered extracellular concentrations of calcium and sodium have been known to influence myocardial contractility since the 1880s. At that time Ringer found that when distilled water was used to make up various salt solutions with which to perfuse the heart, the heart was often unable to contract. This finding, which

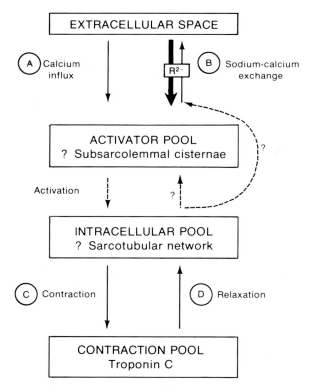

FIG. 11.6. Enhancement of myocardial contractility by an intervention that increases calcium influx via the sodium-calcium exchange mechanism. The increased influx of calcium (B) that occurs when extracellular Ca^{2+} is increased or when extracellular Na^+ is decreased allows greater filling of calcium stores within the myocardial cell.

contradicted earlier experiments in which contraction was regularly seen when tap water was used to make up the perfusate, led to a search for a trace substance in the tap water which sustained the heart's ability to develop tension. In a now classic study, Ringer analyzed the mineral content of the water obtained from the New River Water Company and found that of the many substances present in trace amounts it was the contaminating calcium salts that were essential for the heart to contract. It was subsequently shown that sodium salts had the ability to depress this contractile response. By the mid-1950s it had become apparent that the net effect of the opposing actions of these cations on myocardial contractility could be expressed by the following relationship:

$$\text{Contractility} \sim [Ca^{2+}]_o / [Na^+]_o{}^2 \qquad (11.1)$$

In other words, the tension developed by the heart depended not on the absolute concentrations of sodium or calcium in the fluid bathing the heart but on the ratio between these two cations. This finding can be interpreted to mean that these cations compete for a negatively charged receptor (R^{2-}), which can transport either one calcium or two sodium ions into the cell, and that the nature of the ion transported is determined by their relative concentrations in the extracellular fluid. Thus when calcium is carried into the cell contractility is increased, whereas the inward flux of sodium reduces contractility. The nature and characteristics of this anionic receptor are described in Chapter 9 (Fig. 9.2). In terms of the diagram in Fig. 11.1, this carrier can be considered to mediate calcium influx as shown in Fig. 11.6. It appears likely that the effects of extracellular Ca^{2+} and Na^+ on contractility reflect the operation of the sodium-calcium exchange mechanism described in Chapter 9, a mechanism that is distinct from that which controls the slow inward current.

Cardiac Glycosides.

The cardiac glycosides (e.g., digitalis), like the Bowditch staircase and postextrasystolic potentiation, appear to influence myocardial contractility through an action on calcium fluxes across the sarcolemma. The search for the mechanism of action of these drugs has been one of the classic quests in cardiovascular research. Ever since Withering concluded that the active ingredient in the herb tea prepared by Old Mother Hutton of Shropshire "could be no other than foxglove" *(Digitalis purpurea),* investigators have sought to understand the means by which this agent relieved the symptoms of congestive heart failure. With the advent of modern cardiac physiology it became clear that cardiac glycosides enhanced myocardial contractility. Subsequently attempts were made to explain the positive inotropic effects of these drugs in terms of an action on virtually every subcellular system of the myocardium as these were identified and characterized. In many cases the initial studies tended to suggest that the cardiac glycosides affected the system under study, whereas subsequent attempts to confirm the positive findings proved unsuccessful and attention shifted to the next system to be characterized.

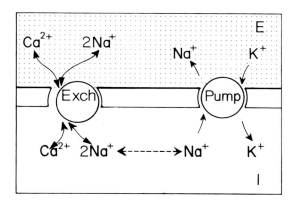

FIG. 11.7. Possible mechanism by which inhibition of the sodium pump enhances myocardial contractility. Inhibition of sodium efflux by way of the sodium pump *(right)* (e.g., by cardiac glycosides) increases the Na⁺ concentration in an intracellular space that also supplies Na⁺ to the sodium-calcium exchange mechanism *(left)*. The increased intracellular Na⁺ concentration reduces calcium efflux by competing with Ca²⁺ for binding to the intracellular site of this exchange mechanism. The resulting decrease in calcium efflux causes an increase in intracellular calcium stores.

There is now universal agreement that the cardiac glycosides inhibit the sodium pump of the sarcolemma. This ATP-dependent cation pump exchanges the sodium which enters the cell during the upstroke of the action potential for extracellular potassium, thereby maintaining the normal transcellular gradients of these two alkali metal ions (Chapters 9 and 14). The inhibitory effects of the cardiac glycosides can be readily seen in studies of the Na-K-ATPase, an enzyme believed to be derived from the sarcolemmal sodium pump.

Sodium pump inhibition and enhancement of myocardial contractility may be related through an effect of increased intracellular sodium concentration to decrease calcium efflux across the plasma membrane (Chapter 9). There is evidence that the sodium entering the cell during the upstroke of the action potential contributes to a subsarcolemmal sodium pool, where it competes with calcium for efflux by the sodium-calcium exchange mechanism. Thus under conditions where the sodium content of this subsarcolemmal pool is increased (e.g., sodium pump inhibition), less calcium is pumped out of the cell. A currently popular hypothesis regarding the mechanism of action of the cardiac glycosides states that these agents, by inhibiting sodium efflux via the sodium pump, cause intracellular sodium concentration to increase. The resulting accumulation of sodium increases the ability of this ion to compete with calcium for efflux via the sodium-calcium exchange that normally carries calcium out of the cell (Fig. 11.7). In this way cardiac glycoside-induced inhibition of sodium efflux can cause more sodium and less calcium to be carried out of the cell via the sodium-calcium exchange. The resulting reduction in calcium efflux results in an increased cellular content of calcium (Fig. 11.8). It should be stressed that this mechanism is not universally

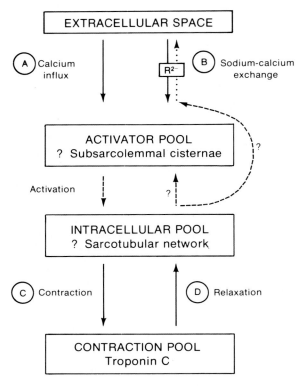

FIG. 11.8. Enhancement of myocardial contractility by an intervention that decreases calcium efflux via the calcium-sodium exchange mechanism. The decreased efflux of calcium (B) allows greater filling of intracellular calcium stores, but it is not known whether this calcium is retained in the activator pool, the intracellular calcium pool which supplies the contractile proteins, or both.

accepted as being responsible for the phasic increase in myocardial contractility brought about by the cardiac glycosides. It is possible, for example, that these agents augment calcium influx by increasing the slow inward current (Fig. 11.5).

The Negative Staircase

The phasic mechanisms for the control of myocardial contractility discussed up to this point appear to enhance tension by increasing the calcium content within the myocardial cell. These positive inotropic responses are believed to occur when the total cellular content of calcium is augmented either by increased calcium influx or decreased calcium efflux. Conversely, a reduction in myocardial contractility by these mechanisms would occur when the amount of calcium in the cell is decreased. At this point we consider a different type of inotropic effect. Unlike those already described, the effects discussed below can be attributed to changes in the *distribution* of calcium within the cell, rather than to changes in the *total content* of cellular calcium.

The complex relationships between stimulation frequency and myocardial contractility that can be explained most readily by retention of calcium in an inaccessible pool were described in 1902 by Woodworth. He observed a second staircase —one in addition to the positive staircase already described by Bowditch. The second staircase, in which tension was found to *decrease* as the rate increased, is called the *negative staircase,* the Woodworth staircase, or the negative inotropic effect of activation (NIEA). When it follows a decrease in stimulation frequency, the negative staircase causes a transient increase in tension. This latter manifestation of the negative staircase, which can heighten tension after a long diastole, is called the *recuperative effect of a pause.*

The negative (Woodworth) staircase is generally seen at higher stimulation frequencies than is the positive (Bowditch) staircase. The negative staircase therefore manifests as a fall in tension at an increased stimulation frequency and a rise in tension as the cardiac rate decreases (Fig. 11.9).

The rate changes that elicit a negative staircase also can cause concurrent changes in tension that are attributable to the positive staircase. The changes in tension produced by the negative staircase, however, evolve more rapidly than the positive staircase. As a result (Fig. 11.10), the first and possibly the second beat after an increase in stimulation frequency shows a decline in tension (*1,* Fig. 11.10). This rapidly evolving fall in tension, which represents the operation of the negative staircase, is then overcome by a more slowly developing enhancement of tension due to the positive staircase (*2,* Fig. 11.10). Similarly, the recuperative effect of a pause (also a manifestation of the negative staircase—in this case an enhancement of tension seen when stimulation frequency is decreased) causes an increase in the tension developed by the first beat following a reduction in stimulation frequency. This manifestation of the negative staircase is shown as *3* in Fig. 11.10. Again, this positive inotropic effect of the negative staircase is overcome as tension declines owing to the slower disappearance of the positive

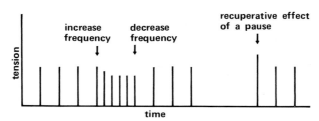

FIG. 11.9. The negative (Woodworth) staircase. The tension developed by a strip of cardiac muscle during a series of isometric contractions decreases during the first few beats after the stimulation frequency is increased, and increases when the stimulation frequency is decreased. The effects of the positive staircase, which usually develops concurrently, are not shown here. Another manifestation of the negative staircase is the recuperative effect of a pause *(right)* in which the tension developed during the first beat after stimulation of the muscle is interrupted shows potentiation of tension.

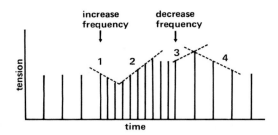

FIG. 11.10. Simultaneous evolution of the positive and negative staircases. The initial response to an increase in the frequency of stimulation is a transient fall in tension (1, the negative staircase), which is then overcome by a rise in tension associated with the more slowly evolving positive staircase (2). Similarly, the initial response to a decrease in stimulation frequency is a transient rise in tension (3, the negative staircase) followed by a fall in tension as the effects of the positive staircase wear off (4).

staircase which, as discussed earlier, causes tension to decline as stimulation frequency is decreased (*4*, Fig. 11.10; see also Fig. 11.2).

The rapidly developing inotropic effects of the negative staircase may be due to trapping of calcium in an inaccessible intracellular pool from which it cannot be released to bind to troponin. This hypothesis is attractive as the rapid time course of the negative staircase is easily explained as the result of an altered distribution of calcium between intracellular pools, in contrast to the more slowly developing positive staircase, which is now believed to result from movements of calcium between the inside and outside of the cell. A relatively slow transport of calcium from a relaxation site to an excitation site could, when stimulation frequency is increased, cause calcium stores in the latter to become depleted. As a result, less calcium would be available at the excitation site for release to the contractile proteins. Conversely, a pause or reduction in stimulation frequency would allow calcium accumulated in the relaxation site to flow in increased amounts to the excitation site, thereby augmenting tension in subsequent contractions. Another equally plausible explanation for the negative staircase is that the recovery of the ability of calcium channels in the sarcoplasmic reticulum to open is so slow that at high stimulation frequencies calcium permeability does not reach its maximum. In this way, calcium efflux from the sarcoplasmic reticulum would be reduced at high heart rates (Fig. 11.11). Regardless of the mechanism, the effects of the negative staircase are eventually overwhelmed by opposing rate-dependent changes in calcium fluxes across the sarcolemma (the positive staircase). In the case of an increase in rate, the augmented filling of the sarcoplasmic reticulum by the calcium influx shown in Fig. 11.5 ultimately overcomes the effects of reduced calcium release and so increases the quantity of calcium available for release to troponin C. Conversely, the increased calcium release from internal stores that occurs during the recuperative effect of a pause (also a manifestation of the negative staircase) is eventually overcome when, at lower stimulation frequencies, the excess calcium flows out of the cell.

It should be emphasized that the present analysis of force-frequency relation-

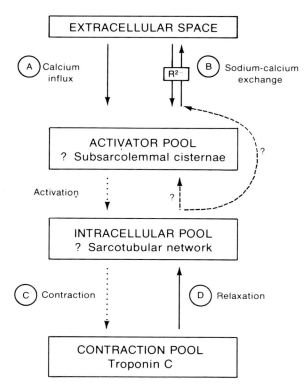

FIG. 11.11. Reduction of myocardial contractility by an intervention that decreases calcium efflux from the intracellular pool. The negative staircase which accompanies increased stimulation frequency can be attributed to decreased calcium flux (C) that results from trapping of calcium in an inaccessible site in the sarcoplasmic reticulum or from slow recovery of the ability of this structure to release calcium following the preceding contraction.

ships such as those illustrated in Fig. 11.10 remains somewhat conjectural. These interpretations fit well with several indirect lines of evidence regarding the control of calcium fluxes within the cell, but many gaps in our knowledge remain to be filled, especially regarding the genesis of the negative staircase.

Changes in the Rates of Intracellular Calcium Fluxes

The functional significance and possible mechanism of the control of the ATP-dependent calcium pump of the sarcoplasmic reticulum by the cyclic AMP-protein kinase system were discussed at some length in Chapter 9. Accelerated calcium removal from troponin C caused by an increased rate of calcium transport into the relaxation site can be shown to be initiated by the cyclic AMP-protein kinase system according to the reaction scheme shown in Fig. 9.5. The resulting acceleration of relaxation partly explains the abbreviation of systole that

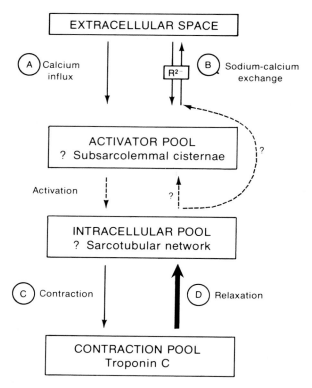

FIG. 11.12. Acceleration of myocardial relaxation by an intervention that activates the calcium pump of the sarcoplasmic reticulum. The resulting increased rate of calcium removal from the cytosol (D) accelerates the rate at which calcium is dissociated from its binding sites on troponin. Stimulation of the calcium pump may also increase calcium stores in the intracellular pool.

accompanies the cardiac response to catecholamines, e.g., epinephrine (Fig. 11.12). In addition to accelerating relaxation, the effects of phosphorylation of phospholamban in the sarcoplasmic reticulum may contribute to the inotropic response to catecholamines because phosphorylation of the sarcoplasmic reticulum appears to increase the Ca^{2+} affinity of the calcium pump. The resulting increase in the Ca^{2+} gradient across this membrane system would allow more calcium to be retained within the sarcoplasmic reticulum during diastole, thereby leading to enhanced contractility by providing more calcium for release during subsequent systoles.

The mechanisms by which myocardial contractility is controlled undoubtedly include many additional factors not discussed in this chapter. Furthermore, some of the interpretations presented in the preceding pages are based on incomplete and often contradictory findings. It is hoped that the reader excuses the errors of both omission and commission that have inevitably crept into this chapter.

It seems appropriate to attempt to systematize our knowledge of this subject if only to enhance our ability to absorb the significance of new experimental findings and new approaches to these important cellular control mechanisms.

BIBLIOGRAPHY

Awan, M. Z., and Goldspink, G. (1972): Energetics of the development and maintenance of isometric tension by mammalian fast and slow muscles. *J. Mechanochem. Cell Motil.,* 1:97–108.

Katz, A. M. (1965): The descending limb of the Starling curve and the failing heart. *Circulation,* 32:871–875.

Langer, G. A. (1972): Effects of digitalis on myocardial ionic exchange. *Circulation,* 46:180–187.

Ray, K. P., and England, P. J. (1976): Phosphorylation of the inhibitory subunit of troponin and its effects on the calcium dependence of cardiac myofibril adenosine triphosphatase. *FEBS Lett.,* 70:11–16.

Reuter, H. (1974): Exchange of calcium ions in the mammalian myocardium: Mechanisms and physiological significance. *Circ. Res.,* 34:599–605.

Swynghedauw, B., Léger, J. J., and Schwartz, K. (1976): The myosin isozyme hypothesis in chronic heart overloading. *J. Mol. Cell. Cardiol.,* 8:915–924.

Wollenberger, A. (1975): The role of cyclic AMP in the adrenergic control of the heart. In: *Contraction and Relaxation in the Myocardium,* edited by W. G. Nayler, pp. 113–190. Academic Press, New York.

Wood, E. H., Hepner, R. L., and Weidmann, S. (1969): Inotropic effects of electric currents. *Circ. Res.,* 24:409–445.

Woodworth, R. S. (1902): Maximal contraction, "staircase" contraction, refractory period, and compensatory pause of the heart. *Am. J. Physiol.,* 8:213–249.

12

The Heart as a Muscular Pump

Cardiac action is usually measured in hemodynamic terms (e.g., stroke volume, cardiac output, and blood pressure), but it should not be forgotten that these hemodynamic effects are manifestations of the processes of muscular contraction. In skeletal and isolated cardiac muscle preparations (e.g., papillary muscle), contractile behavior is described in terms of tension development and changes in muscle length. Similarly, during the pumping of the heart, the muscle fibers in the walls of the ventricles develop tension and undergo shortening. Yet as an organ the heart generates *pressure* not *tension;* and the shortening of its muscular fibers is manifest as the ejection of a *volume* of blood rather than *shortening* while bearing a load. During contraction of the myocardial fibers in the intact heart, therefore, changes in force and muscle length are transformed into changes in pressure and volume.

WORK DIAGRAM

During each cardiac cycle the walls of the ventricle undergo a sequence of changes in tension and length. These changes can most simply be understood by first examining the changing mechanical state in an afterloaded skeletal muscle, i.e., a muscle in which the load is not initially borne by the resting muscle. Such an afterloaded contraction can be divided into five phases (Fig. 12.1).

At rest the muscle is not bearing the load, which rests on a support such as a table top. During *isometric contraction* (A, Fig. 12.1) the muscle has not yet developed enough tension to lift the load so the muscle does not shorten. When active tension equals the load, the muscle begins to shorten, causing the load to be lifted during an *isotonic contraction* (B, Fig. 12.1). At the end of the isotonic contraction the muscle begins to relax. Initially the muscle lengthens while still holding the load. During this period of *isotonic relaxation* (C, Fig. 12.1) the load returns to its original position on the tabletop. Subsequently the muscle dissipates its tension during *isometric relaxation* (D, Fig. 12.1). From these analyses one can construct a "work diagram" that defines the conditions of force and length during the contraction cycle just described (Fig. 12.2).

This work diagram shows four phases: two of contraction (A, isometric contraction; and B, isotonic contraction) and two of relaxation (C, isotonic relaxation; and D, isometric relaxation). Because contraction and relaxation take place under identical conditions of loading, the curves for contraction and relaxation are superimposed.

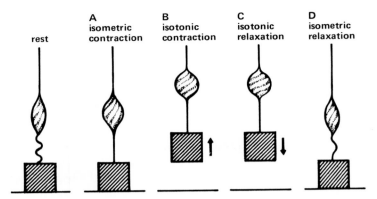

FIG. 12.1. Cycle of contraction and relaxation in an afterloaded skeletal muscle. At rest the load is not borne by the muscle but rests on a support. During isometric contraction (A) the tension within the muscle rises until it equals the load, after which the load is lifted during an isotonic contraction (B). Relaxation is initially isotonic, during which the load is lowered to the support (C). When the load reaches the support, isometric relaxation (D) begins and continues until the tension within the muscle falls to zero.

Suppose that instead of relaxing under the same loading conditions present during contraction the muscle was relieved of its load at the end of the period of shortening (*B*, Fig. 12.1). The load on the muscle would then fall to zero prior to lengthening, so that the phase of isometric relaxation would precede the return to initial length. Subsequently the muscle would lengthen at zero load. Under these conditions the work diagram would resemble that in Fig. 12.3. This diagram is analogous to that of the heart, which relaxes at almost zero load because closure of the semilunar (aortic and pulmonic) valves disengages the load (i.e., pressure in aorta and pulmonary artery) from the ventricles.

The work diagram of the heart shown in Fig. 12.4 for the left ventricle is generally similar to that shown in Fig. 12.3 except for several important differences. The first is that the ordinate and abscissa represent pressure and volume rather than load and length. Although pressure and volume in the ventricle are

FIG. 12.2. Work diagram of the contraction-relaxation cycle depicted in Fig. 12.1: isometric contraction (A); isotonic contraction (B); isotonic relaxation (C); and isometric relaxation (D). The curves for contraction and relaxation, which are in fact superimposed, have been separated in this figure for clarity.

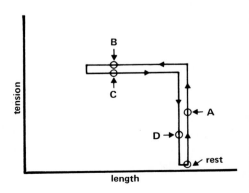

FIG. 12.3. Work diagram of a muscle from which the load is disengaged prior to relaxation. Isometric contraction (A) and isotonic contraction (B) occur as in the afterloaded contractions depicted in Figs. 12.1 and 12.2. However, the load is removed from the muscle just before it begins to relax so muscle tension falls to zero during isometric relaxation (C), after which the muscle lengthens (isotonic relaxation; D) at zero load.

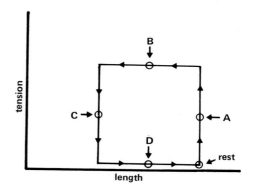

analogous to load and length, they are not the same (see below). Yet for the purposes of this illustration the analogy is sufficiently close to permit a useful comparison between the work diagram of the left ventricle (Fig. 12.4) and that of skeletal muscle (Fig. 12.3).

The second difference between the work diagrams of skeletal muscle and the left ventricle is the condition of loading at the start of contraction. The left ventricle begins to contract not at zero load but with a measurable end-diastolic pressure, so that to a small but significant extent ventricular contraction is *preloaded*. As the left ventricle develops tension, the mitral valve closes and until

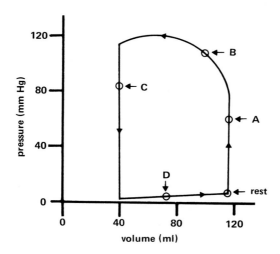

FIG. 12.4. Work diagram of the left ventricle. Unlike the contraction depicted in Fig. 12.3, a small preload is borne by the resting muscle at the onset of contraction (rest). Isovolumic contraction (A) proceeds until the venticle begins to empty (ejection, B), after which pressure rises and then falls. Closure of the aortic valve at the end of systole removes the load (i.e., aortic pressure) from the ventricle, so the initial phase of relaxation occurs under isovolumic conditions (C). When left ventricular pressure falls below that in the left atrium, intraventricular pressure rises as the atrium empties into the ventricle (D).

the aortic valve opens contraction is *isovolumic* (i.e., there is no change in volume). The term isometric contraction as applied to this phase of systole is a misnomer as the shape of the left ventricle changes: The apex-base diameter shortens and the circumference increases, giving a more rounded contour to the cavity. When left ventricular pressure exceeds that in the aorta, the aortic valve opens and *ejection* begins. Although aortic pressure rises and then falls, the actual tension on the walls of the left ventricle decreases throughout ejection owing to the operation of the law of Laplace (see below). At the end of systole, when the ventricular myocardium begins to relax, aortic valve closure marks the end of the period of ejection. By preventing the load (the aortic pressure) from acting on the left ventricle during relaxation, the aortic valve relieves the ventricular myocardium of its afterload during the subsequent phases of relaxation. As a result, the initial phase of ventricular relaxation, like that of the skeletal muscle contraction shown in Fig. 12.3, takes place at zero load. Because there is no volume change (both inflow and outflow being prevented by valve closure), this initial phase of ventricular relaxation is one of *isovolumic relaxation*. Like isovolumic contraction, isovolumic relaxation is associated with shape changes in the ventricle and so is not isometric. When pressure in the left ventricle falls below that in the left atrium, blood begins to flow into the ventricle during the period of *filling*. This influx of blood from the left atrium generates the preload for the next contraction. The events in the right ventricle are similar during the cardiac cycle.

The comparison between Figs. 12.3 and 12.4 is valid only in general terms since the skeletal muscle contraction is characterized by changes in length and tension whereas that of the ventricle is measured as changes in volume and pressure. While volume is not the same as length, it is related to length; similarly, pressure is not the same as tension, although the two entities are closely related.

VOLUME AND LENGTH: A GEOMETRIC RELATIONSHIP

The relationship between length and volume is determined by the laws of geometry. In a sphere, for example, volume is defined by the equation:

$$V = \frac{4}{3}\pi R^3 \tag{12.1}$$

where V = volume and R = radius. Because the circumference is equal to $2\pi R$, volume is also related to the third power of circumference, so that a 50% reduction of the circumference of a sphere is accompanied by a reduction in volume to one-eighth its original value.

The complex architecture of the ventricles, and especially that of the left ventricle, can be represented as an ellipsoid in which D_A, D_L, and L_M are, respectively: anterior-posterior diameter, lateral diameter, and maximal length (Fig. 12.5). The left ventricle is not truly ellipsoidal, however, so that utilization of D_A, D_L, and L_M (which are shown for orientation in Fig. 12.5) also involves a

FIG. 12.5. Outline of the cavity of the left ventricle during diastole in anteroposterior and lateral projections. The volume of the ventricle can be approximated by assuming its cavity to be an ellipse whose long axis is L_M and whose short axes are D_A and D_L.

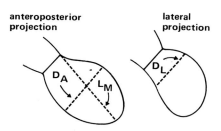

anteroposterior projection   lateral projection

number of assumptions. The estimated lengths D_A, D_L, and L_M can be then used in the equation for the volume of an ellipse to estimate left ventricular volume:

$$V = \frac{4}{3}\pi \left(\frac{D_A}{2}\right) \times \left(\frac{D_L}{2}\right) \times \left(\frac{L_M}{2}\right) \qquad (12.2)$$

Other methods for determining the left ventricular volume are also used in clinical cardiology but are beyond the scope of this text. These complex relationships should not obscure the fact that relatively small changes in ventricular fiber length produce proportionately much greater changes in volume.

PRESSURE AND TENSION: LAW OF LAPLACE

The relationship between the tension in the walls of the ventricle and the pressure within its cavity (intraventricular pressure) is as complex as the relationship between the circumference of the ventricle and its volume. *Tension* is the force exerted along a line (e.g., dynes per centimeter), whereas *pressure* is the force that acts on a surface (e.g., dynes per square centimeter). The units used for measurement of pressure in cardiovascular hemodynamics are usually millimeters of mercury or centimeters of water. These units represent the height of a column of mercury or water that exerts the corresponding force per unit of surface area. The conversions of these hemodynamic terms to gram-centimeter-second units are given in Table 12.1.

Like the relationship between length and volume, that between tension and pressure is influenced by the size and shape of the ventricle. Those relationships are defined by the law of Laplace, which takes into account the radius of curvature of the ventricular walls in the interconversions of pressure and wall tension. In its simplest form, as applied to a cylinder having infinitely thin walls, the law

TABLE 12.1. *Units of pressure*

Unit	Dynes/cm²
1 mm Hg	1,330
1 cm H₂O	980

FIG. 12.6. The law of Laplace. The tension on the walls of a thin-walled cylinder *(T)* is equal to the pressure with the cylinder *(P)* × the radius of curvature *(R)*.

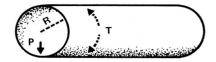

of Laplace states that wall tension is equal to the pressure within the cylinder times the radius of curvature of the wall:

$$T = P \times R \tag{12.3}$$

where T = wall tension (e.g., dynes per centimeter), P = pressure (e.g., dynes per square centimeter), and R = radius (e.g., centimeters) (Fig. 12.6). This relationship states that *wall tension at any given pressure increases as the radius of the cylinder increases and vice versa.* One application of the law of Laplace is seen in the tank trucks used to transport fluids and gases under pressure (Fig. 12.7). In order to minimize the hazard of bursting, tanks subject to high internal pressures are constructed with smaller radii of curvature than are tanks which carry material at low pressures. Similarly, in the ventricle the tension on the walls increases as ventricular chamber volume increases, even when the intraventricular pressure remains constant.

The tendency of a tank to burst can also be reduced by increasing the thickness of its walls. In the heart with thickened ventricular walls, wall tension is distributed over a larger number of muscle fibers, thereby reducing tension on each. The equation defining the operation of the law of Laplace in a thick-walled cylinder is written:

$$T = \frac{P \times R}{h} \tag{12.4}$$

where h = wall thickness. [T in Eq. (12.4) is, more correctly, a *stress*, i.e. the force exerted across an area.] As the geometry of the ventricles is more complex than that of a cylinder (see, for example, Fig. 12.5) ventricular wall tension cannot

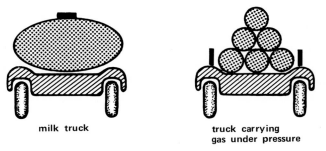

milk truck

truck carrying
gas under pressure

FIG. 12.7. A practical application of the law of Laplace. In a truck carrying gas under high pressure *(right)* several cylindrical tanks, each having a very short radius of curvature, are used. A single tank with a large radius of curvature is used in a milk truck, where the pressure within the tank is low *(left)*.

be measured with precision. A number of complex formulas used to approximate this parameter are beyond the scope of this text.

The complexity of the relationship between the geometry of the ventricular cavity and the tension on its muscular walls should not obscure two fundamental facts. The first is that dilation of the ventricles leads directly to an increase in the tension on each muscle fiber in its walls. This follows both from the law of Laplace [Eq. (12.3)], which defines a direct relationship between the diameter of a hollow organ and the tension on its walls at any given pressure, and from the thinning of the walls of the ventricle which occurs as the heart dilates. Referring to Eq. (12.4), ventricular dilation increases wall tension T, even when intraventricular pressure P is constant, both by increasing the radius R and decreasing the wall thickness h. The second major consequence of these geometric and physical laws is that an increase in wall thickness reduces the tension on any individual muscle fiber. Hence ventricular hypertrophy in the overloaded heart serves not only to increase the number of active sarcomeres but reduces the load on each by distributing tension among a greater number of muscle fibers. Both of these considerations are of central importance in understanding the impact of disease on the heart (Chapter 21).

Tension is not distributed uniformly in all layers of the muscular walls of the heart. This is especially true in the thick-walled left ventricle. Analyses of the properties of a series of concentric spheres enclosing a cavity under pressure show that the tension is highest near the *inner* surface. (At first glance this may appear to contradict the law of Laplace, which states that for an infinitely thin sphere tension is greater as diameter increases. There is, however, no contradiction as the present discussion is concerned with the *distribution* of tension within the thick-walled organ.) In the heart, therefore, the endocardial regions of the ventricular walls contract against higher tension than the epicardial regions. This fact accounts, at least in part, for the greater vulnerability of the endocardial regions of the left ventricle to the detrimental effects of the increased tension which accompanies a sudden increase in intraventricular pressure. Because of the higher tensions developed in the endocardial region of the ventricle this region is more vulnerable to reduction of coronary flow. (Another reason for the vulnerability of the endocardial regions to imbalances between energy demands and energy supply is the relatively lower inflow of arterial blood. This occurs because the coronary arteries penetrate the ventricles from the epicardium and so must traverse a greater distance of contracting myocardium to supply the endocardial portion of the ventricles; see Chapter 1.)

END-DIASTOLIC VOLUME AS A DETERMINANT OF VENTRICULAR FUNCTION: FRANK-STARLING RELATIONSHIP AND STARLING'S LAW OF THE HEART

The relationship between the volume of blood in the ventricles at the moment they begin to contract (the *end-diastolic volume*) and the systolic pressure developed by the ventricle was first described in 1895 by Frank and later more completely in the mammalian heart by Starling in 1914. This relationship, which is

FIG. 12.8. The Frank-Starling relationship (Starling's law of the heart). The systolic pressure developed during isovolumic contraction at any of a series of end-diastolic volumes *(vertical arrows)* increases with increasing end-diastolic volume. At very large end-diastolic volumes, systolic pressure declines with increasing end-diastolic volume.

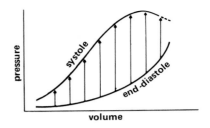

a manifestation of the length-tension relationship already described for skeletal muscle, is referred to either as the *Frank-Starling relationship* or *Starling's law of the heart.* The operation of this physiological law is most clearly seen when a balloon placed within the left ventricle is filled with different volumes of an incompressible fluid such as saline. As the volume of the balloon is increased, both diastolic and systolic pressures vary as a function of end-diastolic volume (Fig. 12.8). The pressure and volume at the end of diastole are increased directly by filling of the balloon. As end-diastolic volume increases, the pressure developed during systole first increases then decreases as a result of the operation of the Frank-Starling relationship. The arrows in Fig. 12.8 connecting values of end-diastolic pressure to pressures at the end of systole, which represent developed or "active" pressure, are vertical because the balloon filled with incompressible fluid precludes any volume change; i.e., the ventricle is contracting under *isovolumic* conditions. If these net pressures developed during systole (i.e., systolic pressure *minus* diastolic pressure) are plotted as a function of the end-diastolic volume, a curve (often called the Starling curve) is obtained that is reminiscent of the length-tension diagram of skeletal muscle (Fig. 12.9).

The curves shown in Figs. 12.8 and 12.9 differ from the length-tension diagrams of skeletal muscle in two important respects: First, the diagrams in Figs. 12.8 and 12.9 deal with volume and pressure, not length and tension. Second, increasing ventricular volume causes the development of relatively high resting tension, manifest in Fig. 12.8 as a high end-diastolic pressure. This resistance to stretch represents a *low diastolic compliance,* a general property of cardiac muscle that is also seen in studies with simpler papillary muscle preparations (Chapter 8).

The intrinsic resistance of cardiac muscle to stretch, along with the noncompliant pericardium, can restrict extreme dilation of the ventricle, thereby serving

FIG. 12.9. The ascending and descending limbs of the Starling curve. The rise of systolic pressure that results from increased end-diastolic volume constitutes the ascending limb of the Starling curve; a fall in systolic pressure as volume is increased further, at very high end-diastolic volumes is the descending limb of this curve.

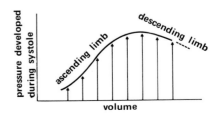

to protect the ventricle from overfilling. It is in fact very unlikely that the normal ventricle can dilate to the point where it enters on the "descending limb" of the Starling curve (Fig. 12.9). This phenomenon is extremely important because operation of a ventricle on this descending limb would represent a *negative feedback* in which an increased preload (manifest as increased end-diastolic volume) would reduce the pumping ability of the ventricle. As a result, the response to an increased load in the heart operating on the descending limb of the Starling curve would be a decrease in work performance. This situation represents a highly unstable state because when decreasing work performance reduces the pumping action of the ventricle, it increases the preload because the ventricle becomes less able to be empty. Operation of the ventricle in the face of the negative feedback of the descending limb thus provides the setting for a vicious cycle from which the heart has no simple means of recovery. This situation is quite different from that in a skeletal muscle, which, even if it comes to operate on the descending limb of its length-tension curve, has synergistic muscles that can reverse any negative feedback. Furthermore, unlike the heart, skeletal muscle does not itself determine the preload, so that functioning of a skeletal muscle on the descending limb of its length-tension curve does not necessarily increase the load on the muscle at the start of the next contraction.

The heart normally operates on the ascending limb of the Starling curve of the developed pressure-volume curve (Fig. 12.9), a situation in which increasing load enhances the ability of the ventricle to develop pressure and thus to empty itself. This follows because the enhanced ability to develop tension that results from an increased end-diastolic volume is translated into an increased ability to eject blood. The ascending limb of the Starling curve thus allows the heart either to increase ejection pressure, increase stroke volume, or both when end-diastolic volume is increased. The exact way in which this increased potential to do work is translated into an actual increase in work performance depends on the hemodynamics of the circulation (Chapter 13).

Basis for the Frank-Starling Relationship

The similarity between the Frank-Starling relationship of the heart (Fig. 12.9) and the length-tension relationship of a skeletal muscle suggests that both reflect the operation of a single mechanism. In view of the current uncertainties regarding the mechanism of the length-tension curve in cardiac muscle (Chapter 8), it is not possible to provide a clear explanation for the Frank-Starling relationship in the intact heart. It is clear, however, that the latter reflects, at least in part, the shape of the sarcomere length-tension relationship in cardiac muscle. This resembles that of skeletal muscle except that in the heart extremely high resting tensions are required to stretch the sarcomeres to lengths which put them on their descending limb. The ability of the heart to increase its work performance in response to an increased load while on the ascending limb of the Starling curve therefore reflects a property intrinsic to the sarcomeres. The mechanism responsible for the intrinsic resistance of cardiac muscle to overstretching, which is also expressed in the low resting compliance of the heart, remains unknown.

In addition to the sarcomere length-tension curve, there is another mechanism that can account for the ascending limb of the Starling curve. It is based on the fact that not all muscle fibers in the walls of the ventricle run in a circumferential direction (Fig. 1.3). Because of the branching of myocardial fibers, the longitudinal axes of many fibers are not parallel to the axis of shortening (Fig. 12.10). As a result, the force vectors generated by the fibers that are not parallel to the axis of shortening (b, Fig. 12.10) are only partially effective in generating tension. Stretching the branched fibers tends to increase the extent to which the fibers become parallel to the axis of shortening, allowing a greater portion of the tension developed by the nonparallel fibers (b, Fig. 12.10) to be available for generating pressure in the ventricle, even if there is no increase in the intrinsic ability of the fiber to develop tension. In addition to providing a partial explanation for the ability of increased end-diastolic volume to increase pressure development by the heart, this mechanism illustrates one factor which contributes to the relatively low cardiac efficiency. That component of the force vector which is not parallel to the axis of shortening does not contribute to the ejection of blood, but serves only to deform the wall of the ventricle during systole. When the ventricle relaxes, the latter energy reappears as heat and thus represents a "wastage" which reduces overall efficiency (Chapter 13).

The significance of this possible mechanism for the Frank-Starling relationship is not fully known. In some cardiac muscle preparations a large number of fibers have been found to be "wavy," so that reorientation of force vectors to parallel the axis of shortening when the tissue is stretched may contribute significantly to developed tension. In most preparations, however, this mechanism is probably

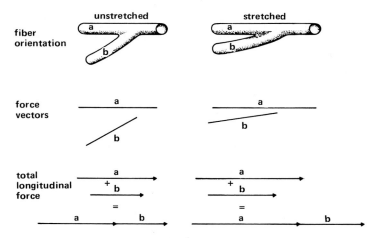

FIG. 12.10. Relationship of fiber orientation to the appearance of systolic force at the ends of a branched strand of cardiac muscle. In the unstretched muscle *(left)*, the branch b is oriented so it is not perpendicular to the long axis of the strand. As a result, only a portion of the force it develops is oriented longitudinally. Stretching the fiber *(right)* causes the branch b to become oriented in a more longitudinal direction. As a result, a larger component of the force it develops is oriented longitudinally.

of little functional importance, so that the sarcomere length-tension curve probably provides the most important basis for the Frank-Starling relationship in the heart.

ATRIUM AS A PRIMER PUMP

The role of end-diastolic volume in determining the contractile properties of ventricular contraction provides an important starting point for understanding the role of atrial systole in the regulation of cardiac performance. The fact that atrial systole normally occurs immediately before ventricular systole allows atrial contraction to augment the volume of blood in the ventricles at that instant (end-diastole) when ventricular volume determines the strength of ventricular contraction. For this reason loss of atrial systole (such as occurs when the atria fibrillate) can reduce ventricular function by abolishing this increment in end-diastolic volume (Chapter 20).

The overall hemodynamic consequences of loss of atrial systole include a rise in mean atrial pressure as well as a decline in cardiac performance. The rise in mean atrial pressure, which impedes the return of blood to the heart and thus gives rise to clinical symptoms of heart failure (Chapter 21), results from reduction in the ability of the ventricle to eject blood caused by the lowered end-diastolic volume.

These effects can be understood if one views atrial systole as a mechanism for increasing diastolic volume *at that instant (end-diastole) when diastolic volume determines ventricular performance* (Fig. 12.11). Atrial systole (*a,* Fig. 12.11) allows the ventricle the "luxury" of a high end-diastolic pressure without the need to "pay the price" of a high pressure throughout diastole. Loss of atrial systole (e.g., in atrial fibrillation) requires that ventricular pressure remain high throughout diastole in order to approach the normal level of end-diastolic pressure (and thus end-diastolic volume) that exists when there is effective atrial contraction. The effects of atrial systole are thus twofold: (a) It augments end-diastolic volume

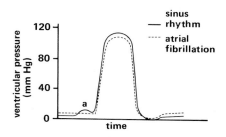

FIG. 12.11. Effects of loss of atrial systole. In a normal left ventricular contraction *(solid line)* atrial contraction (a) increases the left ventricular end-diastolic pressure to a level higher than that during the prior phases of diastole. Loss of atrial systole, which occurs when the atria fibrillate *(dashed line),* is generally accompanied by a decline in left ventricular end-diastolic pressure. Because the ventricle is denied a mechanism (atrial systole) to elevate end-diastolic pressure only in late diastole, the mean left ventricular diastolic pressure is abnormally high in spite of the lower end-diastolic pressure within the ventricle. The fall in ventricular end-diastolic pressure causes left ventricular performance to decline.

and thereby enhances cardiac performance; and (b) it allows the ventricle to enjoy the beneficial effects of a high end-diastolic volume without requiring pressure elevation throughout diastole.

In this chapter we described the operation of two laws which govern the relationship between ventricular volume and the mechanical characteristics of cardiac contraction. The first, the law of Laplace, is a *physical law,* which states that when the ventricle dilates the tension on its walls needed to achieve a given intraventricular pressure is increased. Secondly, there is a *physiological law,* the Frank-Starling relationship, which states that when the ventricle dilates the ability to perform work increases. Within limits (i.e., in the normal range of ventricular volumes) the operation of the physiological law is predominant, so that when the ventricle dilates the increased capacity to generate tension more than compensates for the increased wall tension. As becomes apparent in the next chapter, these consequences of ventricular dilation modify the energy cost of cardiac contraction, so that in certain pathological states the detrimental effects of ventricular dilation can assume greater importance than the beneficial effects.

BIBLIOGRAPHY

Burton, A. C. (1962): Physical principles of circulatory phenomena: The physical equilibria of the heart and blood vessels. In: *Handbook of Physiology, Section 2: Circulation,* Vol. 1, edited by W. F. Hamilton and P. Dow, pp. 85–106. American Physiological Society, Washington, D.C.
Katz, L. N. (1960): The performance of the heart. *Circulation,* 21:483–498.
Rackley, C. E. (1976): Quantitative evaluation of left ventricular function by radiographic techniques. *Circulation,* 54:862–879.
Sandler, H., and Dodge, H. T. (1974): Angiocardiographic methods for determination of left ventricular geometry and volume. In: *Cardiac Mechanics,* edited by I. Mirsky, D. N. Ghista, and H. Sandler, pp. 141–170. Wiley, New York.
Sarnoff, S. J., and Mitchell, J. H. (1962): The control of the function of the heart. In: *Handbook of Physiology, Section 2: Circulation,* Vol. 1, edited by W. F. Hamilton and P. Dow, pp. 489–532. American Physiological Society, Washington, D.C.

13

The Working Heart

The description of cardiac function in Chapter 12 highlighted the muscular basis for the pumping action of the heart and presented certain laws which govern the relationship between length and volume, tension and pressure, and the response of the heart to alterations in preload (i.e., end-diastolic volume). The left ventricle contracting on a fluid-filled balloon under the isovolumic conditions described in Chapter 12, however, represents a highly artificial model of the working heart. Although useful in defining the operation of the law of Laplace and the Frank-Starling relationship, this preparation fails to describe the ejection of blood under pressure, which is the physiological function of the heart. To visualize this property, the preparation described in Chapter 12 must be modified so that blood is ejected during systole.

The ejection of a volume of blood under pressure represents *work,* and the product of *pressure $\times$ volume* has the correct units for work (dynes/cm^2 $\times$ cm^3 = dynes cm). Thus the work of the heart during each beat can be calculated by multiplying the volume of blood ejected during each stroke (the *stroke volume,* usually abbreviated as *SV*) by the pressure *(P)* at which the blood is ejected. Stroke work (the work per beat) can be estimated as:

$$\text{Stroke work} = P \times SV \tag{13.1}$$

Because pressure changes during the phase of ejection (Fig. 1.16), stroke work is more accurately the integral of pressure and volume change:

$$\text{Stroke work} = \int P dV \tag{13.2}$$

where *P* is the pressure under which each increment *(dV)* of the stroke volume is ejected. For most practical purposes, the product $P \times SV$ is sufficiently accurate to characterize stroke work.

Equation (13.1) can be rewritten

$$\text{Stroke work} = P \times (EDV - ESV) \tag{13.3}$$

because stroke volume (i.e., the blood ejected during each cardiac cycle) is equal to end-diastolic volume *(EDV)* minus the volume remaining in the ventricle at the end of systole, the end-systolic volume *(ESV).* Stroke work can thus be increased when *EDV* increases, *ESV* decreases, or both. These represent quite different mechanisms for the augmentation of cardiac work.

The product $P \times SV$ (or the integral $\int P dV$) represents the *pressure-volume work* of the heart. This is the work performed in moving blood under pressure from the left ventricle to the aorta, and from the right ventricle to the pulmonary artery. Under most conditions pressure-volume work represents the great majority of the useful work of the heart.

The work of the atria, which is generated in transporting blood into the ventricles, is usually negligible in that most ventricular filling occurs before atrial contraction, and normal atrial systole develops only low levels of pressure. Even though atrial systole contributes little to the energy requirements of the heart, its importance in governing ventricular systole is large (Chapter 12).

The stroke volumes of the two ventricles are normally the same, whereas pulmonary artery pressure is approximately one-fifth that of aortic pressure. For this reason the pressure-volume work of the right ventricle is approximately one-fifth that of the left ventricle.

In addition to the pressure-volume work, the ventricles also perform work in accelerating the blood as it passes into the aorta and pulmonary artery. The acceleration of blood leaving the ventricles is a form of *kinetic work,* which according to the laws of physics is equal to $\frac{1}{2} mv^2$:

$$\text{Kinetic work} = \frac{1}{2} mv^2 \qquad (13.4)$$

where m is the mass of blood passing from the left ventricle to the aorta or from the right ventricle to the pulmonary artery, and v is the velocity at which this blood passes through the aortic and pulmonic valves. The kinetic work of the left ventricle is normally a small fraction of the pressure-volume work, usually considerably less than 5% of the latter. As pressure-volume work is less in the right ventricle (see above), kinetic work represents a greater proportion of total right ventricular work.

Inasmuch as kinetic work increases as the square of the velocity at which blood leaves the ventricle, and since velocity increases when stroke volume increases, kinetic work increases roughly in proportion to the cube of stroke volume because the volume of blood ejected appears in both the terms m and v^2 of Eq. (13.4). For this reason, in diseases where stroke volume is abnormally high (e.g., aortic insufficiency or severe anemia), kinetic work can represent a significant portion (although rarely more than 10%) of the work of the left ventricle.

Together the pressure-volume work and kinetic work of the ventricles represent *useful work* in that both forms of energy contribute to the movement of blood through the capillaries, kinetic energy being converted to pressure when movement of the ejected blood slows as it passes down the aorta. In addition to this useful work, the heart expends a significant amount of energy in the performance of *internal work* during the cardiac cycle. This internal work is expended both to stretch elastic elements within the muscle ("series elasticity") and to effect rearrangements within the muscular architecture of the ventricle. While there is growing evidence that the series elasticity of cardiac muscle is small, the shape changes which occur during isovolumic contraction and with the changing orien-

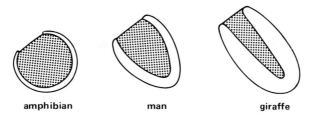

amphibian   man   giraffe

FIG. 13.1. Relationship between the shape of the ventricular cavity and the pressure it develops. The shape of the thin-walled ventricle of the amphibian heart, which develops little pressure, is almost spherical; that of the thicker human left ventricle, which develops a much higher pressure, is elongated. In the heart of the giraffe, where left ventricular systolic pressure is extremely high, the cavity of the thick-walled ventricle is almost tubular.

tation of the branching muscle bundles in the walls of the ventricles (Figs. 1.3, 1.4, and 12.10) require the expenditure of a significant amount of energy during systole. This energy does not contribute to the transfer of blood under pressure to the aorta and pulmonary artery during systole. Instead, internal work is degraded into heat at the end of the cardiac cycle, much as the lowering of a load increases recovery heat (Chapter 5). For this reason internal work represents a wastage of energy. Under some conditions this wastage in the performance of internal work by the heart can become highly significant.

ARCHITECTURE OF THE VENTRICLE

The right ventricle has been stated to operate primarily as a volume pump in that ejection pressure is low, whereas the left ventricle is more of a pressure pump. The architecture of the two ventricles differs in accord with these functional specializations. The radius of curvature of the walls of the more elongated left ventricle is less than that in the right ventricle (Fig. 1.2), and the left ventricular wall is thicker. These represent adaptations by which the left ventricle can generate high intraventricular pressures with relatively low wall tensions [Eq. (12.4)]. In the heart of the giraffe, whose left ventricular systolic pressure often exceeds 300 mm Hg, this adaptation is carried further; whereas the amphibian left ventricle, which generates low pressures, is almost spherical (Fig. 13.1). The right ventricle, which ejects the same stroke volume but against a lower pressure, is crescentic in shape, and the right ventricular free wall is relatively thin (Fig. 13.2) so that, as in the left ventricle, architecture is adapted to function.

STROKE WORK

Pressure-volume work, which has already been indicated to represent the majority of the work performed during each cardiac cycle, can be calculated as the integral $\int P dV$ [Eq. (13.2)]. This integral can be obtained from "work diagrams" (such as that presented in Fig. 12.4) and is the area under the systolic

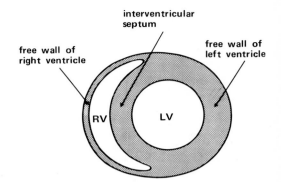

FIG. 13.2. Cross section of the human heart showing the thin-walled, crescentic right ventricle (RV) in which systolic pressure is approximately one-fifth that of the thick-walled, narrower left ventricle (LV).

portion of the curve (Fig. 13.3). The entire shaded area, including the darkly shaded area *(B)* beneath the work diagram, represents the integral $\int PdV$ for the left ventricle and thus the total pressure-volume work. In estimating the work of the ventricle, it is customary to subtract the work done on the left ventricle during diastole, i.e., the work due to ventricular filling. This work, corresponding to the darkly shaded area *B* in Fig. 13.3 is not due to left ventricular systole but represents instead the work of atrial contraction and the inertia of the venous return, both of which contribute to the preload on the ventricle. The majority of left ventricular work (area *A,* Fig. 13.3) is of course the direct consequence of ventricular systole.

In a sense, the two areas *A* and *B* in Fig. 13.3 can be compared to the effort of pulling against a stiff spring after an initial portion of the work has been performed by a partner who pulled the spring partly taut. In this way only part of the work would be performed by the individual who pulled the spring out to the maximum of tension, although it is this individual who generates maximal tension. Similarly, the work contributed by the atria during ventricular filling *(B),* reduces the *total work* of the ventricle but not *maximal tension generated.* Because maximal tension rather than total work is the major determinant of the energy requirements of the heart (see below), variations in the preload (area *B*) can be shown to be of relatively less importance than the absolute level of afterload determining the energy needs of the heart.

FIG. 13.3. Work diagram of the left ventricle. The pressure-volume work performed during each beat is equal to the area A + B, which represents the integral $\int PdV$. A small portion of this work (B) represents work contributed by atrial contraction and the inertia of the venous return, while the majority (A) is the work of the left ventricle.

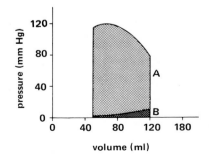

At the outset of this chapter, pressure-volume work per beat was shown to be approximately equal to the product $P \times SV$. Mean ejection pressure is normally ~105 mm Hg, while stroke volume normally is approximately 70 ml so that stroke work is usually ~7,000 mm Hg ml. In centimeter-gram-second units, this corresponds to ~9.3 $\times$ 10^6 dyne cm per stroke.

MINUTE WORK

Cardiac work performance is commonly related to a fixed period of time, generally defined as minute work, i.e., the work performed per minute. Minute work can be estimated by multiplying the work per beat (stroke work) by the number of beats per minute (HR = heart rate):

$$\text{Minute work} = P \times HR \times SV \qquad (13.5)$$

The product $HR \times SV$ is the *cardiac output (CO)*, which is normally approximately 5–6 liters/min. Minute work can thus be calculated as the product

$$\text{Minute work} = P \times CO \qquad (13.6)$$

The foregoing analysis, and especially Eq. (13.5), defines three independent variables, each of which contributes to the minute work of the heart. An increase in left ventricular work, for example, can be effected by an increase in systemic blood pressure, in heart rate, in stroke volume, or all three. Because stroke

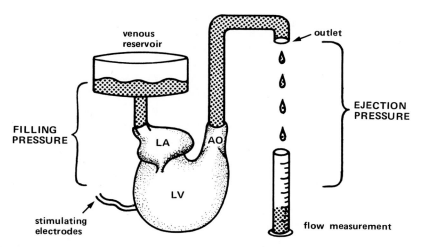

FIG. 13.4. Isolated left heart preparation. Blood flowing from the venous reservoir enters the left atrium under a head of pressure determined by the height of the reservoir relative to that of the atrium. The ventricle, when stimulated to contract, pumps the blood through the aorta into a tube. The height of the outlet of this tube, relative to that of the center of the ventricle, constitutes the ejection pressure. Stroke volume can be determined by measuring the amount of blood ejected during each beat.

volume $= EDV - ESV$ [Eq. (13.3)], minute work is increased when the end-diastolic volume is increased, the end-systolic volume decreased, or both:

$$\text{Minute work} = P \times HR \times (EDV - ESV) \qquad (13.7)$$

Each of the four parameters which contribute to minute work has a different impact on the energetics of cardiac contraction, so that the relationship between minute work and the energy needs of the heart is complex.

The influence of each of the parameters of minute work on the characteristics of cardiac contraction can be evaluated in the isolated heart preparation in which the hemodynamic properties of the system are subject to rigid control. Figure 13.4 illustrates an isolated heart preparation in which only the left ventricle is working. Filling pressure (preload) can be varied by adjusting the height of the venous reservoir. Ejection pressure (afterload) can be varied by raising or lowering the outlet connected to the aorta so as to achieve any desired pressure increment, measured from a "zero" level at the center of the left ventricle. Heart rate can be controlled by stimulating electrodes applied either to the atrium or to the ventricle itself. In this way the effects of independent alterations in *stroke volume, ejection pressure,* and *heart rate* can be examined while keeping constant the other two determinants of minute work.

Variations in Stroke Volume

The stroke volume of the preparation illustrated in Fig. 13.4 can be varied by raising or lowering the venous reservoir, keeping constant the stimulation rate and the level of the outlet connected to the aorta. Raising the venous reservoir increases the pressure within the left ventricle during diastole, thereby causing the heart to dilate. A series of graded changes in the level of the venous reservoir therefore is translated into a series of changes in end-diastolic volume. The resulting effects on cardiac performance can be predicted from the Frank-Starling relationship; i.e., stroke volume increases with increasing filling pressure as long as the heart is functioning on the ascending limb of the Starling curve (Fig. 12.9). The manifestations of the Frank-Starling relationship under conditions where only stroke volume is allowed to vary are shown in Fig. 13.5. Because stroke work is equal to stroke volume times ejection pressure [Eq. (13.1)], stroke work can

FIG. 13.5. Operation of the Frank-Starling relationship under conditions where only stroke volume is allowed to vary. At constant heart rate and ejection pressure, stroke volume rises with increasing end-diastolic pressure. The descending limb shown at high end-diastolic volumes here is not always seen and is probably absent in the normal mammalian heart.

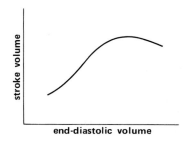

be substituted for stroke volume on the ordinate in Fig. 13.5. Furthermore, as minute work equals the product of stroke work and heart rate [Eq. (13.5)], when the heart rate is kept constant the ordinate in Fig. 13.5 can also be given as minute work. (The kinetic work, which normally represents less than 5% of the total external work, is ignored for simplicity in this discussion.) The Frank-Starling relationship thus can be seen to predict the effects of changing end-diastolic volume on stroke work and minute work.

Variations in Ejection Pressure

In the experimental preparation shown in Fig. 13.4, ejection pressure can be varied by raising or lowering the outlet of the tube connected to the aorta. Controlling the rate of stimulation maintains the heart rate constant in the face of these changes in outflow pressure, but in order to prevent changes in stroke volume the level of the venous reservoir must be changed, because, for example, elevation of ejection pressure impairs the ability of the ventricle to empty, thereby tending to decrease stroke volume. Conversely, reduction in ejection pressure increases stroke volume when heart rate and end-diastolic pressure are maintained constant. Thus in order to maintain stroke volume constant in the face of changes in outflow pressure, the experimenter must raise the level of the venous reservoir when ejection pressure is increased, and lower the venous reservoir when ejection pressure is reduced. In view of the direct relationship between the pressure in the venous reservoir and end-diastolic volume, the latter increases when ejection pressure is elevated at constant stroke volume and heart rate, and falls when ejection pressure is reduced (Fig. 13.6). Figure 13.6, like Fig. 13.5, is a manifestation of the Frank-Starling relationship. As both stroke volume and heart rate are maintained constant, either stroke work or minute work can be substituted for ejection pressure on the ordinate in Fig. 13.6.

Variations in Heart Rate

In the experimental situation described in Fig. 13.4, heart rate can be varied at constant ejection pressure and venous pressure. Under these conditions, as long as the myocardium is not overstressed and diastole lasts long enough to allow

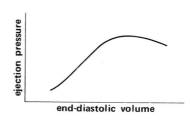

FIG. 13.6. Operation of the Frank-Starling relationship under conditions where only ejection pressure is allowed to vary. At constant heart rate and stroke volume, ejection pressure rises with increasing end-diastolic pressure. A descending limb at high end-diastolic volumes is not always seen unless one plots the dependence of net ejection pressure (systolic minus end-diastolic pressures) on end-diastolic volume. Under these conditions subtraction of the high end-diastolic pressure that accompanies high end-diastolic volumes causes the descending limb of this curve.

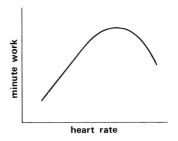

FIG. 13.7. Effects of varying the heart rate on the minute work of the left ventricle under conditions where the stroke volume and ejection pressure are maintained constant. Minute work increases with an increasing heart rate only in the lower range of heart rates. At higher heart rates diastole becomes so shortened that minute work declines as the heart rate is increased further. This curve is not a depiction of the Frank-Starling relationship.

adequate filling of the ventricle, stroke work remains constant. Minute work therefore is proportional to heart rate (Fig. 13.7) as predicted by Eq. (13.5). It should be emphasized that the basis for this curve, unlike those in Fig. 13.5 and 13.6, is *not* the Frank-Starling relationship because ventricular performance during each cardiac cycle is not changed. Instead only the number of contractions per unit of time is altered.

At extremely rapid heart rates, diastole becomes shortened to a point where ventricular filling cannot be completed in the short time the ventricle is in a relaxed state. As a result, the curve shown in Fig. 13.7 deviates downward. The fall in cardiac work at high heart rates is not a manifestation of the descending limb of the Starling curve. Instead, when the heart rate increases at high rates the decreased cardiac work results mainly from a reduction in the period during which the ventricle is able to fill. This occurs because, although the duration of systole is reduced with increasing heart rates (due to the interval-duration relationship discussed in Chapter 14), the duration of systole shortens much less than that of diastole.

Rapid heart rates, when extreme, can increase the energy requirements for cardiac contraction to a level that exceeds the ability of coronary blood flow to deliver substrates, and especially oxygen, to the working myocardium. Under such conditions, a resulting decline in contractility can also cause minute work to decline as the heart rate is increased.

ENERGY COST OF WORK PERFORMED

The importance of oxidative metabolism in the generation of chemical energy for cardiac contraction was emphasized in Chapter 2. The unremitting demand for ATP by the cardiac contractile proteins is met almost entirely by the oxidation of fat, carbohydrates, and to a very minor extent protein. In view of this central role of oxidative energy production, the utilization of chemical energy by the working heart can be estimated from measurements of cardiac oxygen consumption.

The amount of chemical energy made available when a given amount of oxygen is consumed is virtually independent of the substrate oxidized. Even though oxidation of fat yields approximately 9 calories/g of fat oxidized, while that of carbohydrate and proteins yields only 4 calories/g of substrate, a greater amount of oxygen is consumed during the oxidation of each gram of fat. Thus when the release of chemical energy is expressed per liter of oxygen consumed to metabolize each of these foodstuffs, the average value is 4.8 ± 0.2 calories liberated per liter of oxygen consumed, regardless of the substrate oxidized. Cardiac oxygen consumption thus provides an excellent index of the rate at which chemical energy is made available for cardiac contraction.

It is of interest historically that a direct correlation between cardiac oxygen consumption and the work of the heart was noted in 1915 by Evans and Matsuoka. This observation, which demonstrated an increase in energy consumption when muscular work increased, is a manifestation of the Fenn effect, which was first clearly described in skeletal muscle almost 10 years later. Indeed, as was pointed out by Fenn in his classic 1923 paper on this subject, the direct relationship between muscle work and total energy release which bears his name had been known to cardiac muscle physiologists for almost a decade.

Cardiac efficiency can be estimated by dividing the external work of the heart by the energy equivalent of the oxygen consumed. Both numerator and denominator can be expressed either per beat or per unit of time. The resulting quotient provides a good index of cardiac efficiency:

$$\text{Cardiac efficiency} = \frac{\text{work}}{\text{energy equivalent of oxygen consumption}} \quad (13.8)$$

The overall efficiency of cardiac contraction calculated in this manner has generally been found to range between 5% and 20%, the exact value depending on the nature and amount of work performed.

AMOUNT OF WORK PERFORMED: INFLUENCE ON CARDIAC EFFICIENCY

The importance in determining cardiac efficiency of the amount of work performed is apparent if one recognizes that isovolumic contraction by the heart requires the expenditure of a finite, and not insignificant, amount of energy. Much energy must be expended during left ventricular systole even if too little pressure is developed to open the aortic valve. Under these conditions external work is zero, whereas internal work accounts for the expenditure of sizable amounts of energy. As a result, cardiac efficiency is zero. When left ventricular pressure exceeds aortic pressure and blood is ejected from the left ventricle, external work is performed in the ejection of blood under pressure into the aorta. As a result, the numerator in the equation defining cardiac efficiency [Eq. (13.8)] becomes finite and thus so does efficiency. Even though extra energy is liberated to perform each additional increment of external work, efficiency initially increases with increasing external work because the energy liberated that is not converted to external work represents a decreasing proportion of total energy expenditure. The type of curves obtained when the dependence of oxygen consumption and effi-

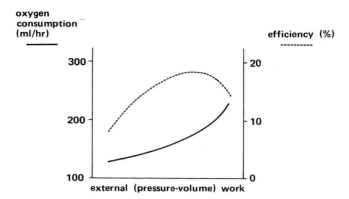

FIG. 13.8. Relationship between the amount of external work performed and the energetics of left ventricular contraction. Oxygen consumption *(solid line)* increases monotonically with increasing work while efficiency *(dashed line)* first rises and then falls.

ciency are plotted as a function of increasing work are shown in Fig. 13.8. Oxygen consumption increases in a monotonic fashion as external work increases, while efficiency first rises then falls. The direct relationship between oxygen consumption and work performance is of course an expression of the Fenn effect. The origin of the biphasic curve relating efficiency to work is more complex, however, and depends on the nature of the work performed.

PRESSURE WORK VERSUS FLOW WORK

The fundamental observations regarding the energetics of cardiac contraction described in this and the preceding sections were first described in 1915 in the classic paper by Evans and Matsuoka already noted. In addition to defining the existence of a direct relationship between cardiac work and the liberation of chemical energy (the Fenn effect), their paper also described interesting and important differences in the energy costs of increasing work by different means. Figure 13.9 shows an experiment of Evans and Matsuoka in which work was increased by increasing either aortic pressure or cardiac output. In Fig. 13.9 increasing work, whether it is brought about by increasing either aortic pressure *(P)* or cardiac output *(CO),* is associated with increased oxygen consumption (solid lines) and efficiency (dotted lines). It is apparent, however, that at a moderate level of work performance (vertical line W_2) energy expenditure is greater when the heart is faced with a high aortic pressure *(P)* than when it is ejecting a larger volume of blood against a lower pressure *(CO)* even though the level of work is the same. This observation means that *a given increment in work is more efficiently performed when it is brought about by raising cardiac output than when it results from increased aortic pressure.* In other words, increased pressure generation by the myocardium is energetically more costly than increased ejection, even when the total increment in external work (pressure × cardiac output) is the same.

The basis for these differences in the energetics of "pressure work" and "flow work" has not been explained fully, but it appears likely that they reflect different amounts of internal work performed by the heart contracting in the face of altered pressures and flows. Even though the product of pressure × cardiac output provides an excellent index of the external work expended in moving blood from the venous system to the high-pressure arterial circuit, energy is also expended during the cardiac cycle to do work within the myocardium. This internal work is due largely to shape changes and the elasticity of the muscular walls of the heart. Thus the absorption of energy within the walls of the ventricle as intraventricular pressure rises during isovolumic contraction represents a form of work which requires an expenditure of chemical energy that is eventually degraded to heat, rather than being used to pump blood.

To understand the mechanism by which internal work is increased disproportionately when ejection pressure is increased, as opposed to the internal work that accompanies a comparable increase in external work associated with an increased cardiac output, it is useful to refer back to the load-energy curves discussed in Chapter 5 (Fig. 5.5). In frog sartorius muscle the curve relating total energy release to load parallels the curve that relates external work to load (Fig. 13.10). Figure 13.10 shows that the amount of heat liberated by the contracting frog sartorius muscle is essentially independent of load. In his early studies on the energetics of muscle, Fenn noted that curves similar to those shown in Fig. 13.10 were quite different when muscles other than the frog sartorius were studied. In the frog gastrocnemius, for example, total energy expenditure did not

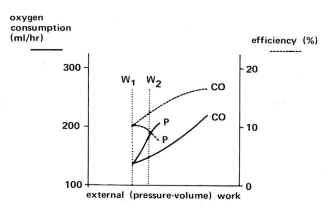

FIG. 13.9. Influence of the nature of the external work performed by a ventricle on oxygen consumption *(solid lines)* and efficiency *(dashed lines)*. When cardiac work is increased from W_1 to W_2 by increasing cardiac output *(CO)* or ejection pressure *(P)*, the resulting effects on oxygen consumption and efficiency differ strikingly. Cardiac efficiency at the higher level of work is much greater when cardiac output is increased than when ejection pressure is increased because of the lower energy requirements of flow work compared to pressure work.

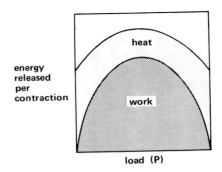

FIG. 13.10. Relationship between load, work, and total energy liberated by a sartorius muscle (Fig. 5.5). Although work and total energy liberation are maximal at intermediate loads, heat production is relatively independent of load.

decline appreciably with increasing load when the load was high (Fig. 13.11). Instead, the liberation of heat increased with load, there being an extra liberation of heat when loads were high. It was possible to show that these differences between the frog sartorius and gastrocnemius muscles could be attributed to differences in the arrangement of fiber bundles in the muscle (Fig. 13.12). The fiber bundles in the sartorius are arranged in a parallel fashion, whereas those in the gastrocnemius muscle have an asymmetrical bipennate arrangement that causes significant shape changes in the muscle, even during isometric contractions. As a result, significant movement of fibers occurs in the gastrocnemius contracting at high loads, even when the ends of the muscle are fixed and the muscle shortens under isometric conditions, i.e., where external work is zero. When fiber shortening occurs, giving rise to these shape changes, the actual distance they shorten is small but high levels of force are required. Small movements therefore are associated with high levels of internal work, which are associated with the expenditure of significant amounts of chemical energy. In the sartorius muscle, where the parallel arrangement of fibers leads to much less shape change during contraction at high load, internal work remains minimal and energy wastage at high loads is much less.

In the heart, in which branching fiber bundles (Fig. 12.10) are arranged in interwoven spiral structures (Fig. 1.3), the energetics of contraction would be expected to resemble those of the frog gastrocnemius muscle more than the sartorius. As a result, one can understand why at higher loads an increasing

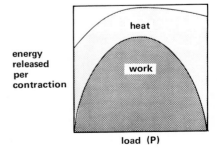

FIG. 13.11. Relationship between load, work, and total energy liberated by the myocardium. In contrast to the frog sartorius muscle (Fig. 13.10), heat production increases disproportionately at high loads.

FIG. 13.12. Arrangement of muscle fibers in two skeletal muscles. In sartorius muscle the fibers are parallel and oriented longitudinally within the muscle. In gastrocnemius, which is geometrically similar to the myocardium, many of the fibers are oriented in directions not parallel to the long axis of the muscle. As a result, when contraction in the gastrocnemius (and in the myocardium) takes place at high loads, the levels of internal work are much higher than are those of the sartorius contracting at a given high load.

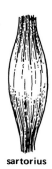

sartorius

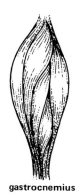

gastrocnemius

proportion of energy is expended in the performance of internal work. The dissipation of this internal work as heat reduces mechanical efficiency, especially when wall tension is high, thereby accounting for the differences in the energetics of pressure work and flow work first observed by Evans and Matsuoka.

LOSS OF EFFICIENCY IN THE DILATED HEART

The energy wastage which occurs at high loads is significant not only when aortic pressure is increased but also when the left ventricle becomes dilated. A loss of mechanical efficiency in the dilated heart occurs because as the ventricular cavity becomes enlarged the radius of curvature of its muscular walls increases. It follows from the law of Laplace that, even when intraventricular pressure remains constant, dilation causes the tension on the walls of the ventricles to increase. For this reason ventricular dilation decreases mechanical efficiency by increasing the load on each muscular fiber (Fig. 13.11).

The loss of efficiency in the dilated heart is augmented by loss of the normal "unloading" of the myocardium during ejection. Normally when the ventricle ejects its stroke volume, the radius decreases significantly. According to the law of Laplace, this reduction in ventricular volume reduces wall tension even though intraventricular pressure remains essentially unchanged. Ejection of the same stroke volume in the dilated heart causes much less of a change in ventricular dimensions, so that the normal decrease in wall tension is reduced. These relationships can be seen in Table 13.1, which gives calculated volumes, radii, circumferences, and wall tensions for a normal and a dilated ventricle. The data in Table 13.1 were calculated assuming the left ventricle to be a thin-walled sphere that ejects at a constant pressure. These assumptions, which obviously represent oversimplifications to facilitate calculations of dimensions and wall tension, do not influence the general validity of the following analysis.

Examination of the effects of ventricular volume on the mechanical characteristics of ejection (Table 13.1) demonstrates that dilation reduces the normal fall in wall tension during ejection. At the start of ejection the effect of ventricular

TABLE 13.1. *Ventricular dimensions*

Parameter	Normal ventricle	Dilated ventricle
At start of ejection		
Pressure (mm Hg)	100[a]	100[a]
Volume (cm³)	92	380
Radius (cm)	2.8	4.5
Circumference (cm)	17.5	28
Wall tension (dynes/cm)	3.72×10^5	5.98×10^5
Stroke volume (cm³)	70	70
At end of ejection		
Pressure (mm Hg)	100[a]	100[a]
Volume (cm³)	22	310
Radius (cm)	1.7	4.2
Circumference (cm)	11	26.5
Wall tension (dynes/cm)	2.26×10^5	5.59×10^5
External stroke work (dyne cm)	9.3×10^6	9.3×10^6
Conditions of external work		
Average wall tension (dynes/cm)	2.99×10^5	5.79×10^5
Change in circumference (cm)	6.5	1.5
As % of end-	~40	~5
diastolic circumference		

[a] equals 1.33×10^5 dynes/cm².

dilatation to increase wall tension (Chapter 12) is already apparent: Wall tension is almost twice normal at any intraventricular pressure owing to operation of the law of Laplace. If one assumes stroke volume to be 70 cm³, and uses the resulting end-systolic volume to calculate dimensions and wall tension, it is found that wall tension falls almost to half its original value in the normal ventricle (from 3.72 $\times 10^5$ to 2.26×10^5 dynes/cm), whereas in the dilated ventricle wall tension decreases only ~10% during systole (from 5.98×10^5 to 5.59×10^5 dynes/cm). External work of course is the same for both ventricles, as the same volume of blood is ejected at the same pressure. The conditions under which this work was performed, however, are quite different. In the normal ventricle average wall tension is much less than that in the dilated ventricle, whereas the change in circumference is much less in the dilated ventricle where there is only a 5% reduction in circumference during systole. This is in contrast to the much greater (almost 40%) reduction in circumference, and thus of wall tension, in the normal ventricle. The significance of these differences can be understood in terms of the preceding discussion of the energetics of pressure work versus flow work. From the data in Table 13.1 it can be seen that to do the same amount of work the dilated ventricle must contract under conditions of sustained high wall tension with little wall shortening (analogous to pressure work), whereas the normal ventricle contracts against a lower, and decreasing, wall tension while undergoing significant fiber shortening (analogous to flow work). For this reason the efficiency of ventricular contraction can be expected to decrease as the ventricle dilates.

ENERGY COST OF ISOVOLUMIC CONTRACTION: ENERGETICS OF VARYING HEART RATE

The high energy cost of increasing the heart rate is apparent from the influence of wall tension on the expenditure of energy by the contracting left ventricle. Because high levels of internal work accompany the development of pressure within the ventricle, and because this work is converted to heat during relaxation, a significant amount of energy is wasted during each systole. An increase in heart rate at constant aortic pressure and cardiac output therefore increases the energy cost of cardiac work simply by increasing the number of times each minute the ventricle must stretch its elastic walls. In addition, energy must be expended during each contraction to set into motion, and to return to the resting state, those processes which trigger contraction. For example, calcium must move out of and be actively pumped back into the sarcoplasmic reticulum with each beat. In terms of the analysis of muscular contraction presented in Chapter 5, more activation energy A and more internal work W_i are expended when the heart rate increases. For this reason tachycardia is a costly although often essential means by which the minute work of the heart can be increased (see below).

EVALUATION OF CARDIAC PERFORMANCE IN THE INTACT ANIMAL AND MAN

The description of the pumping action of the left ventricle in which aortic pressure, stroke volume, and heart rate could be varied independently is extremely important in understanding the energetics of cardiac contraction in the intact animal and humans. Yet the degree of experimental control over the many variables that enter in the expenditure of energy is obviously less in the heart of the intact animal and man in that changes in aortic pressure, stroke volume, and heart rate tend to occur at the same time. For this reason analyses of the independent effects of changing aortic pressure, stroke volume, and heart rate are virtually impossible, especially in a clinical setting. Furthermore, measurements of end-diastolic volume are difficult to obtain and are often inaccurate, whereas end-diastolic pressure is readily recorded. For this reason the Starling curve in the intact animal and man is usually plotted as the dependence of external, pressure-volume work on ventricular end-diastolic pressure (Fig. 13.13). While the relative ease in obtaining data to define these curves is appealing, it is important to remember the approximations and simplifications that underlie such Starling curves. For example, an increase in minute work brought about by an increase in heart rate or aortic pressure is energetically more expensive than a comparable increase brought about by an increased stroke volume and so has a different energetic significance.

Stroke work, instead of minute work, can be used in the construction of Starling curves such as that shown in Fig. 13.13, but such curves still fail to distinguish between the different effects of pressure and flow in determining the energetics of contraction.

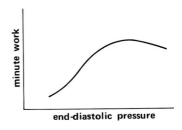

FIG. 13.13. Frank-Starling relationship as it is usually evaluated in man. The ordinate is minute work because precise control of blood pressure and stroke volume is difficult to achieve in cardiac patients. The abscissa is end-diastolic pressure, which is more easily measured than end-diastolic volume.

ESTIMATION OF THE ENERGY REQUIREMENTS OF CARDIAC WORK IN HUMANS

Two indices have been found empirically to be useful in estimating the energy expenditure of the working heart. Most simple is the product *aortic pressure* $\times$ *heart rate,* which has been shown experimentally to correlate well with cardiac oxygen consumption. This product, which includes two of the three terms of the equation for minute work [Eq. (13.5)], omits stroke volume, the most difficult to measure but fortuitously the least important determinant of the energy expended during cardiac contraction. A somewhat more elaborate index of myocardial oxygen consumption is the tension-time index in which the average ejection pressure is multiplied by the duration of ejection (Fig. 13.14). It is apparent from Fig. 13.14 that a better term for this area would be pressure-time index.

Both of these indices correlate well with cardiac oxygen consumption, although the effects of the law of Laplace and of stroke volume are not considered. These indices are thus approximations. In the clinical setting, where precise measurements of blood pressure and heart rate are easily obtained, these two indices do provide a reasonably accurate index of the energy demands of the heart.

CHANGES IN MYOCARDIAL CONTRACTILITY

The significance of changes in the contractile state of the myocardium in the adjustment of the heart to changing physiological, pharmacological, and pathological states was described in Chapters 9 and 11. Although many attempts have been made in the intact heart to define changes in myocardial contractility by construction of force-velocity curves, this approach has not fulfilled its early promise in defining the true state of myocardial contractility. Construction of

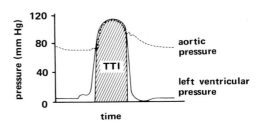

FIG. 13.14. Tension-time index. The oxygen consumption of the heart is roughly proportional to the area under the ejection phase of the left ventricular pressure curve, which represents the tension-time index (TTI).

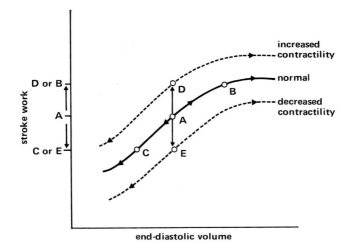

FIG. 13.15. Family of Starling curves. The work of the heart *(ordinate)* varies with changing end-diastolic volume *(abscissa)* according to the Frank-Starling relationship. These length-dependent changes in the work of the heart are described by the three curves here, which represent a family of Starling curves (e.g., Figs. 13.5, 13.6, and 13.13). The work of the heart can also be varied by changes in contractility, which by definition represent increases or decreases in cardiac work that are not the result of changing end-diastolic volume. As depicted here, changes in contractility cause the heart to shift to a new Starling curve.

The solid curve (CAB) describes normal myocardial contractility, and point A represents the basal state. Changes in cardiac work that result from alterations in venous return shift the work of the heart along this "normal" curve; e.g., cardiac work can be increased from A to B by enhanced venous return, or it can be decreased from A to C by a reduction in venous return. These changes in cardiac work are associated with no change in contractility.

The work of the heart can also be changed by interventions that modify myocardial contractility. A positive inotropic agent can increase cardiac work from A to D under conditions where end-diastolic volume remains constant. Conversely, cardiac work can be decreased from A to E by a negative inotropic agent without change in end-diastolic volume. Points D and E fall on different Starling curves *(dashed lines)*, so a change in contractility can modify the work of the heart with no change in end-diastolic volume.

Note that it is not possible to define the mechanism responsible for a change in myocardial function simply by measuring either cardiac work or end-diastolic volume alone. These analyses, instead, require the accumulation of sufficient data to define the relationship between changing cardiac work and end-diastolic volume in terms of the family of Starling curves.

such curves requires a number of assumptions regarding the geometry of the heart, synchrony of fiber contraction, uniformity of contractility, series elasticity, and the time- and length-dependent characteristics of the contractile process. In spite of the difficulties in defining the *absolute level of myocardial contractility,* it is much easier to document *changes in myocardial contractility.* Since a change in myocardial contractility is any change in the ability of the cardiac muscle to do work *at constant end-diastolic fiber length,* the position of a control Starling curve defines a baseline of contractility. Changes in contractility will lead to a shift in the Starling curve. Figure 13.15 shows a "family of Starling curves," in which the curve containing the points *A, B,* and *C* represents the control state.

At a constant level of contractility, pressure-volume work increases when end-diastolic volume rises from *A* to *B;* and, conversely, work decreases when end-diastolic volume falls from *A* to *C.* A positive inotropic intervention, which by definition represents an intervention that increases work capacity at any given end-diastolic volume (or fiber length), does not abolish the Frank-Starling relationship. Instead, a new Starling curve is inscribed in which work at each end-diastolic volume is increased (curve containing *D*). Conversely, a negative inotropic intervention shifts the Starling curve downward (curve containing *E*).

There are therefore two ways by which the heart can increase its stroke work: (a) by increasing end-diastolic volume (*A* → *B*, Fig. 13.15); and (b) by increasing contractility (*A* → *D*, Fig. 13.15). If one considers minute work, an increased heart rate represents a third independent means for increasing the amount of work performed per unit of time. These three mechanisms, while independent, are not mutually exclusive. Nor need they all move in the same direction; i.e., contractility, end-diastolic volume, and heart rate can change discordantly.

The energetic implications of these mechanisms for altering cardiac work are quite dissimilar. By increasing end-diastolic volume (i.e., by utilizing the Frank-Starling relationship), the heart increases its work performance via a mechanism that increases the size of the ventricular cavity, thereby altering the geometry and leverage of the walls of the heart. The law of Laplace states that this mechanism increases wall tension, thereby tending to reduce cardiac efficiency (see above). The energetically detrimental effect of dilatation can be avoided when contractility is increased because this mechanism causes the ventricular cavity to become smaller. These differences can be readily understood under conditions where ejection pressure is maintained constant and only stroke volume is changed. Remember that stroke work equals $P \times (EDV - ESV)$ [Eq. (13.3)]. The Frank-Starling relationship increases work by increasing *EDV:* an increase in contractility increases work by decreasing *ESV*. An increase in heart rate is energetically more costly than a decrease in *ESV* in increasing minute work [which equals $P \times HR \times (EDV - ESV)$; Eq. (13.7)] because of the energy wastage during isovolumic contraction.

Both the Frank-Starling relationship and changes in myocardial contractility serve a regulatory function in the intact animal. These two mechanisms, however, probably serve different physiological roles. The Frank-Starling relationship is most important in beat-to-beat adjustments to changes in circulatory dynamics, e.g., in balancing the outputs of the right and left ventricles and in mediating the responses to minor changes in venous pressure such as are brought about by changing body position. The response of the heart to more drastic changes in circulatory dynamics (e.g., those that accompany exercise) are mediated largely by changes in myocardial contractility; indeed the heart normally becomes *smaller* during exercise carried out in a standing position, even though cardiac output is markedly increased. To a large extent, therefore, the normal heart is able to avoid the energy wastage that accompanies dilation by increasing the intensity of its contractile processes, rather than by relying on changes in end-diastolic volume to meet large increases in the hemodynamic requirements of the body.

BIBLIOGRAPHY

Evans, C. L., and Matsuoka, Y. (1915): The effect of various mechanical conditions on the gaseous metabolism and efficiency of the mammalian heart. *J. Physiol. (Lond.)*, 49:378–405.

Martin, D. S. (1928): The relation between work performed and heat liberated by the isolated gastrocnemius, semitendinosus and tibialis anticus muscles of the frog. *Am. J. Physiol.*, 33:543–547.

Sarnoff, S. J., Braunwald, E., Welch, G. H., Jr., Case, R. B., Stainsby, W. N., and Macruz, R. (1958): Hemodynamic determinants of oxygen consumption of the heart with special reference to the tension-time index. *Am. J. Physiol.*, 192:148–156.

See also References to Chapter 12.

14

Cardiac Action Potential

The generalization that all processes in the heart are at least an order of magnitude more complex and interesting than the corresponding mechanisms in skeletal muscle is clearly illustrated when we examine the form and ionic basis of the cardiac action potential. In skeletal muscle, as in nerve, the action potential is a brief, biphasic event in which rapid depolarization is quickly followed by restoration of the resting potential (Fig. 14.1). With the exception of a low amplitude after-potential, this entire process requires no more than a few milliseconds. In the heart, on the other hand, the action potential lasts longer, consists of several phases, and varies in its characteristics from region to region within the heart. The action potential in the Purkinje fibers, for example, lasts over 300 msec and consists of at least five morphologically defined phases (Fig. 14.2). The upstroke of the action potential *(phase 0)*, which corresponds to depolarization in the skeletal muscle fiber (Fig. 14.1) is extremely rapid, as it is in nerve and skeletal muscle. In most regions of the myocardium, however, depolarization is followed by two phases that do not have clear counterparts in nerve and skeletal muscle. A brief phase of early repolarization *(phase 1)* is followed by a plateau *(phase 2)*, which is largely responsible for the long duration of the cardiac action potential. Repolarization *(phase 3)* corresponds to the repolarization phase of the action potentials in nerve and skeletal muscle, while the resting potential of the cardiac action potential *(phase 4)* is similar to that in other excitable cells. As might be expected, the ionic basis for the complex series of events which produce the cardiac action potential has similarities to the ionic mechanisms responsible for the action potential in nerve and skeletal muscle. Yet many significant differences exist. These reflect specializations in the ionic channels of the cardiac sarcolemma that account for a number of the features of the normal and abnormal electrocardiogram.

Before discussing the mechanisms now believed to be responsible for the cardiac action potential, several terms must be defined. *Membrane potential* (E_m) represents the voltage difference between the interior of the cell and the surrounding medium. In the resting cell a microelectrode inserted through the sarcolemma records a potential more negative than that of the extracellular fluid, so that during diastole the cell interior is stated to have a negative potential (Fig. 14.3). In describing resting potential, one is dealing with a *potential difference*. This potential difference can be viewed from the inside of the cell, in which case the surrounding medium is considered to have a positive charge, or the resting

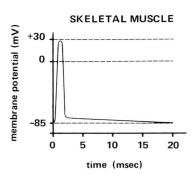

FIG. 14.1. The skeletal muscle action potential is a brief biphasic potential change in which rapid depolarization (upward deflection) is quickly followed by repolarization (downward deflection). A small positive after-potential causes an approximately 10-msec delay prior to return of the membrane potential to its resting level of −85 mV.

potential can be related to the potential at the outside of the cell, in which case resting potential is defined as being negative. The latter convention is generally employed in electrophysiology, where the potential of the interior of the cell relative to that in the surrounding medium is described. An *increase* in resting potential thus represents a greater degree of electronegativity inside the cell; a *decrease* in resting potential represents a reduction in the electronegativity of the cell interior.

Depolarization, as the term states, represents a decrease in the electronegativity of the interior of the resting cell. The amplitude of the action potential therefore defines the extent to which cellular electronegativity decreases from its resting level. In all regions of the heart the inside of the cell becomes electropositive at the peak of the action potential (Fig. 14.2) so that membrane polarity is reversed. An increase in the extent of this reversal in polarity, or "overshoot," can be referred to as a greater degree of depolarization.

Hyperpolarization and repolarization both describe increased electronegativity within the cell. *Hyperpolarization* represents an increase in resting potential, i.e., to more negative levels of potential within the cell. *Repolarization* describes the return of membrane potential to a more negative value after depolarization, i.e., the recovery of resting potential to the normal level after an action potential.

The terminology used to describe *current flow* across the cell membrane is even more complex than that which describes membrane potential. The accepted terminology in electrophysiology describes currents as if they were carried across

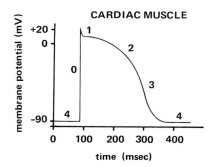

FIG. 14.2. The cardiac action potential (shown here for a Purkinje fiber) lasts over 300 msec and consists of five phases. Phase 0 (upstroke) corresponds to depolarization in skeletal muscle and phase 3 (repolarization) corresponds to repolarization in that tissue. Phases 1 (early repolarization) and 2 (plateau) have no clear counterpart in skeletal muscle, while phase 4 (diastole) corresponds to the resting potential.

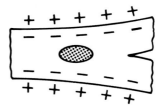

FIG. 14.3. Cardiac muscle cell at rest. The polarity of the normal resting potential is negative inside the cell and positive at the cell exterior.

the cell membrane by positively charged ions (even when they are carried, in fact, by negatively charged ions).

An inward current, according to electrophysiological convention, represents that flux of charge which would result if positive ions moved into the cell. Because an outward movement of negative ions has the same effect on membrane potential as an inward movement of positive ions, the efflux of negative ions also gives rise to an inward current. As the interior of the resting cell is negatively charged (Fig. 14.3), inward currents cause depolarization.

Outward currents can result either from the movement of positively charged ions out of the cell interior to the surrounding medium or from the flux of negatively charged ions into the cell interior. Outward currents therefore increase electroegativity in the cell interior. In the resting cell, mechanisms which increase outward currents cause *hyperpolarization.* Outward currents that occur after depolarization tend to restore the resting potential to its original negative value and so cause *repolarization.*

The definition of a *membrane current* can be confusing because of differences between conditions during stimulation and those after stimulation. Immediately prior to stimulation, when the membrane is still in its resting state, the outside of the cell is positively charged (Fig. 14.3). Under these conditions a cathode (e.g., a stimulating electrode) on the outside of the cell draws a positive charge from its external surface (Fig. 14.4A). The resulting movement of positive charge away from the outer side of the sarcolemma causes the resting cell to depolarize by discharging a capacitor. The corresponding *capacitive current* resembles an outward current (see above) because positive charge has moved away from the outside of the sarcolemma and a negative charge has moved away from the inside of this membrane. For this reason a depolarizing capacitive current resembles an outward current and so is opposite in direction from the depolarizing ionic (or ohmic) inward currents described in the preceding paragraphs.

When depolarization by a cathodal current causes the membrane potential to reach its threshold, an action potential is initiated by changes in the ionic permeability of the sarcolemma. The action potential results from currents produced by the flow of ions through the membrane. These *ionic currents* are quite different from the capacitive currents described in the preceding paragraph. Ionic currents are responsible for the regenerative action potential and the recovery of the resting potential, as well as for the spontaneous electrical activity of the heart (pacemaker activity). In the case of the ionic currents, and in contrast to the capacitive currents, inward currents are depolarizing (Fig. 14.4B). The

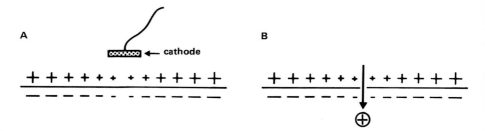

A

← cathode

B

+ + + + + + + + + + + +   + + + + + + + + + + + +

− − − − − − − − − − − −   − − − − − − − − − − − −

⊕

FIG. 14.4. Differences between capacitive and ionic currents. Discharge of membrane potential by a cathode outside the cell **(A)** draws positive charge from the external surface of the membrane and so causes negative charge to move away from the inner surface. This generates a capacitive current that resembles the inward ionic current shown in **B,** where the movement of cations from the outside to the inside of the cell causes a similar decrease in membrane potential.

depolarizing effect of an inward ionic current causes the interior of the cell to lose some of its negativity or to become positive in sign. In this and the following chapters, which focus on the changing properties of the membrane after stimulation, only ionic currents are described; hence inward currents are depolarizing.

Membrane *resistance* defines the relationship between membrane potential and current flow in accord with Ohm's law: $R = E/I$, where R is resistance, E is potential, and I is current flow. Membrane *conductance,* usually designated g, is the reciprocal of membrane resistance, so that $g = I/E$.

The terms permeability and conductance reflect similar properties of the membrane, although they do not, in fact, describe the same thing. *Permeability (P)* is a measure of the ability of a membrane to allow the movement (flux) of a substance from one side to the other. In the case of an uncharged molecule (e.g., sucrose), flux can be determined from the relationship:

$$\text{Sucrose flux} = \text{sucrose concentration} \times P_{sucrose} \qquad (14.1)$$

There can be two such fluxes across a membrane, one in each direction. In the absence of membrane pumps or other factors that influence net movement of the substance, influx and efflux are equal. Under these conditions the system is at a steady state.

The expression relating the flux of a charged molecule to its concentration is more complex in that ion fluxes are modified when there is a membrane potential. Thus a factor must be introduced on the right-hand side of Eq. (14.1) to account for the effects of any electrical field that exists across the membrane. The meaning of permeability in the modified equation, however, remains the same.

Ionic *conductance* g is an index of the ability of a membrane to carry the current i that arises when charge is transferred across the membrane as an ion moves from one side to the other. This current flow is determined by the corresponding conductance and the difference between the equilibrium potential across the membrane for the ion (E in the Nernst equation; see below) and the actual transmembrane potential (E_m). In the case of potassium ion, for example:

$$\text{Current flow } (i_{K+}) = (E - E_m) \times \text{potassium conductance } (gK) \qquad (14.2)$$

Depending on the difference between E and E_m, current can flow in either direction, although not in both directions at any given time.

Conductance provides an index of the ability of the membrane to allow an ion to move from one side to the other, and both conductance and permeability have the dimensions of a velocity (centimeters per second). Unlike permeability, which characterizes ion fluxes in both directions across the membrane at any time, conductance describes the current which flows in only one direction at any time, as described in Eq. (14.2).

IONIC BASIS FOR MEMBRANE POTENTIAL

The cardiac sarcolemma is a semipermeable membrane in which the conductances of different ions change sequentially during the action potential. As a result, each ion is subject to a characteristic sequence of conductance changes during the different phases of the cardiac cycle. At rest, this membrane is highly permeable to potassium and relatively impermeable to sodium, chloride, and calcium, so that gK is high and gNa, gCl, and gCa are low. The remarkable ability of the sarcolemma to undergo sequential changes in these ion conductances accounts for the complex characteristics of the cardiac action potential.

Resting Potential (Phase 4)

The relatively high intracellular concentration of potassium relative to that in the extracellular fluid was known long before membrane potentials were first measured. For this reason the similarity of the electrical potential predicted on the basis of the distribution of potassium ions across the sarcolemma and the resting potential observed in excitable cells was recognized in the earliest studies of membrane potential.

The basis for the resting potential of the myocardial cell can be understood in terms of the electrochemical gradient for potassium that exists across the sarcolemma. The separation of ions across this semipermeable plasma membrane is such that in the resting state potassium ion concentration is much higher within the cell than it is in the extracellular space. [This concentration gradient is due to the operation of the sodium pump (Chapter 9), which utilizes the chemical energy of ATP to pump sodium out of the cell in exchange for potassium, which is thereby concentrated within the cell.] Because the sarcolemma of the resting myocardial cell is permeable to potassium, this ion tends to move down its concentration gradient and so to leak out of the cell. As potassium ions leave the cell interior, however, they carry a positive charge to the outside of the cell, causing an electrical gradient to appear across the sarcolemma in which the outside is positively charged. It is this difference in the density of electrical charge at the two sides of the sarcolemma that gives rise to the resting potential difference between the inside and the outside of the cardiac cell.

The relationship of ion concentration differences to differences in electrical potential is given by the *Nernst equation:*

$$E_m = \frac{RT}{zF} \ln \frac{C_o}{C_i} \qquad (14.3)$$

in which E_m is the membrane potential, R is the gas constant, T is the absolute temperature, z is the valence of the ion, F is the Faraday constant, and C_o and C_i are the concentrations (or more strictly the activities) of the ion at the outside and inside, respectively, of the membrane. In the case of the alkali metal ions, Na^+ and K^+, $z = 1$, so that at 37°C the constants in this equation can be written for ordinary (base 10) logarithms as

$$E_m = 61.5 \log C_o/C_i \qquad (14.4)$$

Equation (14.4) states that a 10-fold difference in the concentration of a monovalent cation, where $C_o/C_i = 10$, produces a potential difference of +61.5 mV. If C_o/C_i is 0.1, E_m is -61.5 mV.

In the case of cardiac muscle at rest, where $[K^+]_o$ is approximately 4.0 mM and $[K^+]_i$ is approximately 140 mM, the value of E_m predicted by the Nernst equation from the ratio $[K^+]_o/[K^+]_i$ is:

$$E_m = \frac{RT}{zF} \ln \frac{4}{140} = 61.5 \times \log 0.029 = -95 \ \text{mV} \qquad (14.5)$$

This estimate is based on the assumption that the cardiac sarcolemma is freely permeable only to K^+ during diastole and is impermeable to other ions for which a concentration gradient exists between the inside and outside of the cell. For most practical purposes these are valid approximations as long as resting potential is in the normal range of -80 to -95 mV.

In those regions of the heart in which diastolic potential is stable (i.e., which do not exhibit spontaneous depolarization or "pacemaker" activity; see below), resting potential is very close to that predicted by the Nernst equation on the basis of the distribution of potassium. Variations in $[K^+]_o$ thus tend to influence directly the resting potential as predicted by Eq. (14.5): Elevation of $[K^+]_o$ causes depolarization, while reduction in $[K^+]_o$ tends to hyperpolarize the membrane. The level of resting potential does not, however, follow the Nernst equation for potassium when $[K^+]_o$ is either very low or very high. When $[K^+]_o$ is very low (less than approximately 3 mM), the extent of hyperpolarization is less than that predicted by the Nernst equation because potassium permeability becomes reduced, allowing permeability to other ions (e.g., sodium) to become important in determining membrane potential (Fig. 14.5). The deviation of E_m at very low $[K^+]_o$ from that predicted from the Nernst equation can thus be attributed to a reduction in membrane permeability to potassium caused by an effect of the low $[K^+]_o$ to expose a "background" sodium current (Chapter 19). Even at normal levels of resting potential, the membrane is not freely permeable to K^+, so that agents which increase potassium conductance (e.g., acetylcholine; Chapter 19) can cause a slight increase in resting potential.

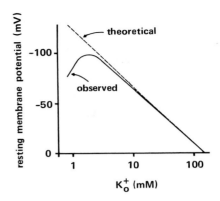

FIG. 14.5. Relationship between K+ concentration outside the myocardial cell (K^+_0) and resting membrane potential. Changes in K^+_0 at normal and high levels cause changes in membrane potential *(solid line)* that closely approximate those predicted by the Nernst equation for potassium *(dashed line)*. At lower levels, however, a fall in K^+_0 causes a decline in observed membrane potential that results from a decrease in potassium conductance.

"TYPICAL" CARDIAC ACTION POTENTIAL

The propagated wave of depolarization which initiates cardiac contraction is carried from cell to cell by regenerative action potentials. Although some regions of the myocardium are specialized for their conductive properties (e.g., the Purkinje fibers of the bundle of His and bundle branches), all impulses in the heart are transmitted by muscle cell to muscle cell communication. The cardiac nerves, which arise from the sympathetic and parasympathetic nervous system (Chapter 1), serve only to modulate myocardial performance and do not participate in the propagation of the wave of excitation through the heart.

A propagated action potential is initiated when membrane potential becomes depolarized beyond a *threshold.* Levels of depolarization that fail to reach this threshold (A and B, Fig. 14.6) do not initiate an action potential; instead the membrane subsequently recovers and no propagated wave of depolarization is initiated. When the extent of depolarization exceeds this threshold, the membrane continues to depolarize even though the initial depolarizing stimulus is turned off. Thus once threshold is reached, subsequent depolarization becomes independent of the initial depolarizing stimulus (C, Fig. 14.6).

The configuration of the cardiac action potential differs between different regions of the heart (see later). In the following discussion we focus on the characteristics of the Purkinje fibers, in which the ionic basis for the electrical events during depolarization has been studied most extensively.

The Upstroke (Phase 0)

The resemblance of resting potential to that potential predicted by the Nernst equation for potassium, coupled with the observation that membrane potential decreases during the upstroke of the action potential, led early investigators to conclude that depolarization of the cell following excitation reflected primarily a fall in potassium permeability. With the advent of intracellular microelectrode recordings of membrane potential, however, it became apparent that membrane

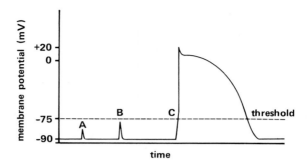

FIG. 14.6. Initiation of an action potential when the membrane potential is depolarized to threshold. Small depolarizing stimuli (A and B) which fail to reach threshold *(dashed line)* are unable to initiate an action potential. When depolarization reaches threshold (C), a regenerative action potential is produced. Once the latter begins, further depolarization becomes independent of the initial stimulus.

potential did not simply decrease toward zero during the action potential, as would be expected if gK fell to a low value. Instead it was found that membrane potential actually became reversed at the height of the action potential, so that the interior of the cell became positively charged relative to the surrounding medium (Figs. 14.1 and 14.2). This effect could not be attributed to changes only in membrane permeability to potassium. It became apparent that the reversal of membrane potential at the peak of the action potential could be explained if the membrane potential at that time was influenced by the transmembrane distribution of sodium ion as predicted by the Nernst equation for sodium. The distribution of this ion, which is present at higher concentrations in the extracellular fluid than in the cell interior, would produce membrane potentials opposite in sign to those caused by the distribution of the potassium ion. In recent years it has been possible to show that this is in fact the case, and that whereas the resting cell exhibits high permeability to potassium and low permeability to sodium, at the height of the action potential potassium permeability becomes low and sodium permeability high.

It is now accepted that the depolarization that occurs during excitation in most—but not all (see below)—regions of the heart is determined to a significant extent by the distribution of sodium across the sarcolemma. Sodium is present at concentrations of approximately 140 mM in the extracellular fluid and 30 mM inside the cell. As a result, a positive membrane potential is predicted by the Nernst equation for sodium:

$$E_m = \frac{RT}{zF} \ln \frac{140}{30} = 61.5 \log 4.6 = +41 \text{ mV} \qquad (14.6)$$

The fact that the action potential does not reach the high level of positivity predicted by Eq. (14.6) reflects both the failure of the membrane to become freely permeable to sodium, even at the height of the action potential, as well as a residual permeability to potassium and chloride.

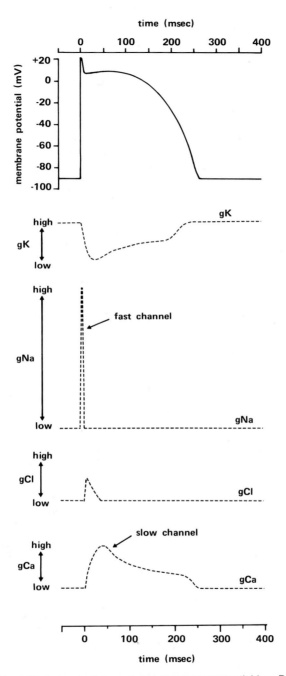

FIG. 14.7. Changes in ionic conductances during the action potential in a Purkinje fiber. Note the typical action potential *(top)* and, reading from top to bottom, the accompanying changes in conductance for potassium (*g*K), sodium (*g*Na), chloride (*g*Cl), and calcium (*g*Ca). An increase in *g*Na or *g*Ca augments inward current flow, whereas increasing *g*K or *g*Cl augments outward current flow.

The rapid upstroke of the action potential in the Purkinje fiber is caused by an extremely rapid inward flow of current across the cell membrane (Fig. 14.7). This fast inward current has been shown experimentally to be carried by sodium ions. Because the cell membrane is lipoprotein in nature, and thus not freely permeable to ions, it is usually postulated that sodium enters the cell by passage through a special "sodium channel" whose opening and closing can be regarded as resembling the opening and closing of a gate (Fig. 14.8). The flux of sodium ions is sometimes stated to involve a "carrier" which allows the charged ion to cross the lipid membrane. Ionic fluxes are extremely complicated and involve special channels for each ion. They are controlled by complex "gating mechanisms" whereby the opening and closing of the channel, and recovery of the ability to reopen, can be varied. A given ion species may cross the sarcolemma by way of more than one channel, and more than one ion species can pass through a single channel (see later). The various ionic channels in the cardiac sarcolemma can be distinguished from each other not only by the ions they carry but by their rates of opening, closing, and recovery, and by the factors which influence their opening, closing, and recovery.

The rate of depolarization *(dV/dt)* and the amplitude of the action potential in most cardiac cells are now believed to be determined largely by the voltage-dependent opening of a channel that allows an extremely rapid increase in sodium conductance. In the resting cell the sodium channel is almost entirely closed, while that for potassium is open. As a result, sodium conductance is low and potassium conductance high. When the membrane is partially depolarized to levels below threshold, sodium channels are partially opened. The degree of opening of these channels increases as membrane potential falls, so that the opening of sodium channels can be said to be *voltage-dependent.*

When resting membrane potential is abruptly changed in a depolarizing direction so as to reach a threshold potential, the opening of the sodium channel becomes regenerative (Fig. 14.6); i.e., the depolarization caused by sodium influx causes still more sodium channels to open. As a result, the inward sodium current promotes the further entry of sodium ions, and so is termed *regenerative.* This is due to the voltage dependence of the opening of the sodium channels described

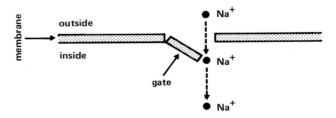

FIG. 14.8. A sodium channel. The influx of sodium ions through the channel is controlled by a gating mechanism. Characterization of any ionic gating mechanism is extremely complex and requires knowledge of its rates of opening and closing, the extent to which it opens and closes, and the time needed for the channel to recover its ability to reopen once it has closed.

at the end of the last paragraph. The resulting explosive increase in sodium conductance and the very rapid flow of sodium ions into the myocardial cell produces a fast inward current and the sharp upstroke of the action potential (Fig. 14.7).

The fact that the fast inward current is carried by sodium ions can be readily demonstrated by replacing sodium in the medium bathing the myocardium by an impermeant ion like choline. Under these conditions the fast inward current does not appear. Tetrodotoxin (TTX), a poison derived from a Japanese puffer fish, has proved to be an extremely useful tool for studying the ionic basis of the action potential because TTX has a specific action to prevent the passage of sodium through the fast channel. Under the influence of TTX, therefore, the fast inward current is abolished.

The voltage dependence of the *opening* of the sodium channel was described in the preceding paragraph. This, as we have seen, gives rise to an extremely rapid process by which partial depolarization causes the development of the regenerative fast inward sodium current. Like the opening of the sodium channels, the *closing* of the sodium channels is also a rapid process. Once the membrane has depolarized, these channels close, thereby terminating the fast inward current (Fig. 14.7). Following closure of the fast channels, the system becomes "inactivated" so that these channels cannot be reopened immediately. Thus although both the opening and closing of the sodium channels are rapid, *recovery* of the ability of these channels to reopen following inactivation is very much slower and depends on the level of membrane voltage and on the time elapsed since the preceding action potential.

The *voltage dependence* of the recovery of the ability of the fast channels to reopen is seen when one tries to stimulate a cardiac muscle cell immediately after the phase of rapid depolarization (phase 0). No significant response is elicited under these conditions. This inability to respond with a second action potential, called *refractoriness,* is due partly to the persistent depolarization during the prolonged plateau phase of the cardiac action potential (Fig. 14.2). Stated another way, the requirement that the membrane potential return toward its resting level before a second action potential can be elicited means that recovery of the ability of the sodium channels to reopen is voltage-dependent. This voltage dependence of the recovery of the sodium channel is reflected in several important phenomena where partial depolarization of the myocardial cell immediately prior to stimulation reduces the fast inward current. These are described in the following paragraphs.

The level of resting potential immediately prior to stimulation influences the rate of depolarization of the cardiac action potential. This relationship results from the influence of membrane voltage on the rate and extent of opening of the sodium channels. If resting potential is high (i.e., in the normal range of approximately -90 mV), rapid depolarization to threshold causes the sodium channels to open rapidly and widely. The result is an action potential with a rapid upstroke and a large amplitude (Fig. 14.9A). If, however, the cell is in a partially depola-

FIG. 14.9. The rate and degree of opening of the fast sodium channels in response to a depolarizing stimulus (S) depends on the resting membrane potential prior to stimulation. A large, rapidly rising action potential is produced when the resting membrane potential is high (a), whereas partial depolarization prior to stimulation (b) causes the stimulus to produce a small, slowly rising action potential. The changes in the upstroke of the action potential reflect effects on the gating mechanism that controls the fast sodium channels.

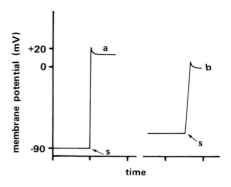

rized state prior to stimulation (e.g., resting potential is in the range of −70 to −80 mV), then a similar depolarizing stimulus produces a more slowly rising action potential whose amplitude is reduced (Fig. 14.9B) because the sodium channels open less widely. In this way the degree of opening of the fast channel can be seen to be voltage-dependent in that partial depolarization prior to stimulation inhibits the opening of the sodium channels. This effect of prior depolarization can also be described as a voltage-dependent reduction in the availability of sodium carrier. Abnormally slow-rising and low-amplitude action potentials, such as that shown in Fig. 14.9, occur not only when the myocardium is activated at low, constant, resting potentials. They are also produced by premature stimulation before full recovery from a prior action potential.

The voltage dependence of the opening of the sodium channels (i.e., its modification by changes in the membrane potential immediately prior to rapid depolarization) is also seen when excitation is effected by depolarizing pulses of different speeds. If threshold is reached quickly, as occurs when the depolarizing stimulus is rapid, there is full development of the sodium conductance (Fig. 14.10) so that the upstroke of the action potential is rapid and the amplitude high (*a,* Fig. 14.10). If threshold is approached very slowly (*b,* Fig. 14.10), however, both the rate of depolarization and the amplitude of the action potential are reduced. These effects of prior depolarization allow a slow depolarization rate or interventions which

FIG. 14.10. The rate and degree of opening of the fast sodium channels in response to a depolarizing stimulus depend on the rate at which membrane potential approaches threshold. A large, rapidly rising action potential is produced when the stimulus reaches threshold rapidly (a), whereas a stimulus that slowly reaches threshold produces a small, slowly rising action potential (b). These changes in the rate of rise and height of the action potential reflect effects on the rate and extent of opening of the fast sodium channels.

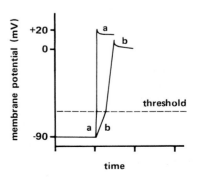

partially depolarize the cell to reduce the rate of rise and amplitude of the action potential. These effects are of considerable importance in the genesis of a number of important arrhythmias (Chapter 16 and 17).

The voltage dependence of the recovery of the ability of the sodium channels to reopen explains many but not all of the phenomena associated with the recovery of excitability after an action potential. It was found recently that a variety of interventions can modify the relationship between membrane voltage and the extent of recovery of the ability of the cell to respond with a fast inward current. These phenomena reflect the fact that the recovery of the ability of the sodium channels to reopen is also *time-dependent*. Thus unlike the rapid *opening* of the sodium channels (which produces the upstroke of the action potential) and the rapid *closing* of these channels (which terminates the fast inward current), the *recovery* of the ability of these channels to reopen can take up to 100 msec or more, even after membrane potential has returned to its resting level. This recovery, like the initial opening of the sodium channels, can be slowed by partial membrane depolarization and by some antiarrhythmic drugs, e.g., quinidine (Chapter 19).

The behavior of membrane permeability to potassium during the action potential is quite different in the myocardium from that described in the classic studies of the squid axon, while those of sodium permeability are quite similar. Note that in Fig. 14.7, gK is shown to decrease during depolarization. This behavior is in contrast to that in nerve, where gK increases during depolarization. This opening of potassium channels during depolarization in nerve allows potassium ions to carry current out of the cell, thereby tending to return membrane potential to its resting level. This phenomenon is called *outward-going rectification*, which is a true rectification, as the depolarization-induced increase in outward current tends to terminate the nerve action potential. In the case of cardiac muscle, on the other hand, the fall in gK with depolarization tends to keep the cell in a depolarized state by preventing potassium ions from carrying enough outward, repolarizing current to restore resting potential. This closure of potassium channels during depolarization in cardiac muscle, which is an *inward-going rectification,* is sometimes called *anomalous rectification.* By retarding the efflux of potassium and thus the generation of an outward current, inward-going rectification prolongs depolarization and so is partly responsible for the plateau of the cardiac action potential.

Early Repolarization (Phase 1)

A brief period of rapid repolarization that follows the upstroke of the cardiac action potential is often called phase 1 of the action potential. This early repolarization, like that in nerve and skeletal muscle, is due mainly to a fall in sodium conductance. A transient increase in chloride conductance during early repolarization contributes to the return of membrane potential toward a plateau level. Because extracellular chloride concentration is approximately 140 mM, or more than four times higher than that inside the cell (approximately 30 mM), increased permeability to chloride allows this anion to flow into the cell, giving rise to an *outward* current (see above). This outward chloride current is voltage-dependent, falling to a low level as membrane potential returns toward zero early in the plateau phase (Fig. 14.7).

The Plateau (Phase 2)

The most distinctive feature of the electrical depolarization of cardiac muscle is the plateau, which is responsible for the prolonged cardiac action potential. The fact that membrane potential is recorded at or near zero for well over 100 msec (compare Fig. 14.2 with 14.1) could be explained by a high membrane resistance, in which case there would be no tendency for current to flow between an electrode inside the cell and one in the extracellular fluid. Alternatively, the plateau of the action potential could occur during a period of low membrane resistance if mutually balanced current flow across the plasma membrane occurred in such a manner as to keep membrane potential in a depolarized state. More than 20 years ago Weidmann showed that membrane conductance was relatively high during the early portion of the plateau, although it fell to low levels later on during the plateau phase. The relative constancy of membrane potential during the initial phases of the plateau therefore can be attributed to ionic currents that neutralize each other so as to maintain the membrane in a depolarized state, whereas the slowness of repolarization later during the plateau is due to decreasing membrane conductance for outward currents.

The fall in membrane conductance during the plateau of the cardiac action potential can be attributed partly to the phenomenon of inward-going (anomalous) rectification, which has already been described. The resulting closure of the potassium channels reduces the efflux of this cation and so decreases both outward current and membrane conductance during the early part of the plateau phase. The observed decline in membrane conductance during the initial period of the plateau occurs because decreasing outward potassium and chloride currents early in the plateau balance a similarly timed decrease in the slow inward current (see below) in such a way that membrane voltage remains virtually constant during this phase of the cardiac action potential.

There is now considerable evidence that a depolarizing (inward) current occurs early during the plateau of the cardiac action potential. This current, called the *slow inward current,* results from the opening of a "slow channel" which allows calcium ions to enter the cell. Unlike the inward sodium current that enters the cell by way of the "fast channel," the slow inward current is seen in sodium-free media, is insensitive to TTX, and is not abolished by partial depolarizations which inactivate the gating mechanism for sodium. On the other hand, the slow inward current is reduced by cations like Mn^{2+} or drugs like verapamil and D-600, which reduce the plateau phase of the cardiac action potential but do not affect the fast inward current carried by sodium. Both the potential recorded during the plateau and the magnitude of the slow inward current depend on $[Ca^{2+}]_o$, increasing with increasing extracellular calcium concentration and vice versa (Chapter 19).

Extracellular calcium ion concentration is approximately 2 mM, whereas during diastole $[Ca^{2+}]_i$ is around 0.1 μM so that the distribution of calcium across the membrane, like that of sodium, causes an inward (depolarizing) current when the membrane becomes permeable to this cation. This 20,000-fold gradient for calcium, according to the Nernst equation, would produce a membrane potential of approximately +132 mV:

$$E_m = \frac{RT}{zF} \ln \ [Ca^{2+}]_o / [Ca^{2+}]_i = \frac{61.5}{2} \log \ 20,000 = +132 \ \text{mV} \qquad (14.7)$$

During systole, when intracellular calcium concentration has increased to approximately 10 μM, this "equilibrium" potential falls to approximately +70 mV.

These estimates of the equilibrium potential for calcium are based on the assumption that the Ca^{2+} concentration immediately beneath the sites on the sarcolemma that contain the slow channels is the same as that in the region of the cell surrounding the myofilaments. As discussed in Chapter 9, however, there is evidence that the calcium which flows into the cell during the slow inward current passes into a special subsarcolemmal region, possibly related to the subsarcolemmal cisternae of the sarcoplasmic reticulum. For this reason the true equilibrium potential for calcium may be more nearly +70 mV than +132 mV. Another explanation for the difference between the observed equilibrium potential during the plateau of the cardiac action potential and that calculated from the differences between intra- and extracellular calcium ion concentrations arises from the fact that the slow channels can also carry sodium. According to this explanation, the measured equilibrium potential reflects not only the value calculated for Ca^{2+} but also that for Na^+, which is much less (see above).

The following mechanisms therefore seem likely to account for the known properties of the plateau of the cardiac action potential. Immediately after the sodium channels open, those for potassium close. Early repolarization occurs when the fast channels close; the membrane conductance remains fairly high because of the development of a net outward current carried by chloride. The latter subsequently comes to be dominated by the slow inward current that is carried by calcium. Both of these currents diminish early during the plateau (Fig. 14.7). The fall in chloride conductance reflects the voltage dependence of this current which decreases as the cell repolarizes, while calcium conductance declines owing to a time-dependent inactivation of the slow channel. Together these changes cause membrane conductance to fall during the plateau phase of the cardiac action potential.

Repolarization (Phase 3)

The repolarization of cardiac muscle, like the return of membrane potential to its resting level in nerve and skeletal muscle, occurs when the membrane permeability to potassium, which initially falls during the phase of rapid depolari-

TABLE 14.1. *Potassium currents in the heart*

Current	Time and occurrence	Characteristics
i_x	Plateau and repolarization	Carries outward, repolarizing, current *Time-dependent*, increasing with time after initial depolarization *Voltage-dependent*, increasing as membrane potential returns toward its resting level (i.e., "regenerative")
i_{x_1} (Early) i_{x_2} (Late)		(Rapid component of i_x) (Slow component of i_x)
i_{K_1}	All phases of the cardiac cycle	A "background" outward current, due in part to potassium efflux and possibly due in part to the electrogenic sodium pump *Time-independent* *Voltage-dependent*, decreasing with increasing depolarization
i_{K_2}	Diastole (only in pacemaker cells)	A diastolic, outward current whose decline causes diastolic depolarization (i.e., spontaneous firing) in pacemaker cells *Time-dependent*, the reduction of this current becoming more marked as diastole proceeds *Voltage-dependent*, this current decreasing as the cell depolarizes from resting potential

zation [due to inward-going (anomalous) rectification], returns at the end of the plateau to the high levels characteristic of the resting cell. The opening of the potassium channels, in combination with closure of the slow channels, allows the return to a state of high potassium conductance, thereby permitting potassium ions to flow out of the cell, generating an outward (repolarizing) current.

The gating mechanisms which allow potassium current to flow out of the cardiac cell during repolarization are quite complex. These repolarizing currents may involve more than one ion-selective channel which facilitates the efflux of potassium ion. The overall net outward current, often called i_x (Table 14.1), follows a time course that has been interpreted as evidence for the existence of two separate channels, one (i_{x_1}) being slightly more rapid than the other (i_{x_2}). The opening of these channels is both time- and voltage-dependent. Their time dependence is manifest by the fact that potassium currents increase with time after the peak of the action potential, even if membrane voltage is held constant experimentally. The fact that they are also voltage-dependent can be shown during interventions that are interposed experimentally so as to drive membrane potential toward more negative (resting) levels during the plateau. These repolarizing interventions are found to increase the opening of the channels that carry i_x, thereby hastening the return to normal levels of resting potential by increasing the outward flow of potassium ion. This ability of membrane repolarization to promote the flow of outward currents—that lead to still further membrane repolarization—allows repolarized areas of myocardium to promote the repolarization of other areas that are still in a depolarized state. This means that repolarization is in some ways regenerative.

Yet another outward current (i_{K_1}) has been found to contribute to repolarization (Table 14.1). Like those currents described as i_{x_1} and i_{x_2}, this one is carried by potassium. Unlike the other ionic currents described in this chapter, however, i_{K_1} appears not to vary with time, although it has been shown to increase as membrane potential becomes more positive, i.e., during depolarization. There is evidence that this "background current" is due partly to the electrogenic nature of the sodium pump, which transports three potassium ions out of the cell in exchange for only two sodium ions (Chapter 9). The resulting net transfer of positive charge from inside to outside by the sodium pump can generate a net outward ionic current that may contribute to i_{K_1}.

Together these potassium ion-selective channels bring membrane potential back to its resting level by allowing potassium ions to carry current out of the myocardial cell (Fig. 14.7). At the same time, they re-establish the normally high conductance for potassium which characterizes the resting myocardium.

ION MOVEMENTS DURING THE ACTION POTENTIAL

From the preceding description it can be appreciated that the changes in membrane voltage which give rise to the rising and falling phases of the cardiac action potential result from the movement of several ions across the plasma membrane. These ion movements, which are responsible for both depolarization and repolarization, are electrogenic in that they give rise to electrical currents. The ion movements that are primarily responsible for the cardiac action potential are summarized in Table 14.2. All these ion fluxes are in a "downhill" direction; i.e., the ions move down an electrochemical gradient and so are not actively transported. Table 14.2 is simplified in that the specificity of some of these ionic channels is not absolute. For example, sodium can enter the cell along with calcium during the slow inward current, and the movement of ions other than potassium may occur when the potassium channels open during repolarization.

Not all ion movements across the cell membrane are electrogenic. For example, most of the sodium that leaves the cell by way of the sodium pump (Chapter 9) is exchanged for potassium, thereby canceling out most of the net movement of electrical charge. Similarly, the transport of calcium out of the cell is now believed to occur largely through a nonelectrogenic process in which each mole of calcium that moves out of the cell is exchanged for 2 moles of sodium (Chapter 9).

The significance of the ion pumps discussed in Chapter 9 can be appreciated by examining Table 14.2. It is apparent that after an action potential has passed along the sarcolemma the chemical composition of the cardiac cell has changed slightly. Sodium, calcium, and chloride have entered the cell, and potassium has been lost. Thus for the ionic composition of the cell to return to its original state, sodium, calcium, and chloride must be eliminated, and the cell must regain potassium. Unlike the "downhill" ion fluxes that produce the action potential, all of the "restorative" ion fluxes are "uphill." Most are nonelectrogenic in that they involve the exchange of one species of cation for another. The fact that active sodium efflux is linked for the most part to potassium influx (by way of the sodium pump) neutralizes the electrical work that would otherwise have to be done to transport positively charged sodium ions out of the electronegative cell interior. Similarly, calcium efflux is affected largely by an exchange for sodium. It is therefore a valid generalization that downhill ion movements in the heart are electrogenic, whereas the pumps that move ions against an electrochemical gradient are nonelectrogenic. From the standpoint of the expenditure of energy by the cell, it can be appreciated that the nonelectrogenic nature of active ion transport

TABLE 14.2. *Ion movements responsible for cardiac action potential*

Ion	Movement	Current	Phase of action potential
Na+	In	Inward	0 (depolarization)
Cl-	In	Outward	1 (early repolarization)
K+	Out	Outward	
Ca2+	In	Inward	2 (plateau)
K+	Out	Outward	
K+	Out	Outward	3 (repolarization)

mechanisms reduces the effective electrochemical gradient against which the ions are moved.

It is a common misconception to assume that during the action potential the concentration gradients for sodium and potassium across the sarcolemma are lost. In fact, only a very small fraction of cellular potassium is exchanged for sodium during a single action potential. As a result, even when the ion pumps are inhibited (e.g., when the sodium-potassium ATPase is poisoned), a large number of action potentials must be generated before the cell gains a significant amount of sodium or loses a measurable amount of the intracellular potassium.

REFRACTORY AND SUPERNORMAL PERIODS

The inability of the myocardium to be re-excited immediately after an action potential is called refractoriness, and the period during which excitability is reduced is called the refractory period. In the case of nerve and skeletal muscle, two kinds of refractory period are commonly described. The "absolute refractory period" is that interval, beginning with the onset of depolarization, where no stimulus, whatever its magnitude, can produce a propagated response. The "relative refractory period" is defined as the interval after the end of the absolute refractory period when only a stimulus stronger than the normal threshold stimulus can initiate a propagated response. The refractory periods are followed by a "supernormal period," during which a stimulus slightly less strong than that which causes depolarization of the fully recovered cell can initiate a propagated response.

In descriptions of the excitability properties of the myocardium, the term absolute refractory period has fallen from use. Instead, the period when no propagated action potential can be initiated by electrical stimulation is called the *effective refractory period* (Fig. 14.11). The choice of this term arises from the fact that electrical stimuli delivered later during the effective refractory period can, if they are strong enough, elicit a local response, i.e., a transient depolarization that is not propagated. Even though the local responses evoked during the effective refractory period do not initiate propagated action potentials, they can influence the properties of subsequent ones (Chapters 16–18). For this reason local responses are important in the genesis of some conduction abnormalities, as is apparent, for example, in the phenomenon of concealed conduction (Chapter 18).

As is the case in nerve and skeletal muscle, the *relative refractory period* is one in which only an abnormally strong stimulus can initiate a propagated action potential. It is important to recognize that the relative refractory period in the heart is an interval not only when stronger than normal stimuli are needed to elicit a propagated response but also when an abnormally slow-rising and low-amplitude response (Fig. 14.9) follows the stimulus after prolonged latency. This long latency, due partly to decremental conduction (Chapter 16), is of considerable importance in the phenomena associated with re-entry (Chapters 17 and 18).

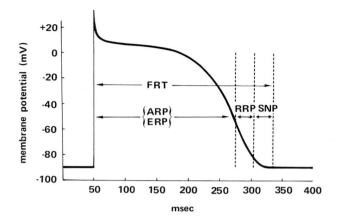

FIG. 14.11. Excitability during the cardiac action potential. The effective refractory period (ARP or ERP), during which stimuli of any strength are unable to initiate a propagated action potential, is followed by the relative refractory period (RRP), during which only stimuli greater than those which normally reach threshold can cause a propagated action potential. This is followed by the supernormal period (SNP), during which stimuli slightly less than those which normally reach threshold can cause a propagated action potential. The action potentials generated during the RRP and SNP usually propagate slowly, so full recovery time (FRT) is the interval following depolarization after which threshold returns to normal and stimulation produces a normally propagated action potential. (From Hoffman and Cranefield, 1960.)

The *supernormal period* that follows the relative refractory period is one in which stimuli that are slightly smaller than threshold stimuli (as measured during diastole) elicit a propagated response. Although excitability is thus supernormal, the action potential which results from excitation of the heart at this time is *not* unusually large; indeed the action potentials elicited during the supernormal phase are usually reduced in amplitude owing to the slow recovery of the sodium channels. A supernormal period is apparently absent in the cells of the AV node. In the cells of the atria and ventricles, as well as in the Purkinje fibers, supernormality occurs at approximately the same time as the "vulnerable period," which is described in Chapter 17. Vulnerability and supernormality occur at about the same phase of the cardiac cycle, but they are *not* directly related to each other (Chapter 17).

The interval between depolarization and the recovery of normal, resting excitability (the *full-recovery time*) encompasses the effective and relative refractory periods, as well as the supernormal period. At the end of the full-recovery time, the myocardial cell responds with a normal threshold to generate a normal action potential.

It is commonly assumed that the phenomena of refractoriness are directly related to those of repolarization, so that recovery of the ability of the myocardium to undergo regenerative depolarization after excitation can be predicted from the degree to which membrane potential has returned to its resting level.

The relationship between these two parameters, however, is more complex than is often appreciated. The ability of the cell to undergo a regenerative sodium-dependent action potential is determined by the degree to which the sodium channel has recovered its ability to open following a prior action potential. As already noted, however, this recovery is both time- and voltage-dependent. Thus although the degree to which the myocardium has repolarized defines the status of the *voltage-dependent* determinant of the recovery of the ability of the sarcolemma to exhibit a sodium-dependent action potential, the fact that this recovery is also *time-dependent* adds another factor that is not directly seen in membrane potential recordings. The discrepancies between the extent of repolarization and the degree to which refractoriness persists can become extremely important, e.g., for understanding the mechanisms of action of antiarrhythmic agents (Chapter 19).

INTERVAL-DURATION RELATIONSHIP

The duration of the cardiac action potential varies with cycle length (i.e., the interval between successive beats) such that when cycle length is reduced at high rates of beating, the duration of the action potential is also reduced. This is a very important physiological adjustment, for if the interval-duration relationship did not exist the ventricles would not have time to fill and so would cease to pump when heart rates became extremely rapid.

> If one assumes the normal action potential duration to be 0.3 sec at a heart rate of 75 beats/minute (cycle length 0.8 sec), then an increase in heart rate to 200 beats/min (cycle length 0.3 sec) would not allow for repetitive responses if the action potential duration remained unchanged. Yet the heart can beat at rates of 200/min, and these rapid heart rates can be tolerated by the normal heart for hours, or even days, with only a modest decrease in cardiac work. This ability of the heart to beat at rapid rates is attributable to the interval-duration relationship, by which a reduction in cycle length causes a decrease in action potential duration.

It is well established that the duration of the cardiac action potential is directly proportional to the duration of the preceding cardiac cycle (Fig. 14.12). The prolongation of the action potential at slow heart rates and the shortening of action potentials when the heart rate becomes rapid probably arise from the characteristics of the gating mechanisms which control the outward movement of potassium (described above as i_x) that normally repolarizes the cell. The slow closure of these potassium channels allows the early arrival of a second action potential to find the potassium channels still partially open. As a result, the repolarization following an action potential that comes very soon after the preceding one is accelerated. Conversely, these channels can close almost fully, and so open more slowly, when heart rates are slow and there is a long interval between successive beats. In this way the ability of potassium channels to reopen can cause

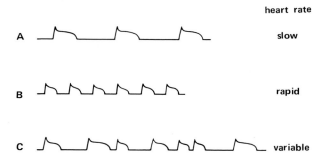

FIG. 14.12. Interval-duration relationship. At slow heart rates **(A)**, where the diastolic interval is long, the action potential duration is long. Where the diastolic interval is short, the action potential duration is also short **(B)**. When the heart rate is variable **(C)**, the action potential duration is directly proportional to the duration of the preceding diastolic interval. The lengths of the refractory periods in these beats are closely correlated to the durations of the action potentials shown here.

the action potential duration to be directly proportional to the length of the preceding cycle.

The interval-duration relationship describes the effects of cycle length on the refractory period as well as on action potential duration. The ability of cycle length to influence refractoriness is well known in electrocardiography in that an abnormally long pause between two beats prolongs the refractory period of the second beat. The interval-duration relationship therefore explains the tendency for impulses arriving soon after the beat following a long diastole to find the conduction system in a partially refractory state. The frequent occurrence of conduction abnormalities in beats closely following the beat after a long diastole (e.g., in Fig. 14.12C, where the third action potential occurs soon after the second, the latter representing the beat following a long diastole), explains some of the patterns seen in the genesis of aberrant conduction (Chapter 17).

MEMBRANE POTENTIALS IN DIFFERENT REGIONS OF THE HEART

The preceding description of the cardiac action potential dealt with the properties of the Purkinje fiber, the most carefully studied of the heart tissues. Special properties of both the diastolic and systolic portions of the action potential are found in other regions of the heart, however (Fig. 14.13). These unique features of the action potential in different cardiac cell types are related to, and in many cases account for, the specific electrophysiological roles served by certain regions of the heart.

Sinoatrial Node

The sinoatrial (SA) node is derived embryologically from the sinus venosus, which is the most rapidly beating chamber of the embryonic heart and so controls

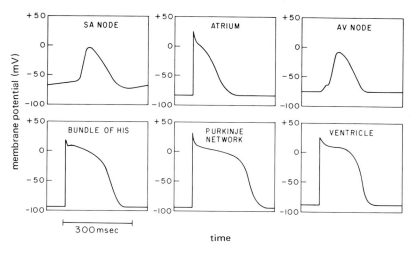

FIG. 14.13. Action potential configurations in different regions of the mammalian heart.

the rate of beating of all its chambers (Chapter 15). In the adult heart as well, the SA node acts as the normal *pacemaker*. Thus the wave of electrical depolarization that initiates both the atrial and ventricular systole originates in this band of specialized myocardial tissue, which is located in the wall of the right atrium near its junction with the superior vena cava (Chapter 1).

Pacemaker activity can be defined as the ability to initiate a propagated action potential, so the hallmark of a pacemaker cell is its intrinsic ability to depolarize spontaneously. From the standpoint of the properties of the cell membrane in a pacemaker cell, the ionic permeabilities during diastole are not constant. Instead, permeability changes occur during diastole that cause membrane potential to decrease spontaneously until threshold is reached, at which time a propagated action potential is initiated (SA node, Fig. 14.13). This spontaneous *diastolic depolarization* of the SA node, sometimes called phase 4 depolarization or the pacemaker potential, is normally responsible for initiating systole in all regions of the heart (Chapter 15).

Pacemaker Activity

The instability of diastolic potential in pacemaker cells was first observed not in the SA node but in spontaneously depolarizing Purkinje fibers. These observations were made in 1951 by Weidmann, who suggested that the slowly decreasing resting potential in diastole could be due to: (a) decreasing potassium conductance; (b) increasing sodium conductance; or (c) decreasing activity of an electrogenic sodium pump. It is now clear that in the Purkinje fiber the first explanation is correct, and that the progressively decreasing resting potential which causes spontaneous pacemaker activity is due to a fall in potassium conductance. While the phenomena underlying pacemaker activity have been studied most extensively in Purkinje fibers, it is now apparent that the properties of these pacemaker cells cannot be extrapolated to other pacemaker cells, notably those in the SA and atrioventricular (AV) nodes. In the Purkinje fibers the slow closing of a potassium channel causes membrane potential to fall during diastole by diminishing the outward flux of potassium. The resulting reduction in outward current occurs at a time when there is a constant inward current, which in the Purkinje fiber is probably carried by sodium. The latter appears not to vary with time and so is thought not to be involved in controlling the rate of pacemaker firing of the Purkinje fiber. Control of pacemaker activity in the Purkinje fiber therefore appears to lie in variations of the rate of spontaneous membrane depolarization that are caused by changes in the rate at which the outward, repolarizing potassium current decreases. The outward potassium current whose spontaneous reduction causes pacemaker activity in the Purkinje fiber is called i_{K_2} (Table 14.1). This outward current is distinct from the repolarizing potassium currents (i_{x_1} and i_{x_2}) and the background current (i_{K_1}) discussed above. Thus the potassium channel whose closure determines pacemaker activity in the Purkinje fiber is not the same as potassium channels which cause membrane repolarization at the end of the action potential.

It is tempting to extrapolate the findings with regard to pacemaker activity in the Purkinje fiber to the more important pacemaker activity in the SA node. Accurate studies of the SA node are extremely difficult because of the small cell size (Chapter 1). At the present time it appears that, as in the Purkinje fiber, diastolic depolarization in the SA node occurs as the result of spontaneous closure of a potassium channel, although there is evidence that an increasing inward current may also contribute to spontaneous depolarization of the SA node. Current knowledge of the ionic channels of the SA node indicate that the channel whose closure causes diastolic depolarization has the characteristics of the channel whose opening causes repolarization (i_x), rather than that which carries i_{K_2} in the Purkinje fiber.

The inward current whose depolarizing effects are "unmasked" as potassium conductance falls in the SA node was initially believed to be carried by sodium. Recently, however, evidence has been obtained that this inward current is carried by calcium. There is also evidence that the major inward current responsible for subsequent depolarization during the action potential of the SA node is also a calcium current. In this way the action potential in the SA node may be calcium-dependent rather than sodium-dependent.

> The diastolic potential of the pacemaker cells of the SA node, even at its maximum, is less than that estimated from the Nernst equation for potassium. This finding indicates that the pacemaker cells in the SA node do not become freely permeable to potassium during diastole. The importance of this phenomenon becomes clear in Chapter 19, when the effects of acetylcholine on the SA node are described.

There are three possible mechanisms which can modify the discharge frequency of the pacemaker cells and thus allow the heart rate to be altered (Fig

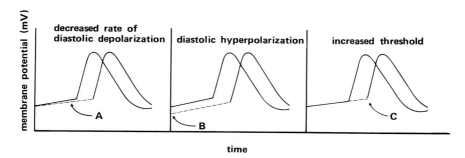

FIG. 14.14. Three possible mechanisms that can slow the rate of pacemaker discharge (*solid line*, control; *dashed line*, slowed): decreased rate of diastolic depolarization *(arrow A)*, diastolic hyperpolarization *(arrow B)*, and increased threshold *(arrow C)*. More than one of these changes may be induced by a given drug. Accelerated pacemaker discharge can occur through the opposite changes in any or all of these parameters (increased rate of diastolic depolarization, diastolic depolarization, lowered threshold).

14.14). In terms of mechanisms that could cause slowing, these are: (a) a decrease in the slope of diastolic depolarization; (b) diastolic hyperpolarization; and (c) an increase in threshold (Fig. 14.14). The actions of specific agents that influence heart rate are discussed in terms of these mechanisms in Chapters 16 and 19.

Atrium

Atrial action potentials are generally similar to the "typical" action potential of the Purkinje fibers except that their durations are shorter (Fig. 14.13). Diastolic potential (phase 4) is constant; hence, pacemaker activity is absent. Depolarization (phase 0) is rapid and is followed by a brief phase of rapid repolarization (phase 1) and then a brief plateau (phase 2) that often merges into repolarization (phase 3) so that separate phases 2 and 3 cannot be identified. The terminal portions of phase 3 tend to return more slowly to the diastolic level than do those in the ventricle or Purkinje fibers. As in the Purkinje fiber, the time course of the atrial action potential and that of the refractory period do not necessarily coincide.

Atrioventricular Node

The AV node, as is discussed more fully in Chapter 16, is a region of slow conduction. This behavior reflects the properties of the action potentials in this region of the heart, which are slowly rising and low in amplitude (Fig. 14.13). Spontaneous (phase 4) depolarization, once thought to be prominent in the AV node, is now believed to be minimal or absent in most regions of this structure, so that the AV node has little or no intrinsic pacemaker activity. Resting potential is approximately −80 mV, and the membrane voltage during depolarization (overshoot) does not usually exceed +5 to +10 mV. Action potential duration in the AV node is longer than in the atrium, but less than in the Purkinje fibers.

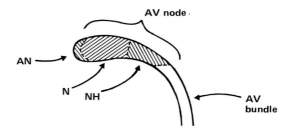

FIG. 14.15. Atrioventricular conduction system. The AV node can be divided functionally into three regions: AN (upper, or atrionodal), N (middle, or nodal), and NH (lower, or nodal-His bundle).

The AV node can be divided functionally into three regions (Fig. 14.15): the AN region (upper or atrionodal portion), the N region (middle or nodal portion), and the NH region (lower, or nodal-His bundle portion). Each of these regions has a distinctive action potential. The amplitude of the overshoot is similar in all regions, but resting potential is lowest in the N region. Action potential duration is shortest in the AN region and increases progressively through the N region to the NH region. The slowest rate of depolarization is found in the N region, where the action potential amplitude is also lowest. Spontaneous pacemaker activity is absent in the N region, but automaticity has been found in both the AN and NH regions.

The low amplitude and slowly rising action potentials recorded in the AV node, which are largely responsible for the slow passage of the wave of depolarization through this structure, have been suggested to reflect the absence of the sodium channel that in other regions of the heart gives rise to the fast inward current. There is now growing evidence that depolarization in the AV node, like that of the SA node, may be due primarily if not entirely to a slow inward current carried by calcium, and that especially in the N region there is no fast inward current. Because of the small size of the AV nodal cells, especially in the N region where the smallest and most slowly rising action potentials are found, it has not yet been possible to test this hypothesis directly by voltage clamp studies.

His-Purkinje System

The "typical" action potential in the Purkinje fiber of the bundle of His has already been described. It generally resembles that in the ventricle except that early repolarization (phase 1) is more prominent and its duration is longer (Fig. 14.13). The action potentials in the more distal regions of the His-Purkinje system are usually longer than those in the bundle of His, so that the cells of the Purkinje network of the ventricles have the longest action potentials found in the mammalian heart (Fig. 14.13). These cells also have very large action potentials, with resting potentials greater than −90 mV and action potential amplitudes greater than +120 mV so that the overshoot is approximately +30 mV. Similarly, the rate of depolarization is very rapid. Normally the cells of the His-Purkinje system have little pacemaker activity, although phase 4 depolarization can be increased under some pharmacological or pathological influences.

Ventricles

The ventricular action potential is similar to that already described for the Purkinje fibers although i_{Cl} and i_{K_2} are of little importance and i_x is of less relevance to repolarization. In relationship to other regions of the heart, the ventricular action potential is of large amplitude, although less than that of the His-Purkinje system (Fig. 14.13). Its duration is longer than that of the atria and shorter than that of the His-Purkinje system. Spontaneous diastolic (phase 4) depolarization is not seen under normal conditions, so that like the working myocardial cells of the atria, those of the ventricle lack pacemaker activity.

PROPERTIES OF THE INTERCALATED DISC

The preceding discussion focused on that region of the cardiac sarcolemma which separates the interior of the myocardial cell from the extracellular fluid. The permeability and conductivity properties of the intercalated disc, which separates the interiors of adjacent myocardial cells (Chapter 1), are quite different

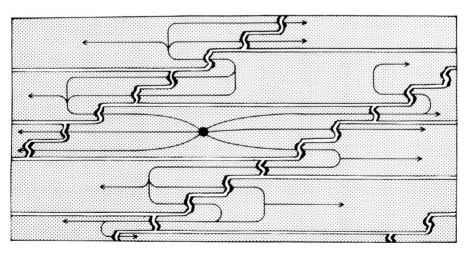

FIG. 14.16. Distribution of current flow in the myocardium (*shaded,* intracellular space; *unshaded,* extracellular spaces). Straight lines represent the sarcolemma, which has a high electrical resistance. Curved heavy lines represent the intercalated discs, which have lower electrical resistance. The flow of current *(thin arrows)* from an intracellular electrode *(dot in center)* is transmitted through the intercalated discs primarily in a longitudinal direction, but current also flows laterally through the branching myocardial syncytium, as shown. Very little current can flow across the sarcolemma. (Modified from Woodbury, 1962.)

from those in the regions of the sarcolemma that were described above. There is no reason to believe that the intercalated disc participates in the complex conductance changes described above. Instead, this specialized cell membrane is freely permeable to charged particles and so represents a low-resistance pathway between adjacent cells. Radioactive potassium injected at one end of a column of myocardial cells, for example, diffuses freely across the intercalated discs from cell to cell almost as rapidly as this ion would diffuse in an aqueous medium. This ability of the intercalated disc to pass charged particles freely from cell to cell allows for the rapid spread of electrical activity between adjacent cells (Fig. 14.16), thereby facilitating propagation of the excitatory impulse throughout the heart.

> The descriptions provided above are valid for most mammalian hearts, including, as far as is known, that of man. Several important species differences have been found, however. In the rat the ventricular action potential is very brief and in some ways resembles that in a skeletal muscle.

While at this point the litany just concluded may seem to represent only "facts to be memorized," it becomes apparent in the following chapters that an understanding of the mechanisms responsible for the genesis and therapy of cardiac arrhythmias requires knowledge of both the ionic basis of the cardiac action potential and the configurations of these action potentials in various regions of the heart. Therefore this descriptive material provides a basis for the discussions on arrhythmias and on the drug actions on cardiac rhythm found in Chapters 16–19.

BIBLIOGRAPHY

Gettes, L. S. (1976): Possible role of ionic changes in the appearance of arrhythmias. *Pharmacol. Ther.* [*B*], 2:787–810.
Hoffman, B. F., and Cranefield, P. (1960): *Electrophysiology of the Heart.* McGraw-Hill, New York.
Katz, B. (1966): *Nerve, Muscle and Synapse.* McGraw-Hill, New York.
Lüttgau, H. C., and Glitsch, H. G. (1976): Membrane physiology of nerve and muscle fibres. *Fortschr. Zool.*, 24:1–32.
McAllister, R. E., Noble, D., and Tsien, R. W. (1975): Reconstruction of the electrical activity of cardiac Purkinje fibers. *J. Physiol. (Lond.)*, 251:1–59.
Noble, D. (1975): *The Initiation of the Heartbeat.* Clarendon Press, Oxford.
Trautwein, W. (1973); Membrane currents in cardiac muscle fibers. *Physiol. Rev.*, 53:793–835.
Woodbury, J. W. (1962): Cellular electrophysiology of the heart. In: *Handbook of Physiology. Section 2: Circulation*, Vol. 1, edited by W. F. Hamilton and P. Dow, pp. 237–286. American Physiological Society, Washington, D.C.

15

The Electrocardiogram

Cardiac muscle can possess at least three major properties: *automaticity,* sometimes called pacemaker activity, which is the ability to initiate an electrical impulse; *conductivity,* the ability to conduct electrical impulses; and *contractility,* the ability to shorten and to do work. All of these properties are found in primitive myocardial cells. With differentiation, three classes of myocardial cells develop, all of which retain the property of conductivity. The first, the ordinary working myocardial cells of the atria and ventricles, have the ability to contract, but under all but the most unusual conditions they lack automaticity. Other cells in the heart, however, remain able to initiate an electrical impulse. These "pacemaker cells," in which contractility is virtually lost, are concentrated in the *SA and lower AV nodes* and in the *His-Purkinje system.* Pacemaker cells are also found as *Purkinje-like cells* in the walls of the atria. A third class of cells, found in the *AV node,* lack both automatic and contractile properties and, in addition, conduct impulses very slowly. The latter cells, which are found mainly in the N region of the AV node, slow the wave of depolarization as it passes from atria to ventricles. The significance of this delay is noted later, when we examine in more detail the normal propagation of the impulse over the heart.

NORMAL SEQUENCE OF ELECTRICAL ACTIVATION

The primary pacemaker of the heart is the SA node, which normally initiates the wave of depolarization that is transmitted through the myocardium to activate all regions of the heart. In adult man a propagated action potential begins in the SA node 60–100 times each minute. The SA node, located in the sulcus formed where the superior vena cava joins the right atrium (Fig. 1.5), is derived from the sinus venosus, the most rapidly beating portion of the tubular heart of the embryo. The latter, which can be divided into four regions—the *sinus venosus, atria, ventricles,* and *truncus arteriosus* (Fig. 15.1)—beats synchronously in response to an impulse initiated in pacemaker cells of the sinus venosus. Even though contraction in the atria, ventricles, and truncus arteriosus is triggered by the impulse transmitted from the sinus venosus, each of these regions contains pacemaker cells. Because the intrinsic rates of the pacemaker cells decrease as one proceeds from the "higher" venous end to the "lower" arterial end of the tubular embryonic heart (i.e., from left to right in Fig. 15.1), the existence of the less rapid, lower pacemaker activities is not seen unless the different regions of the embryonic heart are separated, as was first demonstrated in 1852 by Stannius.

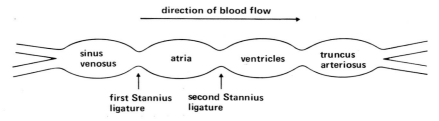

FIG. 15.1. Tubular embryo heart. The flow of blood is from left to right. Intrinsic rates of the pacemaker activity of each chamber also increases from left to right. These different rates of beating were first demonstrated by Stannius, who placed ligatures at the sinoatrial junction (first Stannius ligature) and the AV junction (second Stannius ligature) in the frog heart, which has a functional anatomy similar to that shown here.

By placing tight ligatures between these structures, Stannius showed that when the influence of the more rapid higher pacemakers is abolished the activity of lower pacemakers becomes able to initiate a slow beating of the distal regions of the embryonic heart. A similar situation exists in the adult heart, where the more rapid pacemaker activity of the SA node normally obscures the intrinsic pacemaker activity of lower regions. With some pathological conditions (e.g., where the SA node ceases to function or impulse propagation to the ventricles is blocked) the activity of the lower pacemakers becomes apparent. The most rapid of the lower pacemakers is located in the lower (NH) region of the AV node (Fig. 14.15) and has an intrinsic rate of approximately 40–55 beats/minute. Should a wave of depolarization fail to be transmitted through the AV node and AV bundle into the ventricles, latent pacemaker cells in the Purkinje fibers of the ventricles become able to initiate a propagated action potential within the ventricles. Their intrinsic rate is usually 25–40 beats/minute. Although a large number of potential pacemaker cells is found in the ventricles, these do not always exhibit active pacemaker function when the wave of depolarization fails to reach the ventricles from the atria. The resulting cessation of ventricular contraction represents one mechanism for sudden cardiac death (Chapter 16).

The normal activation sequence in response to an impulse arising in the SA node is shown in Table 15.1. As would be expected from the anatomy and embryology of the adult heart, the impulse which originates in the SA node first activates the atria and then the ventricles. In the latter, the areas surrounding the outflow tracts are last to be activated.

The wave of electrical activation carried to all parts of the heart is transmitted through a functional syncytium of cardiac muscle cells (Chapter 1). This transmission takes place entirely through cardiac muscle and is made possible by the fact that the intercalated discs, the specialized cell-cell junctions of cardiac muscle, contain areas of low electrical resistance (the nexus, or gap junction; Fig. 1.17). Although conduction of the wave of activation throughout the heart takes place only through cardiac muscle, the conduction velocities in all regions of the heart are not the same (Table 15.1). Propagation of the wave of depolarization

TABLE 15.1. *Normal activation sequence*

Normal sequence of activation	Conduction velocity (meters/sec)	Time for impulse to traverse structure (sec)	Rate of pacemaker discharge (min^{-1})
SA node	—		60–100
↓		~0.15	
Atrial Myocardium	1.0–1.2		None
↓			
AV node	0.02–0.05		None, except lower fibers: 40–55
↓			
AV bundle	1.2–2.0		
↓		~0.08	
Bundle branches			
↓	2.0–4.0		25–40
Purkinje network			
↓			
Ventricular myocardium	0.3–1.0	~0.08	None

is fastest in the Purkinje fibers of the bundle branches and the network of conduction tissue in the endocardium of the ventricles. Conduction is less rapid in the AV bundle and atrial and ventricular myocardium, while in the AV and SA nodes the conduction velocity is extremely slow. Although the actual length of the AV node is short, conduction in this structure is so slow it causes a significant delay in the propagation of the excitatory wave from atria to ventricles.

The activation sequence outlined in Table 15.1 is one that is conventionally used in most discussions of electrocardiography, but several additional specialized pathways are now recognized to play a role in impulse transmission in the human heart. Many of these additional pathways have been known for years, but it is only with the more recent interest in the mechanism of arrhythmias that their significance has been recognized.

INTERNODAL TRACTS

The *internodal tracts* (Fig. 15.2), which represent preferred conduction pathways between SA and AV nodes, are defined on a functional, not anatomical, basis. Many electrophysiological studies indicate that rapid internodal conduction takes place along specialized pathways in the atria, although histological studies of the atria fail to demonstrate clearly demarcated bundles of cells through which impulses are carried between the two nodes. It may be that this facilitated conduction occurs when the impulse is transmitted through regions occupied by Purkinje-like cells in the atria.

Three internodal tracts are recognized. The *anterior* internodal tract provides not only a pathway between atria and ventricles but also a tract that passes through the atrial septum to link the two atria electrically. This latter portion of the anterior internodal tract, often called *Bachmann's bundle,* may aid in

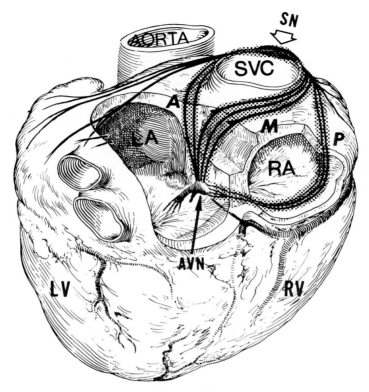

FIG. 15.2. Internodal tracts as seen in a posterior view of the heart in which the right ventricle (RV) is to the right and the left ventricle (LV) to the left of the viewer. The three internodal tracts are anterior (A), middle (M), and posterior (P). Each provides a preferential pathway for conduction between the SA node (SN), located in the wall of the right atrium (RA) near the superior vena cava (SVC), and the AV node (AVN). The anterior internodal tract also provides a conduction pathway to the left atrium (LA). (Modified from James, 1967.)

synchronizing contraction of the two atria, and there is evidence that interruption of Bachmann's bundle is followed by a delay of left atrial contraction relative to that in the right atrium. The *middle and posterior* internodal tracts (named after *Wenckebach* and *Thorel,* respectively) do not branch and serve only as preferential conduction pathways between SA and AV nodes.

ATRIOVENTRICULAR CONDUCTION

The atria and ventricles are separated by connective tissue so that propagation of the wave of depolarization between these chambers depends normally on a single strand of specialized muscle tissue, the AV bundle. Impulses originating in the SA node enter the AV bundle by way of the AV node, a small mass of specialized cardiac muscle located above the coronary sinus on the posterior wall

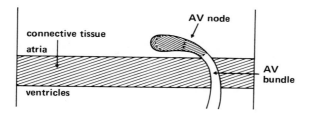

FIG. 15.3. The AV node and AV bundle provide the major conduction pathway traversing the connective tissue barrier between the atria (above) and ventricles (below).

of the right atrium. Thus the AV node and AV bundle normally provide the only electrical pathway that links the atria and ventricles (Fig. 15.3).

Additional strands of cardiac muscle linking the atria and ventricles are sometimes found in normal human hearts. These conduction pathways become functionally active under abnormal conditions or in abnormal hearts (Fig. 15.4). The most important of the additional pathways linking the atria and ventricles is the *bundle of Kent.* This structure, which appears anatomically as a strand of muscle tissue traversing the fibrous barrier between atria and ventricles, can be found at various locations, usually between the right atrium and right ventricle. By allowing impulses arising in the SA node to be conducted rapidly into the ventricles, the bundle of Kent provides an anatomical basis for understanding an arrhythmia called *pre-excitation* [also called the Wolff-Parkinson-White (WPW) syndrome; Chapter 17]. Another conduction pathway, the *bypass fibers of James,* can carry impulses from the atria into the upper portion of the AV bundle, thereby bypassing the normal region of conduction delay in the AV node. The

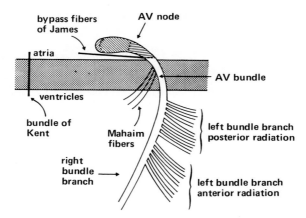

FIG. 15.4. Additional conduction pathways sometimes found to link the atria and ventricles include the bundle of Kent, which is variably located; the bypass fibers of James, which connect the atrial myocardium to the upper portion of the AV node; and the Mahaim fibers, which carry impulses from the AV bundle (or bundle branches) to abnormal sites in the ventricles. These additional pathways do not function in the normal human heart.

Mahaim fibers represent another pathway that permits impulses arising above the ventricles, either from the normal pacemaker in the SA node or from an abnormal site of impulse formation in the atria or AV node, to enter the ventricles. The Mahaim fibers can arise from the AV bundle or either of the bundle branches. It must be emphasized that, with the exception of the AV node and AV bundle, the conduction pathways between atria and ventricles described above normally are not functional.

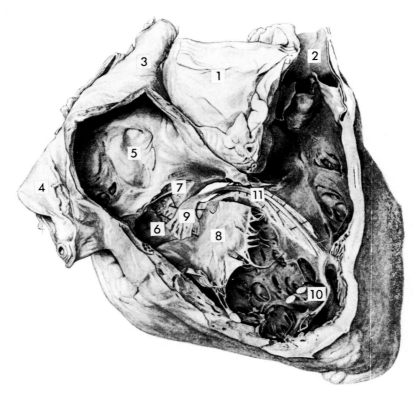

FIG. 15.5. Conduction system of the human right ventricle whose cavity is viewed from the right after removal of a portion of the atrial and ventricular walls. Note the aorta (1); pulmonary artery (2); superior vena cava (3); inferior vena cava (4); fossa ovale of the interatrial septum (5); thebesian valve overlying the coronary sinus (6); false tendon (7); medial leaflet of the tricuspid valve, which has been separated from its point of insertion (8); AV node, dissected free, with finger-like branches radiating proximally toward the coronary sinus (9). The AV bundle arises from the AV node and at the top of the membranous septum (which has been partially opened in this preparation) and divides into the right and left bundle branches. The right bundle branch (11), which can be viewed as a continuation of the common bundle after it gives rise to the left bundle branch, runs beneath the endocardium on the right side of the interventricular septum. The right bundle branch continues, usually without branching, in the direction of the anterior papillary muscle (10), which it reaches by way of the moderator band. (Modified from Wenckebach and Winterberg, 1927.)

VENTRICULAR ACTIVATION

Ventricular depolarization is normally initiated by the Purkinje network, a system of large, specialized, conducting cells that runs just beneath the endocardium of the ventricles. The Purkinje network arises directly from the AV bundle, which divides into the *right* and *left bundle branches* at the top of the interventricular septum (Fig. 1.5). The right bundle branch begins as a distinct bundle of conducting tissue that crosses the endocardial surface of the right ventricle (Fig. 15.5). The left bundle branch, in contrast, does not continue as a distinct bundle but fans out over the endocardium of the left ventricle to impinge on the ventricular myocardium by way of *anterior* and *posterior radiations* (Fig. 15.6). The anterior radiations of the left bundle branch arise more distally, so that partial interruption of the left bundle branch most commonly causes impairment of conduction through the anterior radiation (see *Hemiblocks,* below).

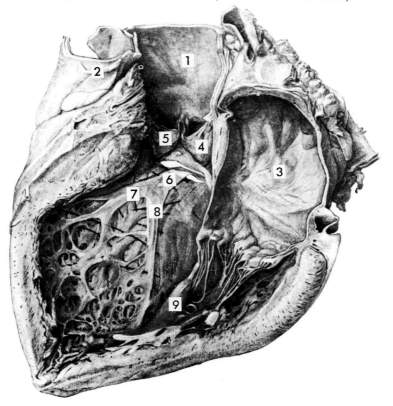

FIG. 15.6. Same preparation as shown in Fig. 15.5 viewed from the left after removal of a portion of the atrial and ventricular walls. Note the aorta (1); pulmonary artery (2); left atrium (3); right posterior (4) and anterior (5) cusps of the aortic valve. The left bundle branch, which emerges through an opening made by removal of a portion of the membranous septum, originates as a wide, flat band (6). The left bundle branch then fans out into anterior (7) and posterior (8) radiations, which run toward the anterior (not shown) and posterior (9) papillary muscles of the left ventricle. (Modified from Wenckebach and Winterberg, 1927.)

The Purkinje network arises from the bundle branches and courses along the endocardial surface of both ventricles where it impinges on the ordinary working myocardium of the ventricular walls. In this way the normal wave of electrical activation is rapidly propagated through the ventricles.

THE ELECTROCARDIOGRAM

The electrocardiogram (ECG), which provides a record of electrical events occurring within the heart, is obtained from electrodes placed on the surface of the body. The ECG plots the sequence of changes in electrical potential differences recorded between different regions of the body surface. Recently it has become possible to record electrical potentials from catheters placed in the cavities of the atria and ventricles. If a bipolar electrode catheter is placed in the right atrium adjacent to the tricuspid valve so that the two recording electrodes are on either side of the AV bundle, an *intracardiac electrogram* is recorded. The deflections of this intracardiac electrogram, often called a His bundle electrogram, are shown along with a representative ECG in Fig. 15.7.

The waves of the ECG were named by Einthoven, who chose to start in the middle of the alphabet with the letter P. Thus the first deflection of the ECG, which represents atrial depolarization, is the P wave. Although depolarization of the SA node precedes atrial depolarization (Table 15.1; Fig. 15.8), no manifestations of this pacemaker activity are seen in the ECG because the SA node is too small to generate electrical potential differences great enough to be recorded from the body surface. The width of the P wave (i.e., its duration) reflects the time taken for the wave of depolarization to spread over the atria.

Following the P wave, the ECG returns to its baseline, indicating that no changes in potential difference between various regions of the heart are apparent at the body surface. Yet during this "silent" interval between the P wave and the QRS complex (see below), the wave of electrical depolarization is being propagated through the AV node, the AV bundle, bundle branches, and the

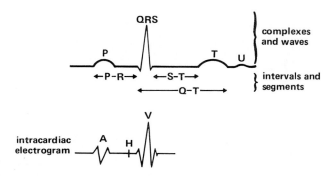

FIG. 15.7. **Top:** ECG recorded from the body surface. **Bottom:** Intracardiac electrogram.

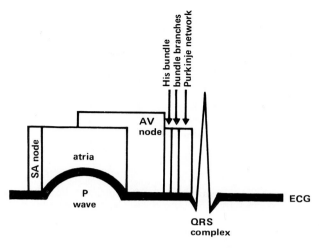

FIG. 15.8. Tissues depolarized by a wave of activation commencing in the SA node are shown in a series of blocks superimposed on the initial deflections of the ECG.

Purkinje network (Fig. 15.8). The lack of any influence of these important electrical events on the ECG, like failure of the ECG to record the activity of the SA node, is due to the small mass of tissue involved.

Analysis of the interval between the P wave and the QRS complex provides much useful information regarding the propagation of the impulse through the AV node, AV bundle, and bundle branches (Fig. 15.8). An index of the time taken for the impulse to pass from the atria to the ventricles is provided by the *P-R interval,* which extends from the beginning of the P wave to the *first* deflection of the QRS complex (whether this initial deflection is an R wave or a Q wave, as defined below). Additional information regarding passage of the wave of depolarization during the P-R interval can be obtained from the intracardiac electrogram, in which the potential difference between two electrodes introduced into the right atrium by an intracardiac catheter is recorded (Fig. 15.9). These recordings exhibit a sharp deflection (*H,* Fig. 15.7) that is generally assumed to arise in the AV bundle (bundle of His; hence the designation *H*). The deflections in the intracardiac electrogram arising from atrial and ventricular depolarization are called *A* and *V,* respectively (Fig. 15.7).

The *QRS complex* records the potentials that appear at the body surface when the wave of depolarization passes through the ventricular myocardium. The amplitude of the QRS complex is much higher than that of the P wave because the mass of ventricular tissue is greater than that of the atria; on the other hand, the duration of the QRS complex is less than that of the P wave, a phenomenon which is readily explained because the wave of depolarization spreads more rapidly through the ventricles via the rapidly conducting Purkinje network (Table 15.1).

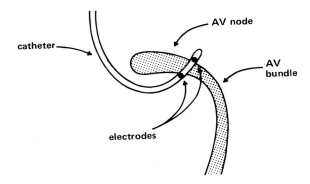

FIG. 15.9. The intracardiac electrogram measures the potential difference between two electrodes on a catheter introduced into the right atrium and placed over the proximal portion of the AV bundle.

The conventions followed in naming the "waves," or deflections, in the QRS complex are as follows. *Q:* any initial downward deflection followed by an upward deflection (if there is only a downward deflection, this is called *QS*). *R:* any upward deflection regardless of whether it is preceded by a Q wave. *S:* any downward deflection preceded by an R wave. If there are additional upward deflections after the S wave, they are designated R', R'', etc.; if additional downward deflections follow the S wave, these are designated S', S'', etc. Whether the deflection in any "lead" (see below) is upward or downward depends on the conventions of electrocardiography.

Following the inscription of the QRS complex, the ECG returns to, or very nearly to, its baseline, where it remains until the inscription of the T wave. This brief isoelectric phase, the *S-T segment* (or RS-T segment), is inscribed at a time during systole when all regions of the ventricle are in a depolarized state. The fact that the potential inscribed on the ECG during the S-T segment is normally the same as that inscribed during the interval after the T wave and before the P wave (the T-P interval), when the ventricles are fully repolarized and in diastole, reflects the absence of potential differences within the ventricles at both times. The isoelectric S-T segment therefore does not indicate that no region of the heart is depolarized, this portion of the normal ECG being inscribed when *all* regions of the ventricles are in a depolarized state. The long duration of the S-T segment reflects the normally prolonged plateau (phase 2) of the cardiac action potential (Chapter 14).

Although the ECG provides a record of the changing potential differences between different parts of the body surface, there is no way of determining the true zero potential of the ECG. For this reason an abnormal potential difference that exists during the S-T segment (ventricular systole) cannot be distinguished from an abnormal potential difference during the T-P interval (ventricular diastole). Both the abnormal presence of a region of nonexcited tissue in the ventricles during systole or the abnormal persistence of depolarization in a portion of the ventricles during diastole causes the potentials recorded during the S-T segment and the T-P interval to differ. As the T-P interval is assumed by convention to represent zero potential, both abnormalities are said to cause a shift in the S-T segment.

Repolarization of the ventricles generates the T wave, which corresponds to the end of phase 2 and phase 3 of the cardiac action potential (Fig. 15.10). The duration of the T wave is considerably longer than that of the QRS complex because, unlike the QRS complex, the T wave is not a rapidly propagated wave. Instead, the duration of the T wave is determined primarily by local factors that influence the duration of the action potentials in each region of the ventricle. Thus the narrow QRS complex arises from the rapidly conducted wave of depolarization that passes over the ventricles, whereas the broader T wave reflects the less synchronous repolarization of the ventricles. The sequence of ventricular repolarization also differs considerably from that during depolarization (see later).

The relationship between the QRS complex and the cardiac action potential is shown in Fig. 15.10. It is apparent that the QRS complex corresponds to the upstroke (phase 0) of the action potential and the S-T segment to the plateau (phase 2), while the T wave reflects repolarization (phase 3). This relationship, however, is much more complex than that shown in Fig. 15.10 because the QRS and T waves represent the *sum* of the effects of all of the action potentials in the millions of ventricular cells that are depolarized in different places and at different times. For this reason the rapidity of the potential changes during the QRS complex also reflects the high velocity with which the wave of depolarization is conducted over the ventricles, whereas the more slowly inscribed T wave also reflects the greater dispersion of action potential duration in the heart.

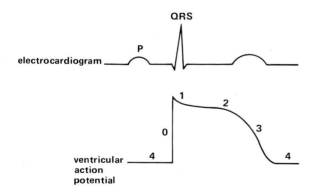

FIG. 15.10. Temporal relationships between the ECG **(top)** and a representative cardiac action potential **(bottom).** The QRS complex is produced by the upstrokes (phase 0) of all of the action potentials throughout the ventricles; the S-T segment corresponds to the plateaus (phase 2), while the T wave is inscribed during repolarization (phase 3) of the ventricular mass. The isoelectric segment which comes after the T wave corresponds to ventricular diastole (phase 4).

The atria, like the ventricles, generate a potential difference during their repolarization. A T_p wave (i.e., the "T" of the P) is not usually seen, however, because its amplitude is small and it is "buried" in the much larger QRS complex. On occasion, such as when P waves are not followed by QRS complexes (heart block; Chapter 16), a T_p wave may become apparent on the ECG.

In some normal ECGs a small deflection is seen after the T wave. This is the U wave, whose mechanism of production is uncertain. It has been postulated that the U wave is related to repolarization of the Purkinje network, in which the action potential duration is greater than that of the ventricular myocardium (Chapter 14), but this explanation is not fully substantiated.

The Q-T interval, which is the time that elapses between the onset of the QRS complex and the end of the T wave, is an index of the duration of the action potential in the ventricular myocardium (Fig. 15.10). Clearly this is only an approximate relationship as both the QRS complex and T wave represent the sum of the potential differences produced by all of the cells of the ventricular myocardium. In spite of the fact that the relationship between the duration of the ventricular action potential and the Q-T interval is only an approximation, measurements of the latter provide a useful index of the effects of drugs and diseases on the time-dependent properties of the electrophysiological properties of the ventricles.

TABLE 15.2. *Durations of waves and intervals in normal adult human heart*

Parameter	Duration (sec)
Intervals	
P-R	0.12–0.20
P-H	0.080–0.140
P-A	0.025–0.045
A-H	0.050–0.120
H-V	0.035–0.055
Q-T	0.30–0.40[a]
Waves	
P	0.08–0.10
QRS	0.06–0.10

[a] Highly dependent on the heart rate, to which the Q-T interval is inversely related.

Table 15.2 provides approximate values for the durations of various waves and intervals in the normal adult human heart. Because many of these time intervals are age-dependent and vary with heart rate, the values in Table 15.2 are presented to give the reader an idea of the relative magnitudes of these intervals rather than as absolute values to be committed to memory.

THE HEART AS A DIPOLE IN A VOLUME CONDUCTOR

The ECG in Fig. 15.7 does not completely represent the electrical potentials generated in the heart during the cardiac cycle. Instead it records the time-dependent changes in electrical potential between points on the surface of the body. The pioneers in the recording of these electrical potentials recognized that the shape and directions of the waves inscribed during the cardiac cycle were entirely dependent on where the electrodes, or *leads,* were placed on the body surface. To understand how the spread of the wave of depolarization over the atria and ventricles produces the potential changes depicted in the ECG, we first examine the far simpler model of a *dipole* in a *volume conductor* (Fig. 15.11).

A dipole is an electrical source, consisting of an asymmetrically distributed electrical charge. The heart can be depicted as a dipole at any instant during the spread of the wave of depolarization because one portion of the myocardium is depolarized while the remaining regions of the heart are still in their resting state. In the resting myocardium the *outside* of the cell is more positively charged than the inside (Chapter 14), whereas in depolarized regions the outside of the cell is negatively charged relative to the inside. For this reason Fig. 15.11—which is analogous to a single frame in a motion picture (e.g., of the ventricles at one instant during depolarization)—shows the partially depolarized heart as an electrical dipole that consists of a resting (positive) region and a depolarized (negative) region.

To generate potentials at the body surface, the cardiac dipole must be in a conducting medium. In Fig. 15.11 this "volume conductor" is provided by placing the dipole in a tray of salt water. The volume conductor therefore is necessary to permit the electrical potentials generated by the dipole to reach the periphery. In man the tissues of the body serve as a volume conductor that transmits the potentials generated by the heart to the body surface.

The model of the heart as a dipole in the center of a volume conductor is of course greatly oversimplified. The heart is not a simple dipole in that the complex pathways of impulse conduction allow multiple dipoles to coexist during depolarization of the ventricles. For the sake of simplicity, however, it is not incorrect

FIG. 15.11. Partially depolarized ventricles within the body depicted as an electrical dipole in a volume conductor. The dipole is seen as the rectangle in the center of the figure, which is positively charged to the right and negatively charged to the left. The volume conductor is shown as a circle *(solid line)* within which are drawn isopotential lines *(dashed lines)*. Potentials (indicated in millivolts) can be recorded from the surface of the volume conductor via electrodes (leads) such as A and B, which face regions of the surface where potentials are −1 and +1 mV, respectively. Also shown is an indifferent lead (V), which records zero potential because it is connected to several electrodes placed on the surface of the volume conductor in such a way that the sum of the recorded potentials is zero.

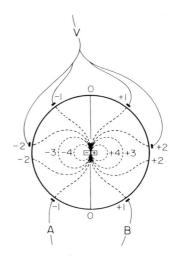

—only oversimplified—to consider the ventricles during depolarization as a single dipole. A more serious oversimplification, in terms of the ECG, is the fact that the body is not a homogeneous volume conductor; e.g., the lungs represent a region of high electrical resistance. Yet the model shown in Fig. 15.11 remains useful in gaining an understanding of the physical principles which govern the genesis of the ECG.

Lines of equal potential can be drawn in the model of the dipole in a homogeneous volume conductor (Fig. 15.11) along which no potential differences exist. Those lines in the half of the volume conductor occupied by the negative pole define negative potentials, and those in the other half positive potentials. The lines of equal potential in Fig. 15.11 illustrate the effects of two physical variables on the potentials generated within the volume conductor. First, the amplitude of the electrical potential falls off in proportion to the square of the distance from the dipole; second, potential decreases as one moves away from the axis of the dipole. Distance, the first variable, can be largely ignored in clinical electrocardiography, so that the differences in potential measured at various points on the body surface are most readily understood as arising from the second variable: the relationship between the electrodes, or leads, on the body surface and the angle defined by the heart's dipole.

ELECTROCARDIOGRAPHIC LEAD SYSTEMS

The potential differences set up by the dipole illustrated in Fig. 15.11, like those resulting from depolarization of the heart, can be sampled using either of two types of *lead systems*. A *bipolar lead* is one in which both recording electrodes are influenced by the dipole (*A* and *B,* Fig. 15.11), so that the potential *difference* between the two leads is recorded. In the example shown in Fig. 15.11, the potential difference between leads *A* and *B* is 2 mV. Whether the recorded potential is +2 mV or −2 mV depends on the conventions chosen by the observer. If one defines electrode *A* as zero, then *B* records +2 mV. If *B* is chosen as zero, then *A* is −2 mV. Because of their simplicity, bipolar lead systems were the first to be used in clinical electrocardiography.

Attempts to define the true zero potential in the human body have led to the use of the so-called *unipolar leads* in which one lead (the *exploring* electrode) is influenced by the dipole, while the other lead (the *indifferent* electrode) is considered to be recording zero potential at all times, i.e., not to be influenced by the dipole. Theoretically such an indifferent electrode can be produced by one of two means. The first involves placement of an electrode so far from the dipole that it records virtually no potential from the dipole simply because the potential declines with increasing distance. This approach to the problem of obtaining an indifferent lead, which can be achieved, for example, by placing an individual in one corner of a saltwater swimming pool and recording from the opposite corner, is obviously impractical for clinical electrocardiography. The second solution, which is a more practical one, is to connect a number of leads, all influenced by the dipole, so that the differences in potential can be assumed to be canceled out. This second type of indifferent electrode, usually called the *V lead,* is assumed to record a potential at or near zero because of mutual cancellation of the potentials recorded by the multiple electrodes, each of which is influenced by the dipole.

The unipolar leads used in clinical electrocardiography measure the potential difference between the V lead, which is assumed to record zero potential (see above) and an *exploring lead,* which is influenced by the cardiac dipole. In the example shown in Fig. 15.11, electrodes *A* and *B* can each be considered to be an exploring lead. Thus the unipolar lead *VA,* which detects the absolute potential at the point of placement of electrode *A,* records a potential of −1 mV. The potential is assigned a negative value because *V* is assumed to be zero. Similarly, the unipolar lead *VB* detects a potential of +1 mV because electrode *B* is located in a region where the potential is equal to +1 mV.

The V lead used in clinical electrocardiography is not, in fact, unaffected by the cardiac dipole throughout the cardiac cycle: As usually constructed, the V lead does not record zero potential (see below). While this limitation presents certain theoretical drawbacks, for all practical purposes the fact that the V leads do not provide true unipolar recordings is of no real clinical significance, as interpretations of electrocardiographic contour are generally *empirical* rather than absolute.

NATURE OF THE CARDIAC DIPOLE

The example of the dipole in a volume conductor depicted in Fig. 15.11 provides a model of the distribution of electrical potential at one instant during depolarization of the ventricles. Yet the ECG is more complex in that the potentials produced by ventricular depolarization change from moment to moment. To understand the genesis of the ECG, which is a graph of the time dependence of the changing electrical potentials set up within the heart, it is useful to consider initially the potential differences that evolve when a simple rectangular strip of cardiac muscle is depolarized (Figs. 15.12–15.16). In the following example note

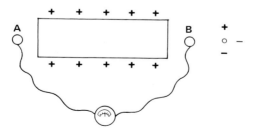

FIG. 15.12. The entire surface of a strip of resting myocardium is positively charged (relative to the interior of the cells of the fiber) so that no potential difference exists between electrodes A and B. A strip chart recording of this bipolar ECG *(right)* records zero potential difference and so remains at its baseline.

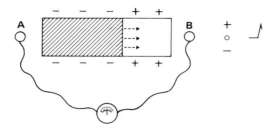

FIG. 15.13. The strip of myocardium depicted in Fig. 15.12 has been stimulated at its left side and is now slightly more than half depolarized *(shaded area)*. The surface of the depolarized area is negatively charged (relative to the interior of the cells of the fiber) so that electrode B is facing a region of greater positivity than is electrode A. The strip chart recorder at the right, which has been wired so that an upward deflection is written when electrode B is more positive than A, thus inscribes an upward deflection. The deflection in this bipolar ECG reaches its maximum when exactly half of the myocardial strip is depolarized. Note that the partially depolarized strip of myocardium represents the dipole shown in Fig. 15.11.

that the polarity of the resting myocardium is depicted as being *positive,* in contrast to the convention used in Chapter 14 where the resting potential is shown to be of the order of *minus* 90 mV. This source of confusion arises because the discussion in Chapter 14 focused mainly on the results of *intracellular* recordings, which at rest are obtained from an area of relative electronegativity. In electrocardiography, however, potentials are recorded from *outside* the cells, which are positively charged in the resting state and become negatively charged during depolarization.

In the resting cell (Fig. 15.12), where all portions of the cell surface are positively charged, no *differences* in potential are recorded, so that the bipolar "ECG" remains at the baseline (zero potential).

When the strip of myocardium shown in Fig. 15.12 is stimulated at its left-hand end, a wave of depolarization is propagated from left to right. As this wave of depolarization passes from left to right across the surface of the myocardium,

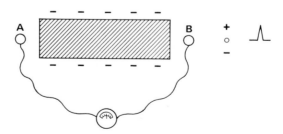

FIG. 15.14. The strip of myocardium depicted in Figs. 15.12 and 15.13 is now fully depolarized. When the action potentials of all cells are in phase 2, their external surfaces are negative relative to their interiors. Because no potential differences exist between the external surfaces of the cells in the strip of myocardium, electrodes A and B both face a similar degree of negativity. The deflection in the bipolar ECG *(right)* thus returns to the baseline.

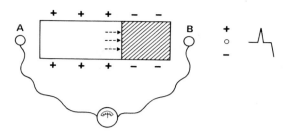

FIG. 15.15. Strip of myocardium depicted in Figs. 15.12–15.14 in which repolarization has begun in the same region that was first to be depolarized, i.e., at the left. Because the cell exteriors in the repolarized region of the strip *(left)* have returned to their normal, resting positivity, electrode B is facing a region of greater negativity than is electrode A. The bipolar ECG at the right thus inscribes a downward deflection (see legend to Fig. 15.13).

a potential difference appears between electrodes *A* and *B* (Fig. 15.13). If electrode *A* is chosen to represent zero potential, electrode *B* records a positive potential relative to electrode *A*. If the polarity of the recording device is set so that an upright deflection is written when *B* is positive relative to *A*, this wave of depolarization causes an upright deflection to appear in the ECG. As the wave of depolarization passes along the strip of myocardium, the potential difference waxes and then wanes, reaching its peak when half of the strip is depolarized.

The potential difference between electrodes *A* and *B* returns to zero when the entire strip is depolarized (Fig. 15.14) because both electrodes now face a similar degree of electronegativity. (Note that the ECG cannot distinguish between wholly depolarized or wholly repolarized myocardial tissue; it records only potential differences.) If repolarization begins at the same point on the strip of myocardium at which the propagated wave of depolarization began, a potential difference opposite in polarity to that seen during depolarization is recorded (Fig. 15.15). That is, electrode *B* faces an area of electronegativity (relative to *A*) and a downward deflection is recorded in the ECG (based on the conventions cited in the preceding paragraph). At the end of the phase of repolarization, the entire strip once again is fully repolarized so that, as in Fig. 15.12, no potential differences are recorded (Fig. 15.16). Thus the ECG record returns to baseline.

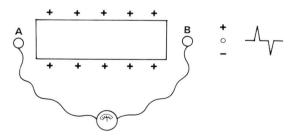

FIG. 15.16. Strip of myocardium depicted in Figs. 15.12–15.15 in its fully repolarized state. The situation is as shown in Fig. 15.12, so that the bipolar ECG *(right)* returns to its baseline.

A simple rule which should be memorized is that an electrode (lead) facing an *approaching* wave of depolarization records a *positive* potential, which inscribes an *upright* deflection in the ECG (where positive potentials are conventionally recorded as upward deflections). If the wave of depolarization moves away from a recording electrode (such as it would if *B*, rather than *A*, was chosen to represent zero in the example just given in Figs. 15.12–15.16), a downward deflection is written.

ELECTRICAL VECTORS

The potential set up by the cardiac dipole at any given instant during depolarization of the ventricles has both magnitude and direction. As seen in the description of Fig. 15.13, the magnitude of the dipole during ventricular depolarization is maximal when approximately half of the ventricular mass is depolarized. The directionality of the cardiac dipole is determined by the relative positions in the body of its positive and negative poles. If the dipole is oriented transversely in the body as shown in Fig. 15.17, *A*, an electrode on the right arm, records a negative potential and *B*, an electrode on the left arm, records a positive potential. This dipole represents a *vector*, having both magnitude and direction. By convention the cardiac dipole is depicted by an arrow, the head of which points toward the positive pole, as shown in Fig. 15.18. The arrow thus points in the direction of propagation of the wave of depolarization, i.e., toward the lead that inscribes an upright deflection. It should be remembered that the arrow points in the direction followed by the wave of depolarization as it passes through the ventricles; its length indicates the magnitude of the potential difference.

QRS Vectors

The ventricles during activation contain a large number of small electrical vectors. Because of the complex geometry of the ventricular mass and the fact that the wave of electrical depolarization normally enters both ventricles at

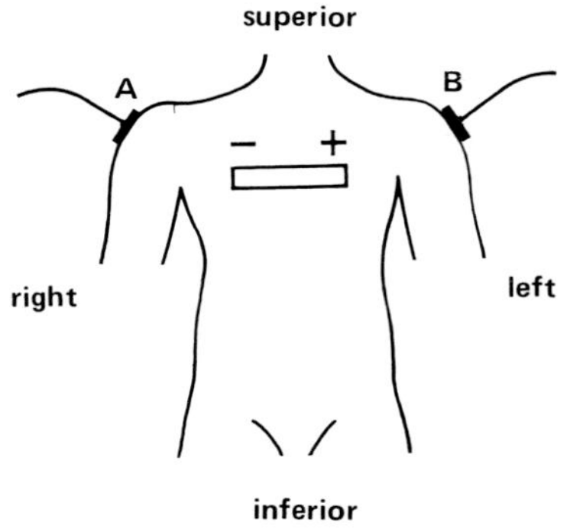

FIG. 15.17. Cardiac dipole in the human body. The ventricles during their depolarization can be viewed in terms of the strip of myocardial tissue described in Fig. 15.13, which establishes a dipole similar to that shown in Fig. 15.11. This analogy is obviously an oversimplification as the heart does not lie in the center of the chest, nor are electrical resistances the same throughout the chest. This analogy remains extremely useful, however, as it simplifies understanding the electrical potential differences recorded between ECG leads on the right (A) and left (B) arms.

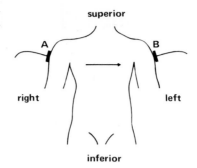

FIG. 15.18. The dipole shown in Fig. 15.17 can be represented as an arrow oriented in the direction of the long axis of the dipole. By convention, the head of the arrow points to the positive pole of the dipole, and so points in the direction of propagation of a wave of depolarization.

almost the same time by way of the right and left bundle branches, many regions of the ventricles are activated simultaneously. At any instant during the spread of the wave of depolarization over the ventricles, therefore, many electrical vectors can be drawn. If all of the vectors that exist at any moment are added together, a *mean electrical vector* can be drawn.

During the period of ventricular depolarization (i.e., during inscription of the QRS complex), a series of such mean electrical vectors occurs. The sequence of these mean electrical vectors is recorded by the ECG; i.e., the deflections in the ECG during the inscription of the QRS complex represent the changing direction and magnitude of the mean electrical vector as it changes during ventricular activation. The *mean QRS vector* is the average over time (i.e., throughout the inscription of the QRS complex) of *all* of the mean electrical vectors that arise during depolarization of the ventricles.

NORMAL SEQUENCE OF VENTRICULAR ACTIVATION

Normal activation of the ventricles can be divided arbitrarily into three phases. The first is activation of the septum, the second activation of the apex, and the third activation of the base of the heart. These three events merge into each other and do *not* represent three distinct events; they are considered separately here only for purposes of illustration.

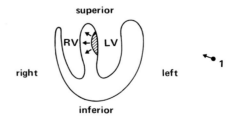

FIG. 15.19. Genesis of the QRS vector: septal activation. The initial portion of the QRS complex is produced when the interventricular septum is activated. Activation begins at the left ventricular surface of the septum and produces an initial QRS vector *(right)* that in the frontal plane is directed to the right and superiorly.

SEPTAL ACTIVATION

FIG. 15.20. Genesis of the QRS vector: activation of the apex. The midportions of the QRS complex are produced when the apex of the heart is activated. Activation begins at the endocardial surfaces of the ventricles and, because left ventricular forces are dominant, produces a frontal vector plane *(right)* directed to the left and inferiorly.

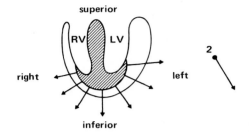

ACTIVATION OF THE APEX OF THE HEART

Septal Activation

The interventricular septum represents the first region of the ventricular mass to be depolarized in the normal sequence of ventricular activation. Activation of the septum begins in the endocardial myocardium of the left ventricle, giving rise to an electrical vector directed to the right. This septal vector is depicted in the frontal plane of the body in Fig. 15.19.

Activation of the Apex

As the wave of depolarization spreads into the ventricles via the Purkinje network, activation of each ventricle proceeds from the endocardial surface toward the epicardium. Because the mass of the left ventricle exceeds that of the right, leftward electrical forces predominate over those directed to the right. As a result, a second arbitrarily defined vector is directed inferiorly and to the left in the frontal plane, as shown in Fig. 15.20.

Activation of the Base

The last portions of the ventricles to be depolarized are the bases of the left and right ventricles. Again, activation proceeds from endocardial to epicardial surface and left ventricular forces dominate, so that this third vector is directed superiorly and to the left, as shown in Fig. 15.21.

FIG. 15.21. Genesis of the QRS complex: activation of the base. The terminal portions of the QRS complex are produced when the base of the heart is activated. Activation begins at the endocardial surfaces and, because left ventricular forces are dominant, produces a frontal plane vector *(right)* directed to the left and superiorly.

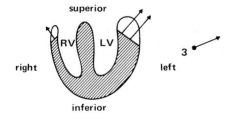

ACTIVATION OF THE BASE OF THE HEART

FIG. 15.22. Projection in a single figure of the three arbitrarily defined QRS vectors shown in Figs. 15.19–15.21. Since the tails of these three frontal plane vector arrows all represent zero potential, the vectors produced by septal activation (1), activation of the apex (2), and activation of the base (3) can be projected in a single figure as shown.

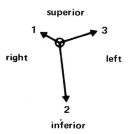

"Vector Loop"

All three of the mean vectors described above are depicted by arrows in the figures. The tips of the arrow tails of each vector correspond to zero potential, and the arrow heads define both the magnitude and direction of the three arbitrarily defined vectors. Since the tails of all three arrows correspond to the same zero potential, they can be connected in a single figure, which depicts the three vectors recorded during the inscription of the QRS complex (Fig. 15.22). The heads of the arrows can be connected by a line that begins at zero when the QRS complex begins, and returns to zero when the QRS complex has ended. If each of the heads of a larger number of vector arrows generated during ventricular depolarization is represented as a dot, the dots describe a loop, as shown in Fig. 15.23A. This vector loop thus represents the "movement" of the arrow head representing the mean electrical vector throughout the QRS complex. The *mean QRS vector* is the sum of *all* of the vector arrows whose heads make up the vector loop (Fig. 15.23B). The mean QRS vector thus represents the average vector resulting from all electrical vectors generated at all times and in all regions of the ventricles during the inscription of the QRS complex.

FIG. 15.23. QRS vector loop and mean QRS vector. The three arrows in Fig. 15.22, shown in **A**, represent only three of the instantaneous vectors generated during inscription of the QRS complex. The loop formed when the heads of all of these instantaneous vectors are connected is shown in **A** by the dashed line. The sum of these instantaneous vectors is the mean QRS vector **(B)**, which thus describes the average of all electrical vectors generated at all times and in all regions of the ventricles during their depolarization.

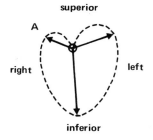

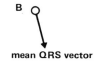

RECORDING THE ELECTROCARDIOGRAM

Bipolar Limb Leads and the Einthoven Triangle

The first systematic approach to interpreting the potential differences set up at the body surface by the cardiac dipole was provided by Einthoven, whose invention of the string galvanometer made possible the high-fidelity recording of the ECG. Einthoven utilized three limb leads—placed on the left arm, right arm, and left leg—to construct an equilateral triangle, and for simplicity he assumed that the heart lay at the center of this triangle (Fig. 15.24). The projections of the potentials set up by the cardiac dipole on the three sides of this "Einthoven triangle" are recorded in three limb leads, as defined in Table 15.3. Each of these is a bipolar lead in that it records the potential difference between two electrodes, both of which are influenced by the cardiac dipole. Each bipolar lead records only that portion of the electrical vector which is parallel to the lead axis (Fig. 15.11).

Einthoven defined the potentials at the right arm electrode as zero in leads I and II, while that at the left arm electrode was chosen as zero in lead III. For this reason positive deflections are recorded in lead I when the left arm is positive relative to the right arm, in lead II when the left leg is positive to the right arm, and in lead III when the left leg is positive to the left arm.

> This choice of the "zero" electrodes was based on Einthoven's desire to obtain upright deflections in all three leads of the normal ECG (see below) rather than on mathematical considerations, which most logically would assign "zero" to electrodes proceeding in a sequence around the sides of the triangle in a single direction. For this reason the sum of the potential differences in leads I and III equal that recorded in lead II.

If one examines the dipole that represents the mean QRS vector of the normal ECG (e.g., that shown in Fig. 15.29), the deflections in leads I–III are determined by the extent to which the potential differences of the dipole parallel each of the respective lead axes (Fig. 15.25). Note in Fig. 15.25 that the greatest potential difference is recorded by lead II, which most nearly parallels the dipole axis;

FIG. 15.24. Einthoven triangle. Einthoven simplified interpretation of the frontal plane ECG by assuming the heart to lie in the center of an equilateral triangle, the corners of which are in contact with electrodes placed on the left arm (LA), right arm (RA), and left leg (LL).

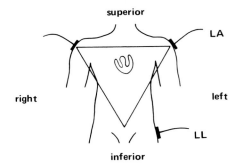

TABLE 15.3. *Standard limb leads*

Lead	Potential between	"Zero electrode"
I	Right and left arms	Right arm
II	Right arm and left leg	Right arm
III	Left arm and left leg	Left arm

whereas the least potential difference is recorded in lead III, which is most nearly perpendicular to the dipole. The smallest QRS complex—which like that in lead III is found in the lead whose axis is most nearly perpendicular to the mean QRS vector—is called the *transitional QRS* because it represents the transition between regions of electronegativity and electropositivity.

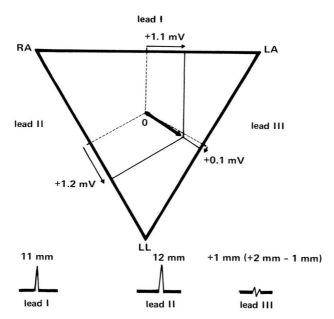

FIG. 15.25. A normal mean QRS vector projected on the Einthoven triangle. The tail of this vector lies in the center of the triangle, which represents zero potential. Each side of the triangle represents one of the three bipolar limb leads, as shown. The magnitude of the mean QRS deflection produced by this vector on each side of the triangle (i.e., in each lead) is determined by dropping perpendiculars *(thin lines)* from the sides of the triangle to the head of the mean QRS vector. (Dashed lines represent the projections on each of the sides of the zero potential.) According to the conventions introduced by Einthoven, upright deflections are produced by the projections of this vector in leads I, II, and III. The estimated QRS deflections are shown at the bottom of the figure, and the original ECG is presented in Fig. 15.29. Note that the QRS complex in lead III of Fig. 15.29 contains both upright and inverted deflections. The sum of these deflections corresponds to the projection of the QRS vector shown here. The QRS in lead III is a transitional complex in that it is almost midway between an upright and an inverted QRS complex. Such transitional QRS complexes are found in that lead whose axis is perpendicular to the mean QRS vector, as shown here.

Figure 15.25 demonstrates that an upright deflection is recorded in the ECG when the recording electrode faces a wave of approaching depolarization. As shown in this example (see also Fig. 15.23B), the wave of depolarization is directed inferiorly and toward the left so that, relative to the right arm, both the left arm (lead I) and left leg (lead II) record upright deflections. The wave of depolarization is nearly perpendicular to lead III, so that there is very little net deflection in the transitional QRS of lead III (the small upright deflection is similar in size to the small inverted deflection in this lead; see Fig. 15.29 for the original of this ECG).

In clinical electrocardiography one does not of course begin with a depiction of electrical vectors arising in the heart. Instead, the deflections obtained in the ECG leads are used to derive these vectors. The mean QRS vector can be defined from the three bipolar limb leads by plotting the magnitude of each deflection on the appropriate side of the Einthoven triangle. The "tail" of the mean QRS vector is placed at the center of the triangle (zero) where the perpendiculars drawn from the midpoints of each of the sides (also zero potential) meet. When perpendiculars are drawn toward the center of the triangle from each of the projections of the vector arrowhead, as determined from the amplitudes and polarities of the QRS complexes in leads I–III, the point of intersection locates the head of the mean QRS vector. (Only two such perpendiculars are in fact necessary to place the head of the vector.)

> It is readily apparent that the Einthoven triangle is only an approximation because the triangle defined by the limb leads is not equilateral, the heart is not in the center of the triangle, and the body is not a homogeneous volume conductor (the lungs, for example, have high electrical resistance). More precise triangles for the analysis of the QRS vector in the frontal plane can be drawn, but even these are not constant from one individual to the next. However, although the Einthoven triangle is only an approximation, it is both clinically useful and clinically used.

Unipolar Limb Leads

Three unipolar limb leads are conventionally employed in clinical electrocardiography. Remember that a unipolar lead measures the potential difference between an *exploring electrode,* which is influenced by the cardiac dipole, and an *indifferent electrode,* which is assumed to record zero potential. The indifferent electrode used in clinical electrocardiography employs the *central terminal* described by Wilson. Wilson's central terminal is made by connecting wires from the electrodes on the three limbs used to obtain the bipolar leads of Einthoven (Fig. 15.24). High resistances (R, Fig. 15.26) are placed in the circuits to overcome the effects of variable resistances where the electrodes are applied to the skin. The resulting lead, called the *V lead,* is assumed to record zero potential throughout the cardiac cycle. Wilson's central terminal does not, in fact, repre-

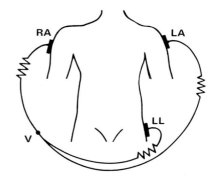

FIG. 15.26. Wilson's central terminal (V) is constructed by connecting the three limb electrodes. Resistances are placed between each electrode and the central terminal to overcome effects of variable resistances where the electrodes are placed on the body.

sent an indifferent electrode, but in spite of this limitation the V lead has become an integral part of clinical electrocardiography.

The three unipolar limb leads are VR, VL, and VF, which record the potential differences between the V lead and the right arm, left arm, and left leg (F = foot), respectively. In each of these leads, the central terminal is assumed to measure zero potential, so that an upright deflection is inscribed when the exploring electrode is positive relative to the central terminal. In lead VF, for example, an upright deflection is recorded when the left leg electrode faces an approaching wave of depolarization, i.e., when the electrical vector is directed inferiorly.

The unipolar limb leads conventionally recorded in the clinical ECG are *augmented* by disconnecting from the central terminal that limb which is the same as that of the exploring electrode. In lead aVF (augmented lead VF), for example, the potential difference recorded is between the leg electrode and a "central terminal" connected only to the right and left arm electrodes. The rationale for disconnecting the leg electrode from the central terminal in the above example is that this procedure augments the amplitude of the recorded potential. This maneuver is easily understood because removal of the "leg" potentials from the central terminal increases the potential difference recorded in lead aVF, compared to that recorded in VF where the leg potentials appear at both sides of the potentiometer. It is apparent that "augmentation" of the unipolar limb leads invalidates the concept that the V leads record a true zero potential. In the example of aVF just cited, for example, the potential recorded at the lead connecting left and right arm electrodes is clearly not zero.

The lack of adherence to theory in the recording of the unipolar ECG emphasizes the fact that interpretations of contour in electrocardiography are empirical. Analysis of arrhythmias, on the other hand, is much more rational (Chapters 16–18).

Chest Leads

The *six chest leads* make up the remainder of the conventional 12–lead ECG. Each chest lead is a unipolar lead in which the Wilson's central terminal (the

TABLE 15.4. *Standard chest leads*

Lead	Position of exploring electrode
V_1	Fourth intercostal space just to the right of the sternum
V_2	Fourth intercostal space just to the left of the sternum
V_3	Midway between V_2 and V_4
V_4	Fifth intercostal space at the left midclavicular line
V_5	Left anterior axillary line horizontally to the left of V_4
V_6	Midaxillary line horizontally to the left of V_4 and V_5

V lead) is compared to an electrode in each of six positions on the chest wall (Table 15.4). In the chest leads, as in the unipolar limb leads, the central terminal is assumed to record zero potential so that an upright deflection is recorded when the electrode on the chest wall is in an area of relative electropositivity, such as would occur when a wave of depolarization approaches the exploring electrode. Thus the QRS complexes in V_1 and V_2 tend to be inverted, and those in V_5 and V_6 are normally upright because depolarization of the left ventricle dominates the normal ECG.

Analysis of Electrical Vectors

The normal electrical vector in the *frontal plane* of the body is usually considered to lie between $-30°$ and $+90°$, where the lead I axis is taken as $0°$ (Fig. 15.27). When the electrical vector is greater than $+90°$, the electrical axis is said to have deviated to the right. Electrical vectors less than $-30°$ are designated as left axis deviation. The applications of these vector analyses to clinical electrocardiography are beyond the scope of the present text. The interested reader is referred to the many excellent texts of electrocardiographic analysis for further details of these analyses and for the interpretation of changes in the contour of the ECG.

The chest leads provide extremely useful information regarding the position of the cardiac dipole in the *horizontal plane* of the body. Analyses of the electrical vectors in this plane, however, are usually less rigorous than those of the projec-

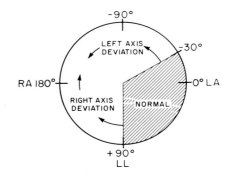

FIG. 15.27. The angle of an ECG vector in the frontal plane is assigned a value according to the convention shown here. A vector directed to the left is assigned an angle of $0°$; one directed to the right is said to have an angle of $180°$. A vector directed inferiorly has an angle of $+90°$; one directed superiorly has an angle of $-90°$. Normal mean QRS vectors range between $-30°$ and $+90°$. Vectors with angles less than $-30°$ exhibit left axis deviation, and those with angles greater than $+90°$ exhibit right axis deviation.

tion of the electrical vector in the frontal plane, which is described by the six limb leads.

Mutual Cancellation of Electrical Vectors in the Heart

The principal reason for the empirical nature of analysis of electrocardiographic contour is the fact that the ECG normally records less than 10% of the total electrical activity of the heart. The failure of the majority of electrical forces arising in the heart to be recorded by the electrodes on the body surface is due to mutual cancellation of electrical vectors oriented in opposite directions. To some extent this cancellation of electrical activity occurs when different regions of the heart are activated in opposite directions (Figs. 15.20 and 15.21), e.g., the electrical vectors in the left and right ventricles are oriented in opposite directions. The large QRS complexes associated with ventricular premature systoles (Chapter 17) show the extent to which loss of synchrony of right and left ventricular activation can augment the potentials recorded at the body surface.

Significant cancellation of the waves of depolarization within the ventricles also results from the fact that depolarization begins not at the surface of the ventricles but within the endocardial surface of the ventricles. Because the Purkinje fibers penetrate the inner third of the ventricular wall, activation of the ventricular myocardium begins at the ends of this rapidly conducting network as a sphere of depolarized tissue within the ventricular wall (Fig. 15.28A). Until a portion of the expanding sphere of depolarization reaches the ventricular surface (Fig. 15.28B), no deflections are seen in recordings from electrodes facing the various surfaces of the heart. This is due to the fact that no potential *differences* exist between electrodes outside the ventricle. For this reason much of the electrical activity resulting from ventricular depolarization is not recorded by electrodes at the body surface.

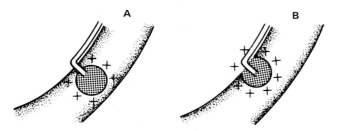

FIG. 15.28. A large portion of the electrical activity generated during ventricular depolarization fails to influence the ECG because of mutual cancellation of waves of depolarization. In the case of a wave of depolarization that begins at the termination of a Purkinje fiber within the ventricular wall, the initial depolarization of a sphere of muscle *(stippled circle)* surrounded by resting tissue produces no potential difference that can be recorded by electrodes outside the heart **(A)**. Only after the sphere of depolarized tissue has expanded to include one surface of the ventricular wall (usually the endocardial surface) does a potential difference appear that can be recorded at the body surface **(B)**.

THE NORMAL ELECTROCARDIOGRAM

A normal 12-lead ECG is shown in Fig. 15.29. Each large "box" in the horizontal direction (time) represents 0.20 sec and is divided into five small boxes of 0.04 sec each. Each large box in the vertical direction (voltage) represents 0.5 mV and is divided into five small boxes of 0.1 mV each. The mean QRS vector, plotted from the amplitudes of the deflections in the three bipolar limb leads, is shown in Fig. 15.25. This ECG illustrates the normal finding that the T wave is inscribed in almost the same direction as the QRS complex (see also Fig. 15.5), and that the duration of the T wave is much longer than that of the QRS complex. This behavior is in contrast to that shown in the simplified set of drawings in Figs. 15.12–15.16.

The shorter duration of the QRS complex, compared to that of the T wave, of the normal ECG stems directly from the fact that the QRS complex arises from a rapidly propagated wave of depolarization, whereas the T wave results from the process of repolarization, which is governed mainly by conditions existing locally in and near each myocardial cell. Although regions of repolarized myocardium tend to promote the repolarization of adjacent, depolarized myocardium (Chapter 14), the time at which repolarization begins in any part of the heart is determined largely by local factors that influence action potential duration.

The temporal dispersion of action potential durations in various regions of the

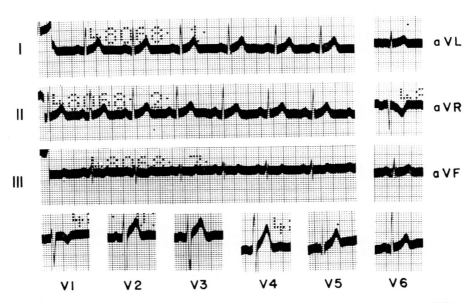

FIG. 15.29. Normal ECG. The mean QRS vector in the frontal plane derived from this ECG is analyzed in Fig. 15.25. The slight changes in QRS configuration in lead III can be attributed to respiratory variations in the position of the heart within the chest. (From Katz and Pick, 1956.)

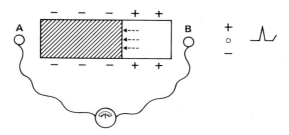

FIG. 15.30. A strip of myocardium, after being fully depolarized (as shown in Fig. 15.14), begins to repolarize in those regions that were depolarized last. In this illustration, which should be contrasted with Fig. 15.15, the deflection in the bipolar lead *(right)* has the same polarity as that seen during depolarization.

ventricular myocardium, which is due mainly to local differences in the length of the plateau (phase 2) of the action potential (see above), also accounts for the usual concordance between the polarities of the QRS complex and the T wave. As shown in Fig. 15.15, these deflections would be discordant if repolarization began in the same region of the heart as did depolarization. The fact that the polarity of the QRS complex is normally the same as that of the T wave can be easily understood if the last areas of the ventricles to be depolarized are the *first* to repolarize, i.e., if the action potential duration is relatively longer in those regions which are first to be depolarized. Thus the concordant polarities of the QRS complex and T wave in the normal ECG (Fig. 15.29) can be explained if repolarization proceeded in a direction *opposite* to that of depolarization (Fig. 15.30). One explanation for relatively longer action potentials in the regions of the ventricles to be depolarized first (i.e., the endocardial surface) is that the action potential duration in the endocardial regions of the ventricles is prolonged relative to that in the epicardial regions by the relatively long action potentials in the Purkinje network, which penetrates only the endocardial regions (Fig. 14.13).

THE ABNORMAL ELECTROCARDIOGRAM

Intraventricular Conduction Delay

The ventricles are normally activated when the wave of depolarization spreads more or less simultaneously through the right and left ventricles. Ventricular activation tends to be synchronous because the impulse passing through the AV bundle is rapidly conducted down both right and left bundle branches after the AV bundle divides at the top of the ventricular septum. Interruption of the AV bundle, or of *both* bundle branches, produces a condition called complete heart block, in which the ventricles are no longer under the influence of the impulse that originates in the SA node (Chapter 16). If conduction in only one of the bundle branches is blocked, the impulse conducted from the atria still reaches the ventricles, although it does so by an abnormal pathway. The resulting conduction abnormality is called bundle branch block. The impulse which eventually depolarizes the ventricle whose bundle branch is blocked follows a circuitous pathway and does not reach the "blocked" ventricle by way of the rapidly conducting His-Purkinje system. Instead, this impulse is conducted more slowly through the ventricular myocardium (Table 15.1), causing the QRS complex in bundle branch block to be *prolonged*. The shape of the QRS complex in bundle branch block is also *bizarre* because the conduction abnormality alters the normal activation sequence of the ventricles.

Right Bundle Branch Block

As illustrated in Fig. 15.4, the right bundle branch can be considered to be the last branch of the AV bundle after the latter has given rise to the anterior and posterior radiations of the left bundle branch. These anatomical characteristics may account for the greater likelihood of selective interruption of the right bundle branch and thus provide an explanation for the greater frequency of right than left bundle branch block. Three features of the ECG of right bundle branch block (Fig. 15.31) are discussed here. As described above, the delayed conduction of the wave of depolarization over the right ventricle causes widening of the QRS

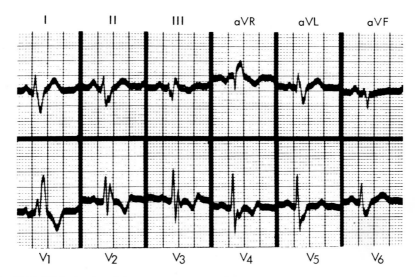

FIG. 15.31. ECG showing right bundle branch block. The broad, slurred, late S waves in leads I and II arise from a terminal QRS vector that is directed to the right, as is also evidenced by the late R wave in lead aVR. The terminal QRS forces, which dominate the main QRS vector, thus exhibit right axis deviation. The diagnosis of right bundle branch block is confirmed by the widening of the QRS complex to 0.14 sec, and by the precordial leads where the rightward orientation of the QRS vector produces a prominent late R wave over the right ventricle, as seen in lead V_1. (From Littman, 1972.)

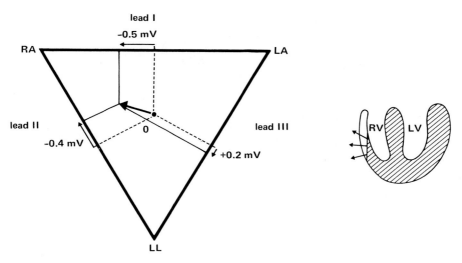

FIG. 15.32. Left: Projection of the mean frontal plane QRS vector of the ECG in Fig. 15.31 on the Einthoven triangle. **Right:** Late activation of the base of the right ventricle produces a mean QRS vector that is directed to the right and slightly superiorly, and so exhibits right axis deviation.

complex. In lead II, for example, the QRS complex extends through 3.5 small boxes, which corresponds to an abnormally long duration of 0.14 sec (Table 15.2). Second, delayed activation of the right ventricle shifts the mean electrical vector of the QRS complex in the frontal plane to the right (Fig. 15.32). This shift in electrical axis occurs because the terminal portions of the QRS complex arise from unbalanced electrical forces in the right ventricle which are directed toward the right (Fig. 15.32). This is reflected in the broad, late S waves seen in leads I, II, and aVL (Fig. 15.31), which indicate that the wave of depolarization is proceeding *away from* the left arm and toward the right arm; hence also the late R wave in lead aVR. Third, examination of the chest leads demonstrates broad, late R waves in the QRS complex recorded in the right precordial leads (V_1 and V_2) and broad, late S waves recorded from the left side of the chest (leads V_5 and V_6). These changes mean that the latter portions of the wave of depolarization are directed anteriorly and toward the right side of the chest, as would be expected in view of the normal anatomical position of the right ventricle to the right of and anterior to the left ventricle. The rightward shift of the mean QRS vector is apparent in the frontal plane vector illustrated in Fig. 15.32. Other abnormal features of this ECG are apparent, notably the fact that the QRS complex and T wave are discordant, e.g., in lead V_1. This discordancy is attributable to the abnormally long conduction path followed by the impulse as it moves through the ventricular mass because the long path tends to overcome the influence of local factors that determine action potential duration and the sequence of repolarization. The reader is referred to standard textbooks of electrocardiography for further details of these abnormalities and their clinical significance.

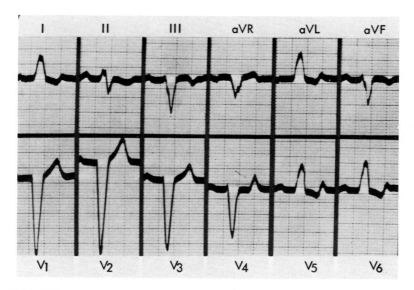

FIG. 15.33. ECG showing left bundle branch block. The broad R wave in lead I and the S wave in lead III arise from a mean QRS vector that is directed to the left and superiorly, as is also evidenced by the tall R wave in lead aVL and the deep S wave in lead aVF. The QRS forces which dominate the mean QRS vector thus exhibit left axis deviation. The diagnosis of left bundle branch block is confirmed by the widening of the QRS complex to 0.17 sec and by the precordial leads where the leftward orientation of the QRS vector produces a broad R wave over the left ventricle, as seen in leads V_5 and V_6. (From Littman, 1972.)

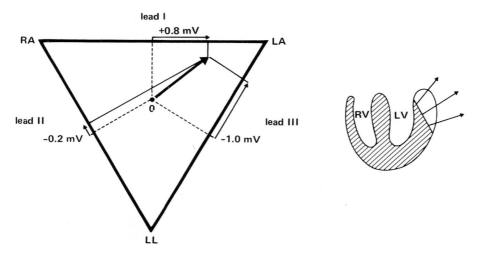

FIG. 15.34. Left: Projection of the mean frontal plane vector of the ECG in Fig. 15.33 on the Einthoven triangle. **Right:** Late activation of the base of the left ventricle produces a mean QRS vector that is directed to the left and superiorly, and so exhibits left axis deviation.

Left Bundle Branch Block

Interruption of both the anterior and posterior radiations of the left bundle branch causes delayed activation of the left ventricle so that, as in right bundle branch block, the QRS complex is widened (Fig. 15.33). The late, unbalanced depolarization of the left ventricular mass causes a leftward shift of the mean QRS vector in the frontal plane, which causes broad, tall R waves to appear in leads I and aVL, and deep, broad S waves to appear in leads III and aVF. The mean QRS vector in the frontal plane is shown in Fig. 15.34. The orientation of the QRS vector recorded in the precordial leads is opposite to that in right bundle branch block, i.e., to the left and posteriorly. For this reason the QRS complex is upright in leads V_5 and V_6, and inverted in leads V_1–V_4. As in right bundle branch block, the T waves tend to be discordant from the polarity of the QRS complexes.

Hemiblocks

Interruption of either the posterior or, more commonly, the anterior radiation of the left bundle branch gives rise to a condition called *hemiblock*. In both left anterior and left posterior hemiblock the QRS complex is ordinarily not abnormally widened because the initial activation of the left ventricular myocardium occurs by way of the Purkinje network; only the terminal phase of left ventricular depolarization is delayed. The hemiblocks therefore are usually manifest as an abnormally directed mean electrical vector which occurs because the direction in which the wave of depolarization traverses the left ventricle has become abnormal. In *left anterior hemiblock* these late electrical forces are deviated to the left (Fig. 15.35),[1] i.e., toward the "blocked" region of the left ventricle. In *left posterior hemiblock* the late unbalanced forces are deviated toward the right (Fig. 15.36).[1]

Ventricular Hypertrophy

As might be predicted, the alterations in the QRS complex produced by right ventricular hypertrophy (Fig. 15.37) [1] and left ventricular hypertrophy (Fig. 15.38) [1] tend to cause the mean QRS axis in the frontal plane to be deviated to the right or to the left, respectively. The direction of the mean electrical vector in the precordial leads also tends to shift so as to point "toward" the hypertrophied ventricle. These shifts in mean QRS vector and the augmentation in voltage that accompanies them are due only partly to the increased muscle mass that characterizes ventricular hypertrophy. Prolongation of the time required for the passage of the wave of depolarization over the enlarged hypertrophied ventricle, rather than the increased muscle mass, is probably the most important determi-

---

[1] No formal vector analyses are provided here for these ECGs; the interested reader is advised to prepare his or her own.

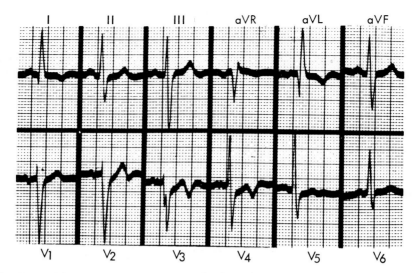

FIG. 15.35. ECG showing left anterior hemiblock. Interrupted conduction through the anterior radiations of the left bundle branch causes late R waves in leads I and aVL, and late S waves in leads III and aVF (left axis deviation) without prolongation of the QRS complex. (From Littman, 1972.)

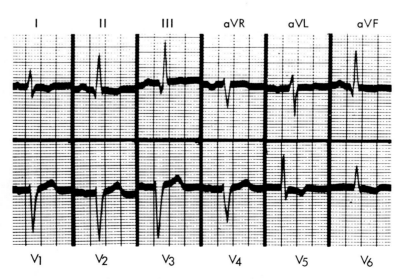

FIG. 15.36. ECG showing left posterior hemiblock. Interrupted conduction through the posterior radiations of the left bundle branch causes late S waves in leads I and aVL, and late R waves in leads III and aVF (right axis deviation) without prolongation of the QRS complex. (From Littman, 1972.)

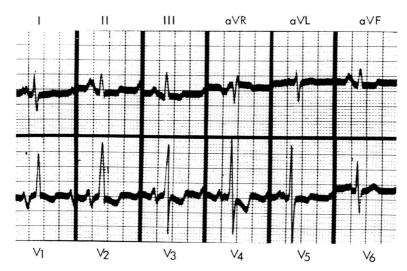

FIG. 15.37. ECG showing right ventricular hypertrophy. There is a slight right axis shift in the limb leads along with tall R waves in the right precordial leads (V_1 and V_2) and prominent S waves in the left precordial leads (V_5 and V_6). The latter indicate a predominance of electrical forces directed toward the right ventricle. There is no prolongation of the QRS complex. Note that the T waves tend to be discordant with the QRS complexes (e.g., lead V_1). The P waves are also abnormal. (From Littman, 1972.)

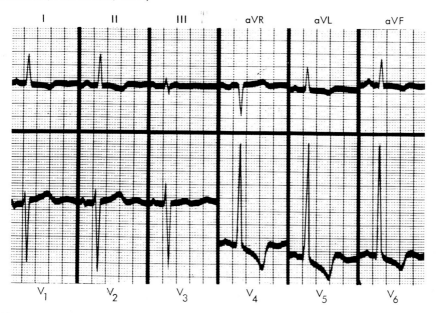

FIG. 15.38. ECG showing left ventricular hypertrophy. Although the frontal plane axis is within normal limits, there are very tall R waves in the left precordial leads (V_5 and V_6) and deep S waves in the right precordial leads (V_1 and V_2). These abnormalities indicate a predominance of electrical forces directed toward the left ventricle. There is no prolongation of the QRS complex. The T waves are discordant with the QRS complexes throughout the ECG. (From Littman, 1972.)

nant of the altered direction of the means QRS vector. Thus the ECG provides only an indirect index of the mass of the ventricles. In this context it should also be emphasized that the ECG provides virtually no information regarding myocardial contractility.

The ECGs shown in this chapter have been selected to illustrate the principles that underlie the electrocardiographic recording of the electrical activity of the normal heart and to demonstrate the type of information that can be obtained from analysis of the QRS vector in the abnormal heart. No attempt has been made to provide a basis for the electrocardiographic diagnosis of cardiac disease, which is appropriate only for textbooks of clinical cardiology and electrocardiography. Instead, the presentation of these "real" ECGs is intended to remind the reader that the physician faced with an unknown ECG can analyze these data in terms of the reasonably well-understood electrophysiological phenomena that have been described in this and the preceding chapter.

BIBLIOGRAPHY

Articles by J. W. Woodbury; A. M. Scher; and H. Schaefer and H. G. Haas (1962): *Handbook of Physiology, Section 2: Circulation,* Vol. 1, edited by W. F. Hamilton and P. Dow. American Physiological Society, Washington, D.C. (Although parts of these articles are now out of date, they express many basic concepts in an extremely lucid manner and so are highly recommended.)

Grant, R. P. (1970): *Grant's Clinical Electrocardiography. The Spatial Vector Approach,* 2nd. ed. rev. by J. R. Beckwith. McGraw-Hill, New York.

James, T. N. (1967): Cardiac innervation: Anatomic and pharmacologic relations. *Bull. NY Acad. Sci.,* 43:1041–1086.

Katz, L. N., and Pick, A. (1956): *Clinical Electrocardiography. Part I: Arrhythmias.* Lea and Febiger, Philadelphia.

Rosenbaum, M. B. (1970): The hemiblocks: Diagnostic criteria and clinical significance. *Mod. Concepts Cardiovasc. Dis.,* 39:141–146.

Wenckebach, K. F., and Winterberg, H. (1927): *Die Unregelmässige Herztätigkeit.* Verlag von Wilhelm Engelmann, Leipzig.

Electrocardiography Textbooks

Burch, G. E., and Winsor, T. (1972): *A Primer of Electrocardiography.* Lea & Febiger, Philadelphia.

Lipman, B. S., and Massie, E. (1965): *Clinical Scaler Electrocardiography.* Year Book Medical Publishers, Chicago.

Littman, D. (1972): *Textbook of Electrocardiography.* Harper & Row, New York.

16

The Arrhythmias

I. Introduction: SA Node, Impaired Conduction, AV Block, Unidirectional Block

The introduction of electrocardiography into clinical medicine at the beginning of the twentieth century greatly facilitated the interpretation of clinical disorders of cardiac rate and rhythm. The availability of precise records of the spread of electrical activity through the atria and ventricles of patients with cardiac arrhythmias led to the production and characterization of similar abnormalities in experimental animals, thereby permitting the rapid and safe testing of a variety of new therapeutic interventions for ultimate use in humans. The growth of knowledge of the clinical features of the arrhythmias has therefore led to a dramatic increase in our understanding of the mechanisms responsible for these disorders. Clinical and experimental electrocardiography remained closely linked during the first decades of this century, so the identification of an increasing number of rules governing the clinical behavior of arrhythmias was paralleled by a growth of basic knowledge of the electrophysiological properties of cardiac muscle. With the advent of intracellular microelectrode recording in the heart, a new dimension was added to the understanding of the mechanisms of the arrhythmias. The identification of the ionic basis of the cardiac action potential (Chapter 14), along with an awareness of the pathogenetic implications of specific abnormalities in the ionic properties of the cardiac sarcolemma, permits a more complete understanding of the causes of a number of clinical disorders of heart rate and rhythm. In view of the growing body of knowledge concerning the interactions of drugs with biological membranes (Chapter 19), these new lines of study promise further advances in the treatment and, more importantly, in the prevention of cardiac arrhythmias in man.

Several of the important physiological principles which underlie our current understanding of cardiac arrhythmias are described in this and the following chapters, and a number of clinical arrhythmias are examined in the light of what is now known about the basic electrophysiology of the heart. These chapters are organized in terms of a simple clinical classification of the arrhythmias, although it must be stressed at the outset that this classification is neither rigorous nor complete. The reader who wishes a comprehensive review of clinical arrhythmias is referred to the many excellent textbooks of electrocardiography. Similarly, these chapters do not represent a comprehensive presentation of modern cardiac electrophysiology. The emphasis is on areas where the interrelationships between clinical electrocardiography and basic electrophysiology are most apparent and so highlight our present understanding of the electrophysiological basis of the arrhythmias. It is hoped that these chapters will allow the reader to appreciate the current understanding of the relationships between electrophysiological abnormalities in the myocardial cell and disorders of heart rate and rhythm that occur in the cardiac patient.

Present methodology does not permit the mechanisms responsible for most clinical arrhythmias to be defined with precision. The ability to reproduce comparable disorders in experimental situations, however, has led to a number of hypotheses regarding the pathogenesis of the abnormalities in man. Direct proof of these hypotheses is lacking in most cases, and it is highly likely that many clinical arrhythmias can be caused by more than one type of electrophysiological abnormality. Chapters 16–18 are intended primarily to provide an understanding of mechanisms which *can* produce the arrhythmias. No claim is made that these mechanisms to be discussed are responsible for *all* or even a major portion of the clinical disorders described. In the case of the tachycardias, for example, there remains no way to determine which are due to abnormalities in pacemaker activity and which arise from disorders in impulse conduction (re-entry). In all probability, both mechanisms occur in clinical practice and are each responsible for an as yet unknown fraction of the clinical tachycardias. This example underlines the tentative nature of the correlation between the arrhythmias and putative pathogenetic mechanisms described in these chapters.

ARRHYTHMIAS DUE TO ALTERED ACTIVITY
OF THE SINUS NODE PACEMAKER

The normal heart rate, which is 60–100 beats/minute (Chapter 15), reflects the frequency of depolarization of the pacemaker cells in the SA (sinus) node. Heart rates greater than 100 [1] that originate within the SA node are designated *sinus tachycardia;* and heart rates less than 60, which reflect slowing of the SA node pacemaker, represent *sinus bradycardia.* Because the SA node is highly susceptible to autonomic influences, most clinical examples of sinus tachycardia and sinus bradycardia arise in response to altered activity of the autonomic nervous system, rather than from primary disorders of function of the SA node.

Sinus Tachycardia

Excessive sympathetic drive is by far the most common cause of sinus tachycardia. This arrhythmia commonly occurs in normal individuals, e.g., during emotional stress and physical exercise (conditions which increase the sympathetic influence on the SA node). In other cases sinus tachycardia occurs under basal

---

[1] The denominator (per minute) is omitted in subsequent discussions, following conventional usage.

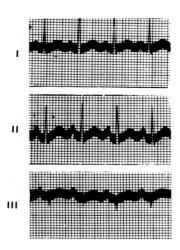

FIG. 16.1. Sinus tachycardia. The rates of atrial and ventricular beating are 125 (P waves and QRS complexes occur every 0.48 sec), and each QRS complex is preceded by a normal P-wave with a P-R interval of 0.16 sec. (From Katz and Pick, 1956.)

physical and emotional conditions because abnormalities outside the heart (e.g., hemorrhagic shock) increase sympathetic drive. The electrocardiographic characteristics of sinus tachycardia include a heart rate greater than 100, with normal P waves followed, after a normal P-R interval, by normal QRS complexes (Fig. 16.1). The mechanism by which catecholamines, which mediate the sympathetic influence on the SA node, increase heart rate are described in Chapter 19, and additional details regarding this arrhythmia are in Chapter 18.

Sinus Bradycardia

By definition, sinus bradycardia occurs when the heart rate falls below 60 and when normal P waves are followed by normal QRS complexes after a normal P-R interval (Fig. 16.2). Many clinical examples of sinus bradycardia result from excessive release of the parasympathetic neurotransmitter acetylcholine at the SA node, as occurs, for example, in vasovagal syncope. The mechanism by which acetylcholine slows pacemaker activity in the SA node is largely attributable to its general effect to increase potassium permeability, which is discussed in Chapter 19.

Sinoatrial Block

There is growing evidence that, especially in the elderly, a condition exists in which some of the impulses generated in the SA node are prevented from depolarizing the atria, giving rise to an arrhythmia sometimes called the *sick sinus syndrome*. When every other impulse leaving the SA node is blocked, this abnormality can give rise to a condition where every other depolarization in the SA node has no influence on other regions of the myocardium. Because the pacemaker activity of the SA node can be detected on the ECG only when the

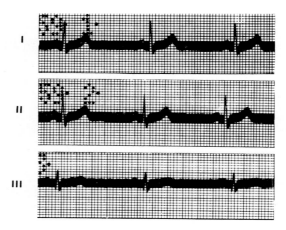

FIG. 16.2. Sinus bradycardia. The rates of atrial and ventricular beating are 54 (P waves and QRS complexes occur every 1.1 sec), and each QRS complex is preceded by a normal P wave with a P-R interval of 0.17 sec. (From Katz and Pick, 1956.)

surrounding atrial tissue is depolarized (Chapter 15), when one of every two sinus impulses fails to activate the atria the resulting abnormality is electrocardiographically indistinguishable from sinus bradycardia at half the normal heart rate. The former represents a condition called 2:1 sinoatrial (SA) block. SA block can also be caused by a high serum potassium level and cardiac glycoside toxicity, both of which tend to prevent the atrial tissue surrounding the sinus node from propagating the action potential generated in the SA node to the remainder of the myocardium.

Sinus Arrhythmia

Variations in the frequency of discharge of the SA node, and thus variations in heart rate, accompany the respiratory cycle in normal individuals. These variations in the frequency of the pacemaker of the SA node, which are characterized by an acceleration of heart rate during inspiration and a slowing during expiration without alterations in the P wave, P-R interval, or QRS complex, give rise to an arrhythmia called sinus arrhythmia (Fig. 16.3). These changes in the frequency of SA node discharge can be attributed to a cyclic decrease in vagal tone and increase in sympathetic tone during inspiration, and an increased vagal tone and decreased sympathetic tone during expiration. Sinus arrhythmia is a sign of a healthy heart in that this response is lost during the early stages of heart failure. Sinus arrhythmia also tends to disappear with advancing age.

Sinus arrhythmia can be conveniently illustrated by a drawing of the conduction of the impulse through the heart called the Lewis diagram (Fig. 16.3), named after Sir Thomas Lewis, one of the pioneers in the study of the ECG. The Lewis diagram consists of four parallel lines delimiting three spaces. It is read from left

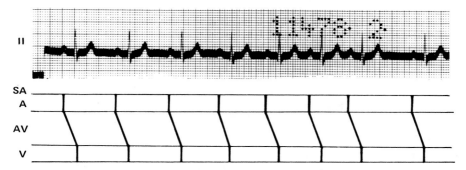

FIG. 16.3. Sinus arrhythmia. The rates of atrial and ventricular beating are variable, but each QRS complex is preceded by a P wave with a P-R interval of 0.19 sec. (The variations in the shape of the P wave suggest a "wandering" pacemaker site in the SA node.) This arrhythmia is diagrammed in a "Lewis diagram," in which the top line (SA) represents the SA node, the upper space (A) the atria, the middle space (AV) the AV node, and the lower space (V) the ventricles. Note that each beat begins in the SA node and is conducted normally through the atria, AV node, and ventricles as depicted by the line, which is read from top to bottom. (ECG from Katz and Pick, 1956.)

to right, the horizontal axis being time. The top line represents the SA node, while the space between the top two lines is used to diagram the passage of the wave of depolarization through the atria. The wider space between the middle lines is used to diagram the AV node, while the lower space indicates the ventricles. A normal sinus beat begins at the top line (SA node), passes rapidly across the top space (atria), more slowly through the middle space (AV node), and again rapidly across the lower space (ventricles). The downward angle of the line drawn on the Lewis diagram thus represents the speed of impulse propagation. In the case of sinus arrhythmia, the speed of impulse propagation through the atria, AV node, and ventricles remains normal, the only change being in the interval between the impulses arising in the SA node that initiates this impulse. Hence as shown in Fig. 16.3, the abnormality consists only of a cyclic variation in the frequency with which the SA node (top line) initiates impulses that are then transmitted normally through the atria (top space), AV node (middle space), and ventricles (lower space).

DETERMINANTS OF CONDUCTION VELOCITY

Knowledge of the factors that influence the speed at which the wave of depolarization is conducted through the myocardium is essential not only for an understanding of the electrocardiographic abnormalities that result from impaired impulse conduction in the heart, but also for understanding the premature systoles and tachycardias to be described in Chapters 17 and 18. Four physiologically important factors that influence conduction velocity in the heart are: (a) action potential amplitude; (b) the rate of rise of the action potential; (c) thresh-

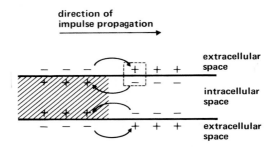

FIG. 16.4. Cable properties of a strand of cardiac muscle transmitting a propagated impulse from left to right. Current flow between the depolarized tissue *(shaded, left)* and resting tissue *(unshaded, right)* is indicated by arrows. Current flows away from the depolarized tissue along the outside of the cell, and the circuit is completed when current flows toward the depolarized region inside the cell. Details of the current flow across the membrane *(dotted rectangle)* are shown in Fig. 16.5.

old; and (d) internal and external electrical resistances. These determinants are often interrelated so that agents that influence conduction velocity may act through more than one of these factors.

The way in which changing electrophysiological properties of the myocardium can alter the velocity of impulse propagation can be understood in terms of the cable properties of the myocardium, which describe the passage of the regenerative action potential along a strand of excitable tissue such as the AV bundle. Propagation of the wave of depolarization results from the depolarizing action of currents flowing from the already depolarized portions of the strand, in which the outside is negatively charged, to the resting and excitable tissue further ahead, where membrane polarity is reversed (i.e., in the normal resting state) as shown in Fig. 16.4. The depolarizing flow of current[2] between depolarized and resting portions of the strand can be represented by arrows that depict the transfer of negative charge between depolarized and resting myocardium. This charge transfer requires that an electrical circuit be established along the strand, in which negative current flows toward the resting tissue along the outside of the cells and returns through the interior of the cells. The requirement for a complete electrical circuit explains the importance of the low-resistance pathway provided by the intercalated disc, which is essential for rapid impulse propagation through the myocardium.

The electrical analog shown in Fig. 16.5, which corresponds to the region of the cell membrane enclosed within the small dotted rectangle in Fig. 16.4, illustrates the way in which the "cable properties" of the membrane can be understood in terms of its resistive and capacitive characteristics. It is important to recognize that as the magnitude of the depolarizing current (light arrows) in-

---

[2] In this discussion of cable properties, current flow is described in terms of the transfer of *negative* charge, in accord with customary usage. This convention is to be contrasted with that used in Chapter 14, where transmembrane ionic currents were described in terms of the transfer of positive charge.

creases, the unexcited regions of the strand are depolarized more rapidly. This relationship allows a larger-amplitude action potential to increase the speed at which the membrane of the unexcited tissue is depolarized and so becomes able to participate in further propagation of the action potential. Similarly, if the resistances to longitudinal current flow (Fig. 16.5) are reduced, propagation of the electrical impulse is facilitated.

The fact that impulse propagation within the myocardium reflects the cable properties that govern the ability of already excited tissue to depolarize the resting tissue ahead gives rise to four physically distinct, although physiologically interdependent, factors which influence conduction velocity. Two of these factors— *action potential amplitude* and *rate of depolarization of the action potential*—are determined by the characteristics of the action potential in the depolarized tissue. *Threshold,* the third of the physiologically important parameters that determine conduction velocity, reflects the properties of the tissue undergoing depolarization. The *electrical resistance* of the medium and, especially of the sarcolemma and cell interior, is the fourth determinant of conduction velocity. While the conductive properties of the extracellular space are probably virtually constant and so cannot play a significant role in controlling conduction velocity in the intact heart, changes in the ability of the cell interior to carry the currents shown in Fig. 16.4 can result from altered resistances at the intercalated discs.

The relationship between the *amplitude* and *rate of depolarization* of the action potential and conduction velocity is readily understood in terms of the cable properties discussed above. Action potential amplitude, by its influence on the flow of depolarizing current (Fig. 16.4), determines the distance ahead that the already depolarized tissue can initiate a propagated action potential. Increasing the magnitude of this depolarizing current permits currents to exceed threshold, and thus to excite the quiescent tissue, a greater distance ahead of the wave front. Viewed another way, the depolarizing effects of a larger-amplitude action potential "reach" further ahead and thus lead to more rapid impulse conduction than those of a smaller action potential. Similarly, an increase in the rate of depolariza-

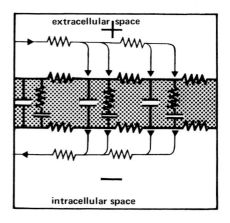

FIG. 16.5. Current flow across the cardiac cell membrane (Fig. 16.4). Current flow *(thin arrows)* in the longitudinal direction is influenced by the resistances in the extra- and intracellular spaces. The membrane *(shaded)* is depicted as containing resistors and capacitors. Resistors are shown in the extra- and intracellular spaces. Conduction velocity in the longitudinal direction is slowed when extra- or intracellular resistance is increased; it is accelerated when membrane resistance is increased.

tion accelerates conduction because the more rapid development of depolarizing currents causes threshold to be reached more rapidly in the excitable, resting tissue ahead of the wave front. An increased rate of depolarization also reduces the extent of voltage-dependent inactivation of the fast sodium channel (see Fig. 14.10).

The role of *threshold* in determining conduction velocity can also be understood in terms of the cable properties described above. Decreased threshold increases conduction velocity by reducing the amount of current flow needed to initiate a propagated action potential in the resting tissue ahead of the wave front. In this way reduction in threshold allows the depolarizing effects produced by the approaching wave of depolarization to activate the resting tissue a greater distance ahead of the wave front.

Changes in the *resistance of the intercalated disc or of the sarcolemma* (Fig. 16.5) can modify conduction velocity. The effects of decreased resistance, however, are quite different at these two locations in the cell. The ability of a decreased resistance to axial current flow (i.e., decreased resistance of the intercalated disc) to accelerate conduction is readily understood, as the resulting enhancement of longitudinal current flow (Fig. 16.5) increases the distance over which a given action potential exerts its depolarizing effect on the unexcited myocardium ahead of the wave of activation. Less obvious is the effect of a decreased resistance of the sarcolemma to slow conduction. This latter effect, by allowing a greater portion of the depolarizing current to flow across the sarcolemma in a direction perpendicular to that of the wave of activation, reduces longitudinal current flow and so slows conduction.

An inverse relationship between fiber diameter and conduction velocity can be explained by the effect of the former on the distribution of current flow just described. In a small fiber, relatively more current flows across the sarcolemma in a direction perpendicular to that of impulse propagation, so that less current flows in the longitudinal direction into the unexcited myocardium ahead of the wave of activation. This altered distribution of current flow in smaller fibers may partly explain the slow conduction velocity in the AV node, where cell size is small.

The operation of the four determinants of conduction velocity described above can be compared to a row of falling dominoes, which in some way illustrates the adherence of the propagated action potential in the heart to the cable properties of the myocardium (Fig. 16.6). Increasing the height of the dominoes, like an increase in *action potential amplitude,* increases the speed at which the "impulse" is transmitted because each domino "reaches further ahead" as it falls. Similarly, if the velocity at which each domino falls is increased (e.g., by pulling each domino downward by means of a magnet in its upper end), the speed of the propagation of the impulse is increased in a manner similar to the effect of increasing the *rate of depolarization* of the heart. Should each domino be tipped slightly to the right in the resting state, the resulting decrease in mechanical threshold for falling, like a decreased *electrical threshold,* would increase the

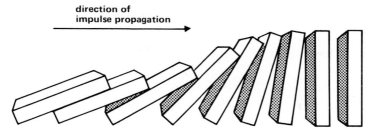

**direction of
impulse propagation**

FIG. 16.6. Row of dominoes falling from left to right. The speed with which this "impulse" is propagated is increased when (a) the height of the dominoes is increased; (b) the velocity at which each domino falls is increased; (c) the inertia needed to be overcome to tip each domino is decreased; and (d) the resistance encountered by the domino as it falls is decreased.

velocity of propagation. Finally, placing the row of dominoes in a vacuum, like reducing the *electrical resistance of the intercalated disc,* increases conduction velocity by decreasing their resistance to falling. Although somewhat fanciful, this analogy may prove useful in understanding the very important relationships between the cable properties just described and conduction velocity in the heart.

One of the major determinants of conduction velocity in the heart is the rate and extent to which sodium channels open at the onset of depolarization. A reduction in the fast inward sodium current by drugs like tetrodotoxin and by incomplete recovery of the fast channel due to partial depolarization of the membrane prior to activation (Fig. 14.9) or to premature depolarization before the cell has recovered from a previous action potential, reduces both the amplitude and rate of rise of the action potential, thereby slowing conduction. This example illustrates the way in which abnormalities in the ionic conductances of the sarcolemma of the cardiac muscle cell can influence the velocity of impulse conduction in the heart.

DECREMENTAL CONDUCTION

The ability of changes in the local properties of one or another region of the heart to influence conduction velocity accounts for the important property of *decremental conduction.* This term, which is self-explanatory, defines the phenomena which occur when a normal action potential enters a region of the myocardium in which conduction velocity becomes slowed. Decremental conduction is seen, for example, when an impulse is propagated into a region of the myocardium in which the opening of the fast sodium channels is impaired, causing the amplitude and rate of rise of the action potential to be decreased (Fig. 16.7). As a result of this change in local electrophysiological properties, propagation of the impulse is slowed when it enters a region of the myocardium exhibiting decremental conduction.

Regions of decremental conduction occur in abnormal hearts, e.g., in ischemic areas where the sodium pump is inhibited by a lack of chemical energy. Such

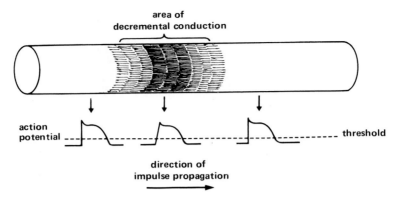

FIG. 16.7. Effects of decremental conduction on the shape of the action potential. When an impulse transmitted from left to right in a strand of cardiac muscle **(top)** encounters a region of decremental conduction *(shaded)*, the action potential **(bottom)** becomes smaller and more slowly rising. If the impulse is transmitted beyond the region of decremental conduction into normal tissue *(right)*, a normal action potential is generated, although its arrival is delayed.

regions are partially depolarized because some of the intracellular potassium is replaced with sodium. The resulting partial depolarization partially inactivates the opening of sodium channels and so decreases both action potential amplitude and the rate of depolarization, thereby slowing conduction. Decremental conduction is also a property of certain regions of the *normal* heart; e.g., in the AV node where decremental conduction can be attributed to the slowly rising, low-amplitude action potentials (Chapter 14), to a relative paucity of gap junctions, and to the small fiber diameter (Chapter 1). The possibility that the AV nodal cells lack a fast inward current (Chapter 14) can account for their small, slowly rising action potentials. An additional cause for slow conduction in the AV node is the high internal resistance that characterizes strands of tissue in which cell diameter is small and in which there are few gap junctions. As described above, high electrical resistance at the intercalated disc impairs the flow of depolarizing currents and so slows conduction.

Conduction velocity can return to normal when the impulse emerges from the area of decremental conduction, and returns to an area where local properties provide for the genesis of large action potentials (Fig. 16.7). This reversion of the slowed impulse to one that is propagated rapidly can occur, for example, in the ischemic heart when the impulse emerges from a depressed ischemic region to penetrate a normally perfused area. Similarly, when an impulse that has been slowed by the normal property of decremental conduction in the AV node reaches the AV bundle, conduction velocity again becomes rapid. In some instances decremental conduction may be so pronounced as to render the action potential too small to serve as an effective stimulus to the excitable tissue ahead (Fig. 16.8). Under these conditions the impulse is not transmitted through the area of decremental conduction but becomes completely *blocked.* In the cardiac patient com-

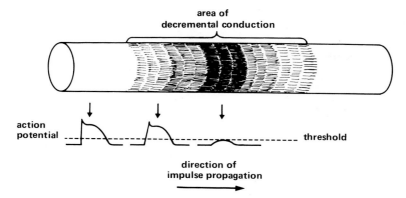

area of
decremental conduction

action
potential

threshold

direction of
impulse propagation

FIG. 16.8. Block of impulse transmission in a strand of cardiac muscle containing a region of marked decremental conduction. If the action potential generated in an area of marked decremental conduction (dark shading) fails to reach threshold, the normal tissue ahead of the impulse (right) is not depolarized, i.e., impulse transmission is blocked.

plete block of impulse transmission can occur in the AV node under conditions where the normal decremental conduction becomes increased by drugs or disease. Impulse propagation can also be blocked at the periphery of the SA node (SA block; see above), or in one or more areas of the Purkinje system (see *Bundle Branch Blocks* and *Hemiblocks,* Chapter 15). Failure of impulse transmission within localized regions of the myocardium is also extremely important in understanding the genesis of premature systoles and tachycardias because such local areas of block can set the stage for the re-entrant arrhythmias, which are described in Chapter 17 and 18.

ATRIOVENTRICULAR BLOCK

The physiological slowing of impulse propagation through the AV node accounts for the normally long P-R interval, which lasts 0.12–0.20 sec. A variety of abnormalities in AV nodal conduction can increase this slowing, thereby giving rise to a condition called AV block. Three degrees of AV block are recognized clinically. First-degree AV block, the mildest of these abnormalities, is manifest electrocardiographically as a prolongation of the P-R interval. Second-degree AV block is more severe in that the depression of impulse conduction through the AV nodes causes some but not all impulses to fail to traverse the AV node. In third-degree AV block, every impulse entering the AV node is blocked so that all electrical connection between the atria and the ventricles is lost.

First-Degree AV Block

First-degree AV block can be recognized on the ECG as a prolongation of the P-R interval (Fig. 16.9). By itself, this abnormality has little effect on the pumping

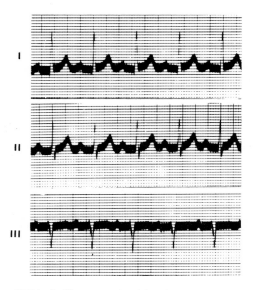

FIG. 16.9. First-degree AV block. The rates of atrial and ventricular beating, which are normal, are the same, so that each P wave is followed by a QRS complex. However, the P-R interval is abnormally prolonged to 0.26 sec, demonstrating an abnormal degree of block in the AV node. (From Katz and Pick, 1956.)

action of the heart, although as a warning of possible increases in AV block it is not without clinical significance. First-degree AV block (as well as higher degrees of AV block) can be caused by a variety of abnormalities including excessive parasympathetic (vagal) tone and cardiac glycosides (both of which slow AV conduction), as well as by damage to the AV node.

Second-Degree AV Block

Second-degree AV block is characterized by the failure of some but not all supraventricular impulses to traverse the AV node. The electrocardiographic features of second-degree AV block are a prolonged P-R interval plus the finding that some P waves are not followed by a QRS complex. In typical cases of second-degree AV block, all ventricular contractions are initiated by impulses that traverse the atria (i.e., all QRS complexes are preceded by a P wave) but not all atrial impulses are conducted to the ventricles (i.e., not all P waves are followed by a QRS complex). As a result, the ratio between atrial impulses and ventricular impulses (i.e., the ratio between P waves and QRS complexes) is greater than one. If every other P wave is blocked, the resulting abnormality is 2:1 AV block (Fig. 16.10).

Other ratios between P waves and QRS complexes are also seen in second-degree AV block. In 4:3 AV block, for example, every fourth P wave is not followed by a QRS complex (Fig. 16.11). When the ECG in Fig. 16.11 is analyzed

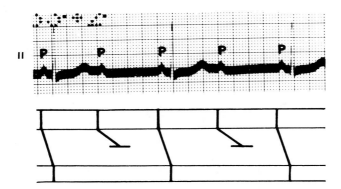

FIG. 16.10. Second-degree AV block with 2 : 1 AV conduction. There are twice as many P waves (P) as QRS complexes in this record, indicating that every second P wave is blocked. In the Lewis diagram *(below)* every other impulse is depicted as being blocked in the AV node *(short horizontal lines)*. (ECG from Katz and Pick, 1956.)

by constructing a Lewis diagram, it can be seen that each fourth impulse reaching the AV node from the atria is blocked, a phenomenon that gives rise to a "dropped beat" when the pulse of such a patient is felt. The extent of block in the AV node is sometimes variable, so that the ratio of P waves to QRS complexes in second-degree AV block can increase and decrease in a given patient.

An interesting and important feature of some cases of second-degree AV block is the *Wenckebach phenomenon,* which is manifest in Fig. 16.11 as a progressive prolongation of the P-R interval leading ultimately to a dropped beat. In Fig. 16.11, the first P-R interval after the initial nonconducted beat (that preceding the first QRS complex) is 0.17 sec; the next P-R intervals are 0.31 and 0.37 sec, and the P-R interval after the fourth P wave following the nonconducted P wave is infinite (i.e., the atrial impulse is not conducted to the ventricles). The progressive increase in P-R interval which precedes a nonconducted beat is characteristic of the Wenckebach phenomenon. An additional feature of this phenomenon is that prior to the nonconducted P wave the *P-R interval increases by decreasing increments.* Thus the first increment in the P-R interval in the ECG illustrated in Fig. 16.11 is 0.14 sec (0.31 sec for the second P-R interval minus 0.17 sec for the first), while the second increment is only 0.06 sec (0.37 sec for the third P-R interval minus 0.31 sec for the second).

The increase in P-R interval described above may be caused primarily by the progressive decrease in the interval between the antecedent beat and the P wave that follows, which causes the impulse to arrive during the relative refractory period of the AV node. In the example shown in Fig. 16.11, almost 2 sec has elapsed between the QRS complex *preceding* the first nonconducted P wave (not shown) and the first conducted P wave *after* the dropped beat (the second P wave, reading from left to right). This long diastolic interval following the successful passage of an impulse throught the AV node allows the AV node to recover fully, so that it is not difficult to understand why the shortest P-R interval is seen after

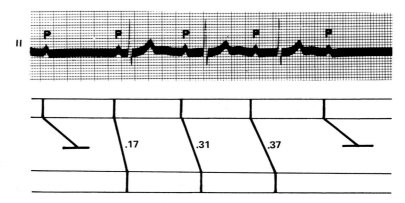

FIG. 16.11. Second-degree AV block demonstrating 4 : 3 AV conduction and the Wenckebach phenomenon. There are four P waves (P) for every three QRS complexes. In the Lewis diagram *(below)* it can be seen that the P-R interval (numbers on diagram) is shortest after the dropped beat. The P-R interval then increases, but by decreasing increments, until the next dropped beat. This ECG demonstrates typical Mobitz type I AV block. (ECG from Katz and Pick, 1956.)

the longest interval following successful AV node conduction. The subsequent P wave (the third, reading from left to right) follows the preceding QRS complex by only 1.13 sec so that the AV node has had less time to recover its excitability following its depolarization by the passage of the impulse that initiated this first QRS complex. The shortened time for recovery of excitability in the abnormally depressed AV node thus can account for the further prolongation of the P-R interval. The next interval, between the second QRS complex and the subsequent P wave, is 0.94 sec, so that when this P wave (the fourth) arrives at the AV node, it encounters tissue that has had much less time to recover. This causes the following P-R interval to be prolonged further. The blocked P wave (the fifth) follows the preceding QRS complex by only 0.70 sec, so that it can be deduced that this short time has not allowed the AV node to have recovered sufficiently from the passage of the preceding impulse to allow for AV conduction. In this way a slow decay of the depressant effect of prior depolarization of the AV node may explain the characteristics of the Wenckebach phenomenon.

Not all cases of second-degree AV block exhibit the Wenckebach phenomenon. In some patients the dropped beat is *not* preceded by prolongation of the P-R interval. In the ECG shown in Fig. 16.12, which shows 6:5 block, the P-R intervals preceding and following the nonconducted P waves are equal at 0.26 sec, so that the Wenckebach phenomenon (i.e., progressive prolongation of the P-R interval prior to the appearance of the dropped beat) is absent. This rarer type of second-degree AV block is commonly defined as *Mobitz type II* AV block, whereas that characterized by the Wenckebach phenomenon (Fig. 16.11) is classified as *Mobitz type I* AV block. The distinction between these two types of second-degree AV block is extremely important because Mobitz type II AV block often heralds the onset of third-degree AV block while the former tends to be more benign. These differences in clinical behavior reflect the fact that Mobitz type I AV block usually results from depressed conduction in the AV node that arises mainly from physiological abnormalities (e.g., vagal depression) rather than from an anatomical lesion. In contrast, Mobitz type II AV block is an indication that AV conduction is impaired by an anatomical lesion that is often located more distally in the conduction system of the ventricles, e.g., in the AV bundle or the bundle branches (bilateral bundle branch block).

> The differences in behavior between the two types of second-degree AV block described above, and especially the property of Mobitz type II AV block either to conduct or not to conduct without gradations in the extent of conduction delay, can be understood on the basis of these anatomical considerations. Thus when an anatomical lesion in the His-Purkinje system is sufficiently severe to allow only a "thread" of tissue to effect AV conduction, it is possible that the ability of the impulse to be propagated from atria to ventricles is so precarious that a slight worsening of the anatomical lesion completely blocks conduction rather than just adding to the conduction delay. In such cases the only effective therapy is usually to insert an electrical pacemaker that can stimulate the ventricles directly. In the case of Mobitz type I AV block, on the other hand, normal sensitivity of the AV node to the inhibitory actions of parasympathetic influences allows the physician to induce a favorable response by simpler forms of therapy, e.g., the administration of vagal blocking agents like atropine, which can improve AV conduction by abolishing the tonic depressant affect of the vagus. A spontaneous remission of Mobitz type I AV block can be expected if the arrhythmia is due to physiological or pharmacological depression of the AV node, as is often true in an acute myocardial infarction where the AV block may be due to a vagal reflex or to drugs used to reduce pain (Chapter 22), or when the arrhythmia is due to an overdose of cardiac glycosides. In these latter cases, pharmacological therapy is often effective and the reversible nature of the conduction abnormality usually does not require insertion of an electrical pacemaker.

The distinction between Mobitz types I and II AV block can often be made with a reasonable degree of probability by careful analysis of the ECG in cases such as those described above. Not all patients with second-degree AV block showing the Wenckebach phenomenon, however, are suffering from the more benign form of AV block. Furthermore, where there is 2:1 AV block, there is

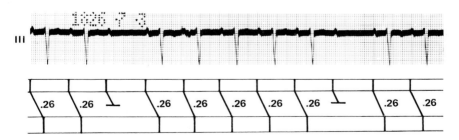

FIG. 16.12. Second-degree AV block, Mobitz type II. The P-R interval is constant at 0.26 sec (numbers in Lewis diagram, *below*). and neither decreases after the nonconducted P waves nor increases prior to the dropped beats. (ECG from Katz and Pick, 1956.)

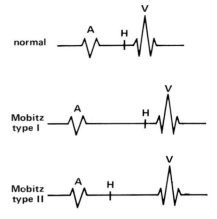

FIG. 16.13. Intracardiac electrograms. **Top:** Normal. **Middle:** AV block, Mobitz type I, showing a normal H-V interval and a prolonged A-H interval indicative of block within the AV node. **Bottom:** AV block, Mobitz type II, showing a normal A-H interval and a prolonged H-V interval indicative of block distal to the AV node.

no opportunity to apply these electrocardiographic criteria to identify the probable site of the conduction disturbance. The intracardiac electrogram is thus often used to distinguish between block within the AV node or the more dangerous block that can occur in the His-Purkinje system. The site of AV block can be defined if an H deflection is recorded from an electrode catheter in the right ventricle that is placed over the AV bundle (Fig. 15.9). Where Mobitz type I AV block results from conduction abnormalities in the AV node, the A-H interval is prolonged and the H-V interval normal, whereas in type II AV block that results from lesions in the more distal regions of the conduction system, the delay is between H and V (Fig. 16.13). These same criteria (i.e., the relationship between the H deflection in the intracardiac electrogram and the A and V waves) can also be used to define the site of block when AV block is complete (see below).

Third-Degree AV Block

Third-degree AV block, also called complete AV block or simply heart block, represents the interruption of all conduction between the atria and ventricles. As a result, the atria and ventricles beat independently of each other, there being no electrical connections between these two regions of the heart. The ECG in third-degree AV block is characterized by P waves and QRS complexes which bear no constant relationship to each other (Fig. 16.14). The regularity of the P waves in complete heart block reflects the fact that atrial contraction is under the normal control of the SA nodal pacemaker. The beating of the ventricles is slower than that of the atria as shown in Fig. 16.14 (unless there is an additional abnormality such as ventricular tachycardia) because the initiation of ventricular systole has reverted to one of the "lower" pacemakers (Table 15.1). In some cases the onset of third-degree AV block is not accompanied by the initiation of ventricular depolarizion by any pacemaker below the site of block. This condition, which is not rare, is a common cause of *cardiac arrest,* which if not treated

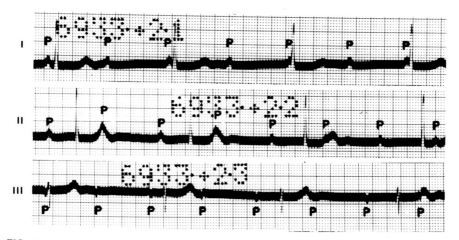

FIG. 16.14. Third-degree AV block (complete heart block). Although the appearance is superficially that of 2 : 1 AV block, careful examination of all leads demonstrates lack of a constant relationship between the P-waves, which come at a basic rate of 78 (P), and the QRS complexes, which are regular at a rate of 36. The apparent P-R interval thus differs markedly between the various leads, indicating that the atria and ventricles are beating independently. The QRS duration is normal (0.07 sec), suggesting that the ventricles are activated by a pacemaker above the bifurcation of the AV bundle. A Lewis diagram for this type of arrhythmia is shown in Fig. 16.15. (From Katz and Pick, 1956.)

promptly is lethal. In some patients several seconds can elapse between the onset of complete heart block and the initiation of pacemaker activity in the ventricles. This latter condition produces syncope and is often called the Stokes-Adams syndrome, after the physicians who first described it.

The site of the pacemaker that controls ventricular systole can be deduced from the configuration of the QRS complex in patients with complete heart block. When the pacemaker is in the AV bundle, the QRS complex is narrow (as it is in Fig. 16.14), and in the absence of additional conduction abnormalities the pattern resembles the QRS complex recorded before the onset of third-degree AV block. This is probably the case in most examples of congenital complete heart block, as the QRS complexes are usually normal and ventricular rates are often only slightly below normal. However, if the ventricles are depolarized by a pacemaker located in one or another of the ventricles, as commonly occurs in acquired complete heart block, the QRS complex is prolonged and bizarre (Fig. 16.15). The appearance of such QRS complexes indicates that the ventricles are activated by an impulse originating below the bifurcation of the AV bundle that activates the ventricles via an abnormal pathway.

The prolonged, bizarre QRS complexes shown in Fig. 16.15 resemble those seen in patients with an intraventricular conduction delay (bundle branch block; Chapter 15). For this reason examination of an ECG such as that in Fig. 16.5 cannot distinguish between complete AV block with a pacemaker below the

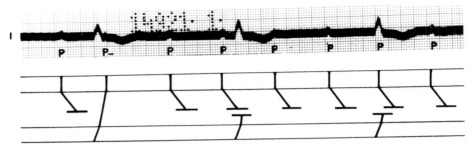

FIG. 16.15. Third-degree AV block (complete heart block) with an atrial "capture." The diagnosis of third-degree AV block is made because there is no fixed relationship between P waves (P), which come at a basic rate of 73, and the QRS complexes, which are regular at a rate of 27. The QRS is prolonged to 0.14 sec, which can be explained if the ventricles are activated by an impulse arising in one of the bundle branches. The second P-wave from the left (P—) illustrates the unusual occurrence of an atrial "capture." This P-wave, which is narrower than the others in this lead, is premature and comes approximately 0.16 sec after the preceding QRS complex. As shown in the Lewis diagram *(below),* this behavior can be explained if the premature P wave was initiated by retrograde conduction of the ventricular beat through the AV node into the atria, i.e., if the ventricular beat "captured" the atria. (ECG from Katz and Pick, 1956.)

bifurcation of the AV bundle and heart block where the ventricular pacemaker is located above this bifurcation but which is complicated by coexistent bundle branch block. This distinction can be made, however, in some circumstances, e.g., where the onset of the QRS abnormality coincides with the appearance of third-degree AV block.

UNIDIRECTIONAL BLOCK

The concept of unidirectional block is extremely important and allows several features of both normal and abnormal impulse conduction to be explained. Furthermore, as is seen in the discussion of re-entry (Chapter 17), unidirectional block can play a major role in the genesis of premature systoles and tachycardias. The term unidirectional block means what it implies: complete block of impulse conduction but in only one direction. In the case of impulse propagation through the AV node, unidirectional block is a feature of *normal* conduction in the heart. Thus antegrade conduction from atria to ventricles through the AV node is normally more rapid than retrograde conduction from ventricles to atria, and conduction is often possible only in the antegrade direction (*ante:* before, i.e., from atria to ventricles) but not in the retrograde direction (*retro:* behind, i.e., from ventricles to atria). Unidirectional block also occurs in diseased regions of the myocardium, e.g., within the ventricles or His-Purkinje system of the ischemic heart.

A simple way to produce unidirectional block in a strand of myocardial tissue is to compress it with a wedge-shaped wooden block (Fig. 16.16). This causes an asymmetrically distributed disturbance of cellular function, as the greater the compression the greater is the depression of conduction. The initial effect of the asymmetrical depression of conduction is often the appearance of unidirectional

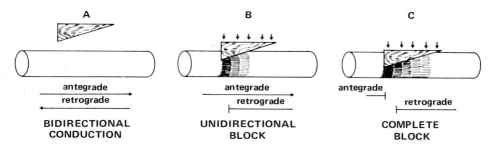

FIG. 16.16. Unidirectional block produced by compression of a strand of cardiac muscle by a wedge-shaped wooden block. **A:** Bidirectional conduction occurs in the normal, uncompressed tissue. **B:** Unidirectional block is produced by moderate compression of the strand, which allows conduction to proceed from left to right (defined here as conduction in the antegrade direction) but not from right to left (retrograde block). (Darker shading indicates a greater degree of decremental conduction.) **C:** Bidirectional (complete) block is produced by more severe compression of the strand. Conduction in both directions is blocked by the marked degree of decremental conduction.

block (Fig. 16.16B) that manifests as failure of conduction only in the retrograde direction (which is arbitrarily defined in Figs. 16.16–16.19 as conduction from right to left) and not in the antegrade direction (left to right). Although mild compression does not block antegrade conduction completely, conduction in this direction is slowed (see below). More severe degrees of compression (Fig. 16.16C) cause complete block, in which conduction is blocked in both directions.

The mechanism responsible for the phenomenon of unidirectional block illustrated in Fig. 16.16B can be understood if one draws a plot of the distribution of the ability of the propagated action potential to excite the tissue ahead of it

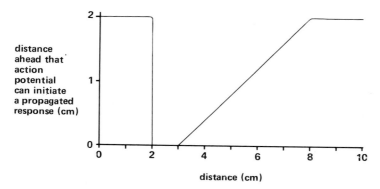

FIG. 16.17. Asymmetrically distributed decremental conduction. The distance ahead that an impulse can be propagated is shown on the ordinate as a function of the distance along the strand of cardiac muscle *(abscissa)*. Normal tissue (0–2 and 8–10 cm) can activate resting muscle up to 2 cm ahead. The ability to initiate a propagated action potential is completely lost from 2 to 3 cm and is depressed from 3 to 8 cm. See Fig. 16.16 for an example of how such an asymmetrical distribution of decremental conduction can be produced.

at various locations in the fiber shown in Fig. 16.16B. As shown in Fig. 16.17, the depression of conduction is asymmetrically distributed. In the uncompressed regions of the tissue, from 0 to 2 cm and from 8 to 10 cm, the normal action potential has arbitrarily been chosen to have the capability of activating tissue up to 2 cm ahead. Between 2 and 3 cm (under the point of the wedge in Fig. 16.16) the tissue is damaged sufficiently to have completely lost the ability to initiate a propagated action potential. In the tissue between 3 and 8 cm (Fig. 16.17), the tissue is only partly damaged so that the distance ahead that can be activated by the impulses arising in this region depends on the degree of compression, as shown in Fig. 16.16B.

If, in the situation depicted in Fig. 16.17, an action potential is initiated at 0 cm, it proceeds in an antegrade direction as defined above. Initially the impulse is propagated normally to 2 cm, at which point it "jumps" over the area of zero conduction as shown by the arrow (*a*) which arises in noncompressed tissue and so can "reach" 2 cm ahead (Fig. 16.18). Thus the normal tissue just to the left of the completely depressed area is able to initiate an action potential at a point 2 cm further to the right, i.e., at 4 cm. At 4 cm the tissue is depressed but retains the ability to depolarize the tissue up to 0.4 cm ahead, i.e., to 4.4 cm (arrow *b*). Here the action potential produced is less depressed and so conducts 0.6 cm to the right, reaching the tissue at 5.0 cm (arrow *c*). At 5.0 cm the ability to conduct is still less depressed and so antegrade conduction continues to gain speed. In this way the antegrade impulse crosses the area of complete depression, emerging after a delay at 8 cm as a normally propagated action potential.

If retrograde condition is initiated in the above example by stimulating the tissue at 10 cm, rather than at 0 cm, the conduction abnormalities arising from the asymmetrical disturbance of conduction are quite different from those seen when conduction proceeds in the antegrade direction. As shown in Fig. 16.19, when the impulse reaches 8 cm, where it first encounters the area of depressed conduction, conduction velocity begins to slow. Up to 8 cm, the impulse is conducted normally to the left, reaching ahead 2 cm to a point at 6 cm (arrow *a'*). Here the impulse depolarizes an area that can propagate an impulse only 1.2 cm, so that the next area to be depolarized is at the tip of arrow *b'*. At this latter point conduction is depressed still further, so that the impulse arising at 4.8 cm conducts only 0.8 cm, to reach this tissue at 4 cm (arrow *c'*). The impulse arising at 4.0 cm (arrow *d'*) conducts less effectively than that depicted by arrow *c'*, so that arrow *d'* is even shorter. This decreasing effectiveness of impulse propagation continues, each impulse becoming less and less effective as it approaches the completely depressed area. Thus when the impulse "trickles" to the point where the ability to initiate a conducted impulse is lost completely (at 3 cm), it ceases to be propagated. In this way the impulse traveling in the retrograde direction is blocked.

The mechanism for unidirectional block shown in Figs. 16.16–16.19 can occur in any bundle of myocardial tissue which sustains an injury that, for example, causes an asymmetrically distributed depression in action potential amplitude.

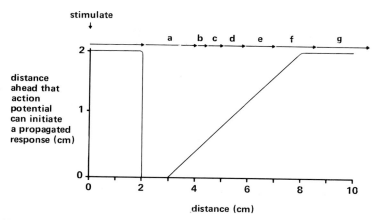

FIG. 16.18. Antegrade conduction in the strand of cardiac muscle in Fig. 16.17. An impulse entering from the left is able to cross the region where the ability to initiate a propagated action potential is completely lost, although the passage of the impulse in the antegrade direction (left to right) is delayed. See text for discussion.

Such an asymmetrical reduction in action potential amplitude or in any of the factors that determine the ability of the action potential to excite the resting myocardium ahead of the propagating wave of depolarization can give rise to unidirectional block, as described in Figs. 16.16–16.19. Thus an asymmetrically distributed decrease in the rate of depolarization has the same effect. Fibrosis, which reduces the ability of the impulse to be propagated by increasing the resistance to the spread of the potentials generated by an action potential, can

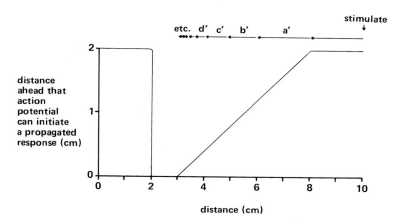

FIG. 16.19. Retrograde block in the strand of cardiac muscle in Fig. 16.17. An impulse entering from the right encounters progressively increasing decremental conduction that renders the impulse unable to initiate an action potential in the normal tissue to the left. The passage of the impulse in the retrograde direction (right to left) is thus blocked. See text for discussion.

also cause unidirectional block when the extent of fibrosis is distributed asymmetrically. Similarly, an asymmetrically distributed increase in threshold can cause unidirectional block but by a slightly more complex mechanism. It is thus apparent that a variety of anatomical and electrophysiological abnormalities can singly or together give rise to unidirectional block. The consequences of this conduction abnormality become apparent in Chapter 17, where the mechanisms responsible for abnormal impulse formation, notably re-entry, are discussed.

BIBLIOGRAPHY

Dreifus, L. S., and Likoff, W., editors (1973): *Cardiac Arrhythmias.* Grune & Stratton, New York.

Ferrer, M. I. (1973): The sick sinus syndrome. *Circulation,* 47:635–641.

Hoffman, B. F., and Cranefield, P. F. (1964): The physiological basis of cardiac arrhythmias. *Am. J. Med.,* 37:670–684.

Katz, B. (1966): *Nerve, Muscle and Synapse,* Chap. 5. McGraw-Hill, New York.

Katz, L. N., and Pick, A. (1956): *Clinical Electrocardiography. Part I; The Arrhythmias.* Lea & Febiger, Philadelphia.

17

The Arrhythmias

II. Abnormal Impulse Formation and Re-entry, Premature Systoles, Pre-excitation

It would seem logical that the mechanisms responsible for arrhythmias caused by abnormal impulse formation would be quite different from those which give rise to the conduction disorders discussed in Chapter 16. For this reason it is not uncommon to find that premature systoles, tachycardia, flutter, and fibrillation are viewed as manifestations of heightened "excitability" within the myocardium. It seems almost obvious that these abnormalities in impulse formation would reflect mechanisms opposite to those leading to disorders like AV block, which result from depressed excitability. Yet it is now quite clear that depressed excitability is responsible for many of the arrhythmias characterized by abnormal impulse formation described in the following pages, as well as the electrocardiographic abnormalities characterized by slow conduction discussed in the preceding chapter.

PREMATURE SYSTOLES

Premature excitation of the atria or ventricles is readily recognized on the ECG by the appearance of abnormally timed P waves or QRS complexes. These premature systoles are often called extrasystoles or ectopic beats, although both of these terms can frequently be misnomers. Premature systoles are not invariably "extra;" i.e., they may sometimes *replace* a beat of the atria or ventricles rather than *adding* to the number of such beats. Nor do premature systoles always arise from ectopic sites in that certain classes of premature systoles originate within the normal conduction pathway, although they do so in an abnormal way. It is true by definition, however, that premature systoles occur when regions of the myocardium become active prior to the time they would normally be depolarized by the normal impulse conducted from the SA node. Premature systoles are thus characterized by the early appearance of a P wave or a QRS complex on the ECG. In some cases even this definition is inadequate as premature systoles can influence the ECG without causing depolarization of the atria or ventricles. In these cases the influence of the premature systole is manifest by its ability to block normal impulse conduction ("concealed conduction;" Chapter 18).

In view of the uncertainties concerning the mechanisms which produce these disorders of impulse formation, this chapter begins with a description of the more common electrocardiographic manifestations of the premature systoles. After a simple classification of these disorders, the mechanisms responsible for their production are discussed.

Several types of premature systoles are recognizable in the ECG, and they are usually named according to their presumed site of origin.

Sinus Premature Systoles

The rather unusual occurrence of premature depolarization of the SA node gives rise to a normal [1] P wave followed by a normal [1] QRS complex after a normal P-R interval. In other words, the only abnormality associated with a sinus premature systole is the premature appearance of the normal conduction sequence.

The example of sinus premature systoles shown in Fig. 17.1 also illustrates a phenomenon called bigeminy, in which the beats are grouped in pairs. The interpretation that this arrhythmia represents the repeated occurrence of sinus premature systoles assumes that the longer P-P intervals reflect the normal rate of discharge of the pacemaker in the SA node, whereas the shorter intervals are caused by premature discharge of the SA node, which then initiates a wave of depolarization that activates the remainder of the heart by way of the normal conduction pathways.

It should be noted that there is another possible interpretation of the ECG shown in Fig. 17.1—i.e., that this represents 3:2 SA block in which every third sinus impulse fails to activate the atria (and thus fails to produce either a P wave or a QRS complex). The fact that the longer P-P interval is not exactly twice the shorter interval (which would at first glance seem to be the expected behavior in 3:2 SA block) can still be explained if the Wenckebach phenomenon is also present, i.e., if the interval between depolarization within the SA node and its conduction into the atria increases prior to the blocked sinus impulse in a manner similar to that which explains the timing of the QRS complexes in 3:2 AV block of Mobitz type I (Chapter 16). Distinction between 3:2 SA block and alternating sinus premature systoles cannot, therefore, be made in this ECG.

Atrial Premature Systoles

The typical electrocardiographic appearance of an atrial premature systole is the premature occurrence of an abnormal P wave followed by a normal QRS complex. The P-R interval after an atrial premature systole is not abnormally short; i.e., it is greater than 0.12 sec (Fig. 17.2). In some cases abnormalities appear in the QRS complex following an atrial premature systole that are caused

---

[1] The term "normal" as used in this chapter to describe the electrocardiographic manifestations of premature excitation means "like the P waves or QRS complexes of the basic ECG." When the basic ECG shows an abnormality (e.g., ventricular hypertrophy), this abnormality also appears in the beats cited here as normal.

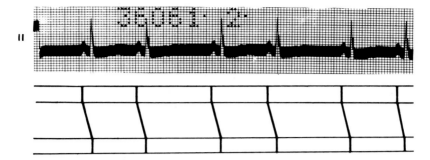

FIG. 17.1. Sinus premature systoles. The second, fourth, and sixth P waves are premature but are normal in contour and are followed by a normal QRS complex after a normal P-R interval. This record also illustrates bigeminy, the beats being grouped in pairs. (An alternative mechanism for this arrhythmia is discussed in the text.) (ECG from Katz and Pick, 1956.)

by the prematurity of ventricular depolarization ("aberrancy;" see below). The fact that the P-R interval and QRS complex associated with the atrial premature systoles are normal is due to the fact that the impulse reaches the ventricles after the normal delay in the AV node and depolarizes the ventricles by the normal pathway. The example of the atrial premature systole presented in Fig. 17.2 illustrates the typical abnormality. The fourth P wave follows the third by an interval considerably shorter than the normal sinus interval; i.e., this P wave is premature. The contour of the fourth P wave, as well as its timing, is abnormal, differing from the remainder of the P waves in this ECG in that the fourth P wave is lower in amplitude and narrower. The third criterion for this diagnosis

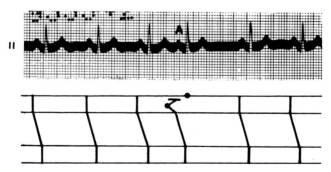

FIG. 17.2. Atrial premature systole. The fourth P wave (A) is premature; is different in contour (smaller) compared to the other P waves, which are sinus P waves; and is followed by a normal QRS complex after a slightly shortened P-R interval (0.16 sec compared to 0.17 sec after the sinus P waves). The interval between the sinus P waves immediately before and after the premature systole is exactly twice the normal sinus interval, indicating that the premature systole did not penetrate the SA node and reset its timing. The small dot on the upper line of the Lewis diagram (below) indicates the timing of a sinus impulse that did not activate the atria because its transmission into the atria was blocked by the premature systole. (ECG from Katz and Pick, 1956.)

is also met because the P-R interval following the fourth P wave is 0.16 sec and thus is not abnormally shortened.

Aberrant Conduction

The QRS complex that follows an atrial premature systole is not always normal in contour, even though the impulse has reached the ventricles by way of the normal conduction pathway via the AV node. In the ECG shown in Fig. 17.3, for example, the fourth QRS complex is prolonged and different in contour from those in the remainder of the record. This QRS complex is premature, but it can be shown to have been produced by an atrial premature systole. (The abnormal P wave of the latter is not distinct but can be identified by the alteration in the shape of the T wave following the preceding QRS complex.) The abnormal contour of the fourth QRS complex is not due to entry of the wave of depolarization into the ventricles by an abnormal path because the impulse which reaches the ventricles from an atrial premature systole is conducted along the normal pathway below the AV node. Instead, the abnormal contour of the fourth QRS complex arises from a conduction abnormality *within* the ventricles that can be attributed to the prematurity of the beat. This abnormality occurs because the impulse conducted from the atrial premature systole has reached the ventricles during the relative refractory period that follows the preceding beat, as is apparent from the very short interval between the third and fourth QRS complexes in Fig. 17.3. As a result, the conduction of the impulse responsible for the fourth

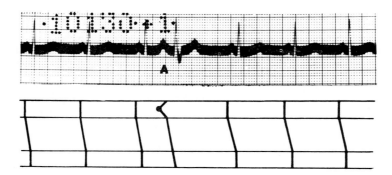

FIG: 17.3. Atrial premature systole with aberrant ventricular conduction. The fourth P wave (A) is premature, falling on the T wave of the preceding ventricular beat where it produces a small notch on its downstroke. The QRS complex that follows the premature P wave is abnormal, being prolonged to 0.12 sec and containing a small, broad S wave not seen in the normal QRS complexes. It is highly probable that this abnormal QRS complex is initiated by the premature P wave, but because of its prematurity exhibits aberrant conduction. Additional evidence for the supraventricular origin of the fourth QRS complex is the fact that the interval between the sinus P waves immediately before and after the premature systole is significantly less than twice the normal sinus interval. This finding indicates that the premature P wave penetrated the SA node where it reset the sinus pacemaker, thereby advancing the timing of the following series of sinus beats. (ECG from Katz and Pick, 1956.)

QRS complex is slightly abnormal—hence the designation "aberrant conduction." The contour abnormalities in an aberrant QRS complex usually appear as changes in its terminal rather than its initial portions. The site of block when the ventricles show aberrant conduction is usually in the His-Purkinje system. This is not unexpected as the action potential, and thus the refractory period, lasts longer in these conduction tissues than in the ventricular myocardium (Chapter 14). For this reason the QRS complex in aberrantly conducted beats resembles that seen in bundle branch block (usually right bundle branch block).

The QRS abnormalities in aberrant conduction resemble not only those of bundle branch block but those associated with ventricular premature systoles as well (see below). Accurate interpretation of these abnormalities in the QRS contour of a premature systole is often difficult and sometimes impossible, although in the example shown in Fig. 17.3 evidence of a premature P wave allows the diagnosis of atrial premature systole with aberrant ventricular conduction to be made with considerable assurance.

The failure of the atria to be activated by the sinus impulse that immediately follows the atrial premature systoles in Figs. 17.2 and 17.3 is readily understood. Such a sinus impulse emerges from the SA node at a time when the atria are in a refractory state following their depolarization by the atrial premature systole, and so is blocked.

The timing of the series of sinus P waves that follows an atrial premature systole is of importance, as this timing can be altered if the atrial premature systole is conducted into the pacemaker region of the SA node. If the wave of depolarization initiated by premature activation of the atria fails to influence the SA node, the subsequent sinus P waves appear at their expected time. Often the premature QRS complex that follows the atrial premature systole occurs at the same time the subsequent sinus P wave is expected, so that the latter is obscured. If sinus rhythm has continued without disturbance from the premature systole, the sinus P wave that comes after the obscured P wave should follow the sinus P wave preceding the premature systole by an interval equal to twice the normal sinus interval. In other words, the regular sequence or "timetable" of sinus P waves would not be altered by the premature systole. In fact, this timetable is upset by the atrial premature systole that is shown in Fig. 17.3. Examination of this ECG reveals that the second sinus impulse after the premature systole, which gives rise to the normal P wave following the atrial premature systole, has come *sooner* than would be expected if the SA node had maintained its normal timetable. (This normal timetable for pacemaker activity in the SA node can easily be determined by simply projecting ahead with a calipers the series of P waves that existed before the atrial premature systole.) The fact that the sinus timetable is altered by the atrial premature systole so as to be moved earlier in time demonstrates that the premature systole has "reset" the sinus pacemaker. The result is a shift of the entire sequence of sinus beats following the premature systole, as can be seen in Fig. 17.3. This behavior is readily explained as being due to penetration into the SA node of the wave of depolariza-

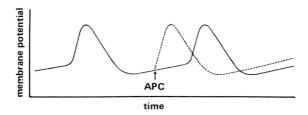

FIG. 17.4. Mechanism by which a premature systole that penetrates the SA node resets the sinus pacemaker. The action potential of a pacemaker cell in the SA node illustrates the normal sinus interval *(solid line)*. The entry of an impulse conducted from an atrial premature systole (APC) causes early depolarization of the pacemaker cell *(dotted line)*, thereby advancing the timing of the following series of action potentials (Fig. 17.3).

tion that was propagated to this structure from the atrial premature systole. The early depolarization of the SA node causes it to fire before diastolic depolarization arising from the normal pacemaker activity has reached threshold. As a result, the subsequent train of sinus impulses is shifted earlier in time (Fig. 17.4). This behavior can readily be identified in Fig. 17.3 because the interval between the two normally generated QRS complexes that includes the atrial premature systole is less than twice the normal R-R interval. (The term "R-R interval" as used here and elsewhere in these chapters means simply the interval between two adjacent QRS complexes.)

Junctional Premature Systoles

Premature depolarization of the AV node or the AV bundle immediately beneath it causes the appearance of a *junctional premature systole* (also called a nodal premature systole). This abnormality results in a premature QRS complex whose contour is normal, or very nearly so, because the premature impulse reaches the ventricles via the normal pathway from the AV node. Junctional premature systoles may or may not be preceded by a P wave. If a P wave is inscribed before the premature QRS complex, the diagnosis of a junctional premature systole requires that the P-R interval be less than 0.12 sec. If this interval is longer than 0.12 sec the diagnosis would instead be an atrial premature systole, as described above.

The relationship between the QRS complex initiated by a junctional premature systole and the accompanying P waves, if present, is variable, but the reason for this variability is not difficult to understand if the mechanism responsible for the basic electrocardiographic abnormality is kept in mind. Because the AV node and associated junctional tissue lie at the only point of electrical connection between the atria and ventricles, a premature impulse arising in this tissue may proceed not only in the antegrade direction to activate the ventricles but also in the retrograde direction to activate the atria. This retrograde conduction does not always take place, however. In cases where the junctional premature systole causes retrograde activation of the atria, the resulting P wave can either precede or follow the QRS complex, depending on the relative speeds of antegrade conduction (which produces the QRS complex) and retrograde conduction (which initiates the P wave). This timing cannot be predicted because the distances traveled by the antegrade and retrograde impulses, as well as their conduction velocities, vary from patient to patient (see below).

The only manifestation of a junctional premature systole when there is no retrograde activation of the atria is the premature appearance of a normal QRS complex without an associated P wave. The ECG in Fig. 17.5 shows two junctional premature systoles, which cause the second and sixth QRS complexes. These two QRS complexes, each of whose contour is similar to that of the remainder of the ventricular complexes in this record, are premature and are not preceded by a P wave; hence they meet the criteria of junctional premature systoles set forth above. The relationship between the junctional premature systoles and the basic sinus rhythm, however, differs in the two examples shown in Fig. 17.5. The second junctional premature systole (the sixth QRS complex) is the more typical as it is followed by a pause. The long R-R interval that follows this junctional premature systole thus results from the inability of the next sinus impulse to penetrate the ventricles. This phenomenon, which results from the refractory state that occurs after the AV node is depolarized by the premature systole, causes the long R-R interval following the sixth QRS complex in Fig. 17.5. The atrial depolarization caused by the sinus impulse immediately following

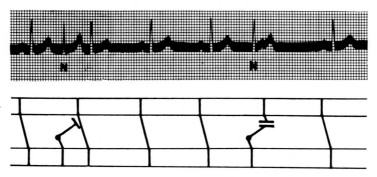

FIG. 17.5. Junctional premature systoles. The second and sixth QRS complexes (N) are premature, normal in contour, and are not preceded by a P wave; they thus meet the criteria for junctional premature systoles. The first junctional premature systole, which produces the second QRS complex, does not interfere with either the initiation or conduction of the following sinus beat, so it is interpolated. (The P wave associated with the third QRS complex falls on the T wave of the junctional premature systole, making it abnormally tall.) The second junctional premature systole, which produces the sixth QRS complex, follows the preceding QRS complex by a longer interval than the first junctional premature systole. This allows the impulse propagated within the AV node from the second junctional premature systole to interfere with passage of the subsequent sinus P wave, which is blocked in the AV node (shown in the Lewis diagram by short horizontal lines). The QRS complex produced by the second junctional premature systole is thus followed by a compensatory pause (see text). (ECG from Katz and Pick, 1956.)

premature systole is evident as an upright P wave (which causes a "notch" on the S-T segment of the premature QRS complex) that is not followed by ventricular depolarization.

Compensatory Pause and Interpolation

The long delay between the premature QRS complex and that caused by the next sinus beat (the seventh in Fig. 17.5) is called a *compensatory pause* because its length is such that the interval between the two QRS complexes enclosing the junctional premature systole is exactly twice that between the normal sinus beats in this record. This means that the timetable of the SA node has not been altered by the premature systole. The term compensatory pause is in some ways a misnomer as the long pause does not really compensate for anything, except to allow the sinus beats to remain on the timetable they would have followed had there not been a premature systole. The fact that the junctional premature systole has not "reset" the SA node is readily understood because, not being conducted in a retrograde manner from the AV node into the atria, this premature systole is not able to influence the timing of pacemaker discharge in the SA node.

The first junctional premature systole in Fig. 17.5, which produces the second QRS complex, is *interpolated* in that it does not block conduction into the ventricles of the sinus beat which follows. Thus the subsequent P wave (which is inscribed on the T wave of the premature systole, causing its peaked appearance) is conducted into the ventricles where it gives rise to the third QRS complex in this record. This normal sinus beat follows the preceding sinus beat after the expected interval. This behavior, where a premature systole is simply added between two normal sinus beats, is called interpolation.

Retrograde P Waves

When junctional premature systoles activate the atria, the resulting P waves arise from *retrograde activation of the atria.* Instead of being activated normally by impulses that begin at the right atrial-superior vena caval junction, retrograde conduction causes the atria to be depolarized by impulses that have penetrated the atria from the AV node. The retrograde P waves produced by junctional premature systoles are therefore abnormal in contour. The characteristic appearance of the retrograde P wave is shown in Fig. 17.6, where an inverted P wave precedes the fourth QRS complex, which is normal in contour, by only 0.08 sec. The shortness of the P-R interval, which in this record is diagnostic of a junctional premature systole, is due to the fact that both the P wave and the QRS complex arise from a single wave of depolarization that originates in the AV node. This allows the emergence of the wave of excitation from the upper (atrial) and lower (ventricular) ends of the AV node to be simultaneous, or nearly so. In Fig. 17.6 the wave of excitation has reached the atrial end of the AV node slightly before it enters the ventricular conduction system—hence the short P-R interval.

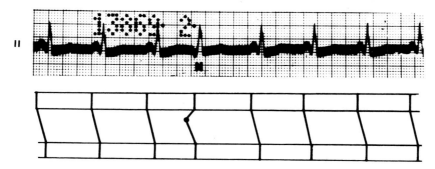

FIG. 17.6. Junctional premature systole with retrograde P wave. The fourth QRS complex is premature but normal in contour and is preceded by an abnormal, inverted P wave. The P-R interval preceding this premature systole is 0.08 sec, so the criteria for a junctional premature systole are met. The P wave preceding the premature systole can be assumed to have arisen from the same junctional focus that produced the premature QRS complex, as shown in the Lewis diagram. The inverted P-wave that precedes the premature systole thus represents a retrograde P wave. (ECG from Katz and Pick, 1956.)

It should be noted that the term P-R interval in this situation is really a misnomer as the impulse has not traveled from atria (P) to ventricles (QRS).

The nature of the abnormality in contour of the retrograde P wave can readily be appreciated by comparing the electrical vectors of normal and retrograde P waves (Fig. 17.7). The normal P wave vector is directed inferiorly and to the left, as would be expected because atrial depolarization normally begins at a site adjacent to the SA node. In contrast, the wave of depolarization initiated by retrograde conduction from a junctional premature systole is directed superiorly because the AV node lies at the inferior border of the atria, near the top of the interventricular septum. For this reason the retrograde P wave is characteristically small in lead I and inverted in lead II.

Junctional premature systoles are sometimes classified according to the temporal relationships between the retrograde P waves and the QRS complexes. In cases in which a retrograde P wave precedes the QRS complex by 0.02–0.12 sec, the beat is classified as an upper nodal beat. When the P wave is presumed to have occurred at the same time as the QRS complex, the beat is designated a middle nodal beat. When a retrograde P wave follows the QRS complex, the beat is called a lower nodal beat. A fourth type of junctional premature systole, called a coronary nodal beat, can be diagnosed when a normal P wave precedes a premature systole by an interval of less than 0.12 sec. These terms are now being discarded, however, because the relationship between the QRS complexes and retrograde P waves associated with junctional premature systole is probably determined more by the relative rates of antegrade and retrograde conduction than by the site in the AV node where the premature systole originated. The term coronary nodal beat is also falling into disuse because the usual explanation for the normal contour of the P waves—that the impulse entered the atria from the upper end of the AV node above the coronary sinus—is now recognized not to provide the only explanation for this behavior. It is also possible that

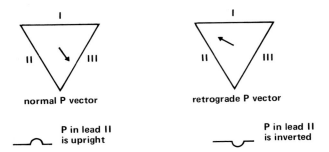

FIG. 17.7. Comparison of normal and retrograde P vectors. The normal P vector in the frontal plane is directed to the left and inferiorly, inscribing an upright deflection in lead II *(left)*. The retrograde P vector, on the other hand, is directed to the right and superiorly, and so inscribes an inverted deflection in lead II *(right)*.

a normal P wave appearing immediately before a junctional premature systole is produced by rapid conduction of a retrograde impulse by way of the SA ring bundles (Chapter 15) to initiate atrial depolarization in the region of the SA node. As in the case of upper, middle, and lower nodal rhythms, therefore, the appearance of the P waves and their relationship to QRS complexes in coronary nodal rhythms is best described in terms of the physiology, rather than the anatomy, of the conduction system.

Ventricular Premature Systoles

When an impulse arising below the bifurcation of the bundle of His causes the ventricles to depolarize prematurely, a ventricular premature systole is seen in the ECG. This type of premature systole is characterized by an abnormal QRS complex that is not preceded by a P wave. The QRS complex produced by a ventricular premature systole differs from the normal QRS complexes that follow the sinus beats, being longer in duration and bizarre in contour (Fig. 17.8). The abnormal contour of the sixth QRS complex in Fig. 17.8, which is a ventricular premature systole, can be explained by the fact that the ventricles are not depolarized by the normal route. Instead of spreading simultaneously over both ventricles from the common bundle, the wave of depolarization is propagated by way of an abnormal pathway in which one ventricle is activated before the other (Fig. 17.9). This asynchrony of ventricular activation is therefore responsible for prolongation of the QRS complex and its abnormal contour.

The mechanism responsible for the prolonged, bizarre QRS complex associated with a ventricular premature systole is in some ways similar to that responsible for the QRS abnormalities seen in bundle branch block. In both cases ventricular activation has lost its synchronization. In the case of bundle branch block, synchrony is lost because the normal wave of depolarization is delayed in its passage to one of the ventricles, whereas in a ventricular premature systole synchrony is lost because the ventricle in which the impulse has arisen prematurely is activated prior to the opposite ventricle.

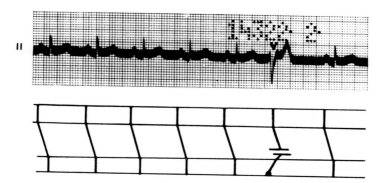

FIG. 17.8. Ventricular premature systole. The sixth QRS complex (V) is premature, not preceded by a P wave, and is prolonged and bizarre compared to the normal QRS complexes in this record, thus meeting the criteria for a ventricular premature systole. This premature systole is followed by a compensatory pause. The sinus P wave that is blocked (shown in the Lewis diagram) is "buried" in the QRS of the ventricular premature systole. (ECG from Katz and Pick, 1956.)

The ventricular premature systole shown in Fig. 17.8 is followed by a compensatory pause because the impulse arising in the ventricles has not been conducted to the atria and so is unable to influence the timing of depolarization in the SA node (the sinus P wave that followed the last normal beat before the premature systole is not seen as it is "buried" in the much larger premature QRS complex). Ventricular premature systoles can also be interpolated (Fig. 17.5), although interpolation is uncommon. If there is retrograde conduction of the ventricular premature systole through the AV node into the atria, a retrograde P wave follows the premature QRS complex. In most cases, however, the behavior of the ventricular systoles is as shown in Fig. 17.8; i.e., there is a full compensatory pause and no evidence of retrograde conduction through the AV node.

Fusion Beats

In the event a ventricular premature systole begins so late in the cardiac cycle that the resulting activation of the ventricles from "below" begins at the same time the normal sinus impulse conducted through the AV node has begun to

FIG. 17.9. Normal conduction pathway followed by an impulse that reaches the ventricles via the AV bundle and bundle branches *(left),* and the abnormal conduction pathway followed by an impulse arising in the left ventricle *(right).* The greater length of the latter pathway explains the prolongation of QRS seen in a ventricular premature systole.

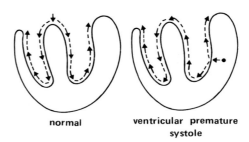

normal   ventricular premature
                        systole

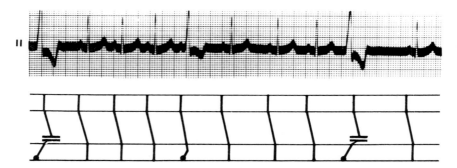

FIG. 17.10. Ventricular premature systoles showing a fusion beat. The first and ninth QRS complexes are premature, not initiated by P-waves, and are prolonged and bizarre. These are typical ventricular premature systoles. The fifth QRS complex is also premature but is less prolonged and less bizarre than the other QRS complexes. The P-R interval preceding this QRS complex is 0.10 sec, so it can be deduced that the later portions of this QRS complex are initiated by the impulse propagated normally into the ventricles by way of the AV bundle and bundle branches. The initial portion of this QRS complex is abnormal, its upstroke being slurred as is that of the other two "typical" ventricular premature systoles. This fifth premature systole thus represents a fusion beat in that it combines the features of both the normal and abnormal QRS complexes. The dual origin of the fusion beat is shown in the lower space (ventricles) of Lewis diagram. (ECG from Katz and Pick, 1956.)

depolarize the ventricles from "above," a *fusion beat* may be seen. The fifth QRS complex in Fig. 17.10 is an example of such a beat: It is midway in contour between the QRS complexes associated with the normal sinus beats (which make up the majority of the ventricular beats in this record) and the ventricular premature systoles which give rise to the first and ninth QRS complexes. In this fusion beat the impulse arising from the sinus node has entered the ventricles very soon after the beginning of the ventricular premature systole, thereby lessening the abnormality of the QRS complex. In other fusion beats, the initial portion of the QRS complex can be initiated by the normally conducted impulse, the ventricular premature systole influencing only its terminal portions. Recognition of fusion beats is of considerable importance in diagnosis, especially in ventricular tachycardia (see below).

PRE-EXCITATION (WOLFF-PARKINSON-WHITE SYNDROME)

When an impulse arising in the SA node is conducted into the ventricles by way of a pathway other than the AV node, an abnormality appears in the QRS complex which may resemble that seen in a ventricular premature systole. Most commonly, such an accessory pathway transmits the wave of depolarization from atria to ventricles more rapidly than the AV node, which is a region of normal conduction delay. As a result, the abnormal QRS complex is preceded by an abnormally short P-R interval. This combination of an abnormal QRS complex preceded by an abnormally short P-R interval (less than 0.12 sec) is called

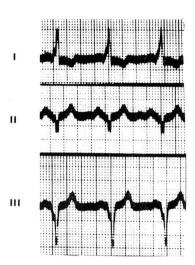

FIG. 17.11. Pre-excitation (Wolff-Parkinson-White syndrome). The P-R intervals are abnormally short (0.11 sec), and the QRS complexes are widened (to 0.14 sec) by the presence of delta waves. The latter are seen as slurring of the beginning of the R wave in lead I and of the beginning of the QS complex in lead III. (The T wave is also abnormally inverted in lead I.) (From Katz and Pick, 1956.)

pre-excitation or the *Wolff-Parkinson-White* (WPW) syndrome after the three cardiologists who first described this abnormality.

The characteristic QRS complex in pre-excitation is abnormally prolonged, mainly because of a slurring during its initial inscription. The slowly rising (or falling) initial deflection in the QRS complex in pre-excitation is called a *delta wave* (Fig. 17.11). The conduction abnormality in pre-excitation is usually confined to the initial part of the QRS complex because of the subsequent entry of the normal wave of excitation into the normal conduction pathways of the AV bundle and Purkinje system. The importance of pre-excitation lies not only in its ability to produce QRS complexes that resemble, and so must be distinguished from, ventricular systoles, but also because the existence of two pathways for AV conduction in patients with pre-excitation causes them to be prone to develop atrial tachycardias (Chapter 18).

MECHANISM OF ORIGIN OF PREMATURE SYSTOLES

Much uncertainty remains regarding the mechanisms responsible for premature systoles in man. These difficulties do not arise from the lack of plausible explanations; instead, several possible mechanisms are suggested from precise analyses of clinical ECGs and from the study of arrhythmias produced experimentally. At least three different mechanisms now appear to account for most of these arrhythmias.

Abnormal Pacemaker Activity

The most easily understood of the mechanisms that can give rise to premature systoles is the early discharge of a pacemaker cell, or groups of cells, "below" the dominant pacemaker of the SA node. This straightforward mechanism can arise from any influence that causes partial depolarization: accelerated decline in gK, an increased depolarizing current, or lowered threshold in any of the potential pacemaker cells that normally are unable to fire as rapidly as the SA node. The acceleration of such a "lower" pacemaker can give rise to a premature systole or, if the accelerated discharge is repetitive, a tachycardia (see below).

Inhomogeneity of Repolarization

The ability of local factors to influence the duration of the cardiac action potential gives rise to the possibility that excitability can recover in one region of the heart before the adjacent areas have fully repolarized after passage of a single wave of depolarization. Under these conditions the tissue that has remained depolarized longer than the neighboring tissue may re-excite the regions of the heart that have regained their excitability. In this way a second wave of depolarization can be initiated in the latter and thereby produce a premature systole. In view of the ability of a number of important pathological states, notably myocardial ischemia, to shorten action potential duration, the following description of this mechanism focuses on the way in which abnormal abbreviation of the action potential can produce a premature systole. However, a similar effect can be produced when the action potential is abnormally prolonged in a local region of the myocardium.

When a localized area of the myocardium repolarizes sooner than the tissue around it, the repolarized myocardium can regain its excitability while the adjacent tissues around it remain depolarized. Electrical currents arising in the surrounding, normally depolarized regions can therefore re-enter the tissue that repolarized prematurely to initiate a propagated action potential (Fig. 17.12). This mechanism is shown in the action potentials at the right in Fig. 17.12, where the shortened action potential allows the abnormal tissue in the center of the figure to be re-excited by the electronegativity still present in the surrounding tissue where the action potential duration is normally prolonged. If the normally depolarized tissue is able to re-excite the tissue with the short action potential,

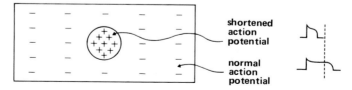

FIG. 17.12. Inhomogeneity of depolarization. This diagram represents potentials outside the cells in a region of the myocardium at an instant, toward the end of the action potential *(vertical dashed line, at right)*. Abnormal shortening of action potential duration in the cells at the center has allowed these cells to recover at a time when the normal tissue is still depolarized. Such an inhomogeneity can allow the cells with the shorter action potential to be reactivated by the surrounding normal tissue, thereby causing a premature systole.

the wave of depolarization propagated through the latter may subsequently re-enter the normal tissue after it has recovered but before the arrival of the next impulse conducted from the normal pacemaker. The result is a premature systole. The electrocardiographic features of such a premature systole depend on the site where this abnormal mechanism is found.

Conduction Abnormalities

Possibly the most important cause of premature systoles, and of tachycardia, is abnormal impulse conduction through regions of the heart where conductivity is depressed. These arrhythmias are produced in areas of decremental conduction by the phenomena of slow conduction and unidirectional block. In experimental preparations it is possible to demonstrate that a single impulse entering a region of decremental conduction can emerge as two (or more) impulses. Microelectrode studies can demonstrate that the second impulse is initiated by the first, which has been delayed in the area of decremental conduction, then conducted by an abnormal pathway back into normal areas of the myocardium. The extra impulses originating in these areas of decremental conduction are sometimes called echoes, and the process responsible for this phenomenon is called re-entry.

A model for the phenomenon of re-entrant excitation, similar to one proposed almost 50 years ago by Schmitt and Erlanger, is shown in Fig. 17.13a. This model, which is based on the anatomy of a point of intersection of a Purkinje fiber and the ventricular myocardium, is equally applicable to the situation in a bundle of conducting or working myocardial fibers (Fig. 17.13b). In both cases the phenomenon of re-entry results from the presence of an area of decremental conduction (unshaded area) in which two properties must be found: (1) slow conduction and (2) unidirectional block. In view of the ease with which the asymmetrical distribution of decremental conduction can give rise to unidirectional block (Chapter 16), the occurrence of these predisposing factors does not appear to be uncommon in the diseased heart or in the heart under the influence of a number of drugs.

A premature systole can be initiated under the conditions shown in Fig. 17.13 when an impulse traversing the tissue encounters the proximal end (*A*, Fig. 17.13) of the area of decremental conduction (unshaded area), where antegrade conduction is blocked. The normal propagation of the impulse through other areas of the functional syncytium of the myocardium continues, however, so that the impulse is eventually conducted to a point beyond the area of decremental conduction. At this point the impulse enters the depressed area from its distal end (*B*), and because the block is only in the antegrade direction the impulse is able to pass through the area of decremental conduction in a retrograde direction, emerging after a delay at the proximal end (*A*). If the impulse has been sufficiently delayed in its passage through the area of decremental conduction, it arrives at (re-enters) *A* after the normal tissue proximal to the depressed area has recovered. In this way a second impulse is initiated in the proximal region of the myocardium

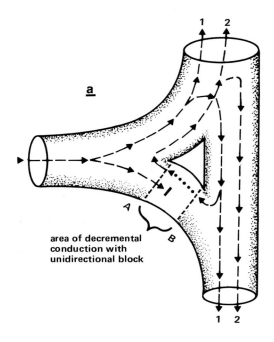

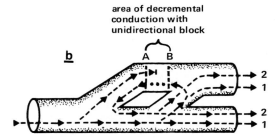

FIG. 17.13. Re-entry at the point of impingement of a Purkinje fiber on the ventricular myocardium **(a)** and within a strand of cardiac muscle **(b)**. In both situations a region of decremental conduction with unidirectional block (A–B) blocks antegrade conduction of the normal impulse (1) but allows this impulse to traverse the depressed region in the retrograde direction *(dotted line)* after a delay. This retrograde impulse re-enters the myocardium proximal to the region of decremental conduction after the proximal tissue has recovered from the normal impulse, thereby allowing the retrograde impulse to initiate a premature systole (2).

that is propagated as a premature systole. The return of the second, premature impulse to point *B* in Fig. 17.13 may produce a second re-entrant premature systole by this mechanism and possibly, through repetition of this mechanism, a run of premature systoles or tachycardia. Alternatively, the first passage of the retrograde impulse through the depressed area may increase its refractoriness so that subsequent conduction is blocked in both directions; hence retrograde conduction is also blocked, and only a single premature systole appears.

Two important conditions are required for re-entry to produce premature systoles and tachycardia by the mechanism shown in Fig. 17.13: slow conduction and unidirectional block. There is little question that unidirectional block can appear readily in regions of the diseased heart in which conduction is asymmetrically depressed (Fig. 16.16). There has been some question, however, concerning the existence of conduction velocities sufficiently low to delay the passage of the impulse through the area of decremental conduction long enough to allow the proximal regions of the heart to regain their excitability. These doubts arose from the need to postulate the existence of action potentials conducted at velocities as low as 1% of normal that still retained the ability to be conducted at all. It is extremely difficult, for example, to postulate a mechanism by which a sodium-dependent action potential (i.e., one due to the fast inward current carried by sodium ions; Chapter 14) could be depressed sufficiently to produce these extremely low conduction velocities without altogether losing its ability to generate a propagated action potential. The recent recognition of the importance of the slow inward current, however, appears to have resolved this question. Indeed, not only do the properties of the slow inward current provide an explanation for the very slow conduction velocity necessary for the genesis of many re-entrant arrhythmias, they also indicate a mechanism whereby such arrhythmias can originate in severely depolarized areas of the myocardium because opening of the slow channel is inhibited less by partial depolarization than is that of the fast channel.

Slow Responses

Depolarization of the myocardium to approximately −50 mV usually completely inactivates the channels that carry the fast inward sodium current (Chapter 14). It is now well documented, however, that such partially depolarized tissues can conduct a propagated action potential, albeit extremely slowly and usually with decrement. These conductive properties, which give rise to slowly propagated waves of depolarization that are often called slow responses, exhibit the features expected of the slow inward current carried mainly by calcium ions (Chapter 14). For example, these slow responses are promoted by catecholamines and methylxanthines, agents which are well known to increase the slow inward current. The characteristics of this slow response are seen in subsequent chapters to provide explanations for a number of the arrhythmias induced by ionic disturbances and drugs, as well as for several features of the abnormal ECGs seen in pathological states.

Summation and Inhibition

Two important phenomena related to the conduction abnormalities discussed in the preceding paragraphs are described at this point, even though they may not be important in the genesis of premature systoles. These phenomena—summation and inhibition—explain instead some of the puzzling features of the

SUMMATION

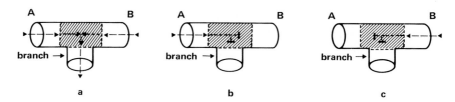

a   b   c

FIG. 17.14. Summation. **a:** The simultaneous arrival of impulses from opposite directions (A and B) in a region of decremental conduction *(cross-hatched)* opposite a branch initiates a propagated action potential in the branch. **b** and **c:** When an impulse enters the area of decremental conduction from only one direction, the impulse fails to be propagated into the branch. Successful propagation into the branch thus requires summation of the impulses entering the region of decremental conduction from both A and B.

arrhythmias related to the premature systoles as they occur singly and repetitively in the clinical ECG. Both of these phenomena, like the re-entry mechanisms described above, occur in depressed regions of the heart which exhibit the property of decremental conduction.

Summation

If two impulses travel from opposite directions toward a branching point in a depressed bundle of myocardial cells, their simultaneous arrival at the branching point can produce a propagated action potential in the branch (Fig. 17.14a). If, on the other hand, an impulse enters only from one direction (Fig. 17.14b and c) it is possible that the area of depressed conduction at the branching point will fail to initiate a propagated action potential in the branch because not enough current is generated to produce an action potential in the branch. The simultaneous arrival of two impulses therefore is necessary to generate an impulse in the branch so that *summation* of the impulses at a point adjacent to the branch is needed to evoke a propagated action potential in the branch. Such an impulse emerges from the branch only after a delay in its passage from *A* and *B* (Fig. 17.14). If this delay is long, the emerging impulse may produce an echo. In this way summation represents a special type of re-entry that may explain the genesis of some examples of premature systoles.

Inhibition

The existence of an area of slow conduction at a branching point in a bundle of myocardial cells can also give rise to a phenomenon in which the *nearly* simultaneous activation of a point in the bundle opposite the branch can *prevent* an impulse from being propagated into the branch. This phenomenon, which is opposite to that seen in summation, has been demonstrated experimentally and may explain certain phenomena seen in the abnormal ECG.

If a region of unidirectional block is present opposite a branching point, an impulse entering from the left (Fig. 17.15a) may be propagated, but not one entering from the right (Fig. 17.15b). This behavior is attributable to unidirectional block, in which conduction of an effective action potential across the point of origin of the branch is possible only when the impulse enters from the left. The existence of unidirectional block at this point can permit an impulse entering from the right to block conduction into the branch of an impulse entering from

INHIBITION

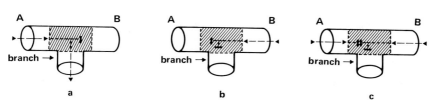

FIG. 17.15. Inhibition. **a:** An impulse entering a region of decremental conduction *(cross-hatched)* from A is able to initiate a propagated action potential in the adjacent branch, whereas **(b)** an impulse entering the region of decremental conduction from B is blocked. **c:** If the arrival of an impulse in the region of decremental conduction from B immediately precedes the arrival of the impulse from A, it can block (inhibit) the ability of the latter to activate the branch.

the left (Fig. 17.15c). The ability of the impulse entering from the right to be propagated into a region it can depolarize, but which when depolarized cannot then generate a propagated action potential, was discussed in Chapter 16 (Fig. 16.19). Recall that an impulse can be conducted into and depolarize an area where action potentials are so poor they cannot serve as effective stimuli to the excitable tissue ahead. In a similar way the impulse reaching the point of origin of the branch shown in Fig. 17.15 from the right can produce action potentials so poor their only effect is to depress conduction at the origin of the branch. As a result, an impulse arriving a short time later from the left is unable to generate an effective action potential in the branch beyond this area of depressed conduction. In this way prior depolarization of an area of decremental conduction can, by increasing the decrement, *inhibit* the transmission of a propagated action potential.

The importance of the phenomenon of inhibition becomes apparent in the description of paroxysmal supraventricular tachycardia (below). Inhibition provides one explanation for the apparently paradoxical ability of an intervention that improves conduction to *stop* a tachycardia.

The preceding discussion should serve to illustrate the point made at the outset of this chapter, i.e., that mechanisms which depress conduction in the heart can cause not only various forms of block but also abnormal impulse formation. The relative importance of depressed conduction in the genesis of the clinical arrhythmias, compared to that of accelerated pacemaker activity, is not yet known. There is now little question, however, that both of these basic mechanisms must be understood by those who wish to deal rationally with the arrhythmias associated with abnormal impulse formation.

BIBLIOGRAPHY

Cranefield, P. F., Wit, A. L., and Hoffman, B. F. (1973): Genesis of cardiac arrhythmias. *Circulation,* 47:190–204.
Katz, L. N., and Pick, A. (1956): *Clinical Electrocardiography. Part I: The Arrhythmias.* Lea & Febiger, Philadelphia.

18

The Arrhythmias

III. Tachycardia, Flutter and Fibrillation, Concealed Conduction

TACHYCARDIA

By definition, any increase in the rate of ventricular beating (i.e., a heart rate greater than 100 beats/minute) represents a tachycardia (Chapter 15). Tachycardias can arise from a number of mechanisms that are, in general, similar to those which cause the premature systoles. These include both accelerated pacemaker depolarization and the various types of re-entry mechanisms discussed in Chapter 17. It has already been pointed out that no fundamental difference exists between a re-entrant pathway that produces a single premature systole and one which gives rise to a tachycardia; the difference is only one of degree, depending largely on the extent to which the passage of the first premature impulse depresses conductivity and thus the ability of the re-entrant pathway to transmit additional premature impulses.

Tachycardias can arise in any part of the heart. Accelerated impulse formation in a specific region of the heart not only gives rise to characteristic electrocardiographic features, but the different types of tachycardia also have distinctive physiological properties. Certain of the more common forms of tachycardia are described in the following pages. It must be remembered, however, that these descriptions are presented from a physiological rather than an electrocardiographic standpoint, so that the reader who wishes a more rigorous treatment of the diagnostic features of these arrhythmias is referred to standard textbooks of electrocardiography cited at the end of Chapter 15.

Sinus Tachycardia

Acceleration of the normal pacemaker in the SA node causes a tachycardia characterized electrocardiographically by normal QRS complexes that follow normal P waves after a normal P-R interval (Chapter 16; Fig. 16.1) Thus like the much less common sinus premature systole, the only abnormality in the ECG associated with a sinus tachycardia is the accelerated rate.

Sinus tachycardia is much more often due to abnormalities that are *extrinsic* to the heart, rather than representing a manifestation of *intrinsic* heart disease. In contrast, the other tachycardias (described later) are almost always caused by an abnormality within the heart.

The normal responsiveness of the SA node to autonomic influences allows overactivity of the sympathetic nervous system to accelerate the sinus pacemaker and thus to cause sinus tachycardia. For this reason a large number of systemic abnormalities can give rise to sinus tachycardia. These include physiological (e.g., exercise, excitement), pharmacological (e.g., catecholamine administration), and pathological (e.g., shock, anemia) conditions that lead to excessive influence of the sympathetic nervous system or its neurotransmitter on the SA node. Sinus tachycardias also can arise from other causes, e.g., fever. As these effects tend to develop over several seconds, or even more slowly, the onset of sinus tachycardia is characteristically gradual, rather than abrupt. Furthermore, as the SA node remains under autonomic control, even in the presence of sinus tachycardia, this arrhythmia is characteristically slowed by vagal stimulation, e.g., that produced by carotid sinus pressure. Although heart rates in sinus tachycardia can exceed 200, they are usually less than 140. All of these features serve to distinguish this extrinsic form of tachycardia from the atrial and junctional tachycardias (see below) that result from disorders intrinsic to the heart.

Atrial Tachycardia

The rapid initiation of electrical activity in the atria might be expected to cause a tachycardia characterized by abnormal P waves followed by normal QRS

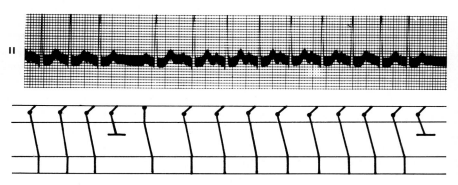

FIG. 18.1. Atrial tachycardia. Following the third QRS complex, which represents the final beat of a paroxysm of the tachycardia, a sinus beat produces the fourth QRS complex in this record. The fifth QRS complex is premature, normal in contour, and is preceded by an abnormal (narrow) P wave. The P-R interval in this beat is normal (0.16 sec), so the beat is typical of an atrial premature systole. The following seven QRS complexes in this series are also preceded by abnormal P waves and occur at a rapid rate that gradually accelerates from 110 to 150. This represents a paroxysm of atrial tachycardia as each beat meets the criteria for an atrial premature systole. Because of the acceleration of the tachycardia during the paroxysm, the later P waves become superimposed on the T waves of the preceding beats. This increasing prematurity eventually causes an impulse entering the AV node from the premature P waves to arrive during the refractory period set up by the preceding beat, thereby causing it to be blocked within the AV node and so terminating the paroxysmal tachycardia. (ECG from Katz and Pick, 1956.)

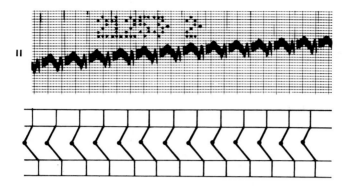

FIG. 18.2. Junctional tachycardia. There is a rapid tachycardia (rate = 170) in which the QRS complexes are normal. Each QRS complex is preceded by an inverted (retrograde) P wave and the P-R interval is short (0.08 sec), so the criteria for junctional tachycardia are met. The ability of each impuse arising in the AV node to depolarize first the atria and then the ventricles is shown in the Lewis diagram. (ECG from Katz and Pick, 1956.)

complexes after a normal P-R interval (see description of the atrial premature systole, Chapter 17). In practice, however, the P waves in atrial tachycardias are difficult to identify because they are often superimposed on T waves. Furthermore, the QRS complexes in atrial tachycardia can be abnormal due to aberrant conduction. For these reasons the ECG in an atrial tachycardia may resemble superficially that of a junctional or a ventricular tachycardia. The clearly recognizable pattern of atrial tachycardia (Fig. 18.1) is therefore not always seen.

A number of important characteristics of the atrial tachycardias relate to their physiological behavior, which is similar to that of the junctional tachycardias. These features are described in the following section: paroxysmal supraventricular tachycardia.

Junctional Tachycardia

The electrocardiographic features of the junctional tachycardias, like those of the junctional premature systoles, depend on the relative timing and the characteristics of both atrial and ventricular activation. The QRS complexes in the junctional tachycardias are not prolonged unless there is aberrant conduction, as may also be the case in the atrial tachycardia (see above). P waves, when discernible as in Fig. 18.2, resemble the "retrograde" P waves described in relation to junctional premature systoles, and may either precede or follow the QRS complex. In other cases there may be no retrograde activation of the atria, or else the P waves may be "buried" in the QRS complexes.

Paroxysmal Supraventricular Tachycardia

Because it is difficult to distinguish atrial and junctional tachycardias on the ECG, and because these tachycardias share similar physiological and clinical features, they are commonly considered together as *paroxysmal supraventricular tachycardias.* This term, which reflects one of the key clinical characteristics of this group of tachycardias, serves to differentiate these arrhythmias that arise above the bifurcation of the bundle of His from the less benign ventricular tachycardias.

Paroxysmal supraventricular tachycardias may last as briefly as a few seconds or up to several days, but they almost always start and stop abruptly. As they tend to come in paroxysms, or bursts, the atrial and junctional tachycardias are often designated together as paroxysmal supraventricular tachycardia or, alternatively, paroxysmal atrial tachycardia (PAT). Figure 18.1 shows an example of such a paroxysmal tachycardia, in this case clearly of atrial origin, in which two sinus beats (with the longer R-R intervals) enclose a paroxysm of eight supraventricular beats. The rhythm of the paroxysmal supraventricular tachycardias is characteristically very regular, although a "warming up" phenomenon can occur in which the first few beats are slightly less rapid than those which follow (Fig. 18.1). The rates of these tachycardias are usually 160 and 200, although they may be as low as 100 or as high as 250.

The usual abrupt termination of a paroxysmal supraventricular tachycardia is shown in Fig. 18.3, where the arrhythmia has been terminated by vagal stimulation, produced in this patient by carotid sinus pressure. Although it is commonly taught that strong vagal stimulation is without effect on the rate of the tachycardia, the slight slowing of the tachycardia prior to its cessation (Fig. 18.3) is characteristic. It is true, however, that the heart rate during the paroxysmal

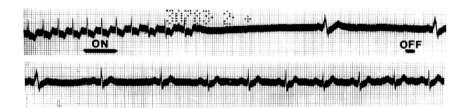

FIG. 18.3. Termination of a supraventricular tachycardia by carotid sinus pressure. A supraventricular tachycardia is seen at the left in the top strip (rate = 188). The horizontal bar (ON) marks the onset of carotid sinus pressure, which initially causes the tachycardia to slow and then to stop abruptly. A pause of slightly more than 3 sec ("standstill") follows, after which a slightly prolonged QRS complex appears. This is preceded by a short P-R interval (0.13 sec); this QRS complex is thus probably junctional in origin (a "junctional escape" beat), conducted aberrantly through the ventricles via an abnormal pathway. Carotid sinus pressure is released at the time of the short bar (OFF). The rate of the junctional escape beats increases (the lower strip is a continuation of the upper strip in which the final QRS complex of the upper strip is repeated) until a sinus beat occurs (the second in the lower strip). The sinus pacemaker then slowly accelerates until (at the right in the lower strip) sinus rhythm (rate = 80) is established. The salient features of this record are: (a) slight slowing of the supraventricular tachycardia prior to its abrupt cessation during carotid sinus pressure; (b) a delay in the re-establishment of normal sinus rhythm due partly to the vagal response to carotid sinus pressure and partly to overdrive suppression; and (c) the escape of a junctional pacemaker during the period when the sinus pacemaker is severely depressed. (ECG from Katz and Pick, 1956.)

supraventricular tachycardias is less responsive to the effects of vagal stimulation than is that during sinus tachycardias. The mechanism that gives rise to paroxysmal supraventricular tachycardia is thus relatively insensitive to vagal stimulation. This behavior can be clearly seen in Fig. 18.3, where powerful vagal stimulation resulting from pressure on the carotid sinus that slows the tachycardia only slightly causes almost complete inhibition of the sinus pacemaker. This inhibition is evident by the facts that more than 3 sec elapse before the next beat follows the termination of the tachycardia, and that the first two beats after the tachycardia ends probably arise in junctional tissue, as evidenced by their short P-R interval. Marked depression of the SA node, which accounts for the long pause prior to the re-establishment of sinus rhythm, is characteristic of the behavior when this arrhythmia is terminated by strong vagal stimulation and so represents one hazard of this form of therapy.

Overdrive Suppression

Following the termination of a tachycardia, normal pacemaker activity is slow to commence, even when the tachycardia is terminated by methods that also do not directly slow pacemaker activity. Furthermore, this initial pacemaker activity commonly shows a "warming up" phenomenon in which its discharge slowly increases during the first few seconds following termination of the tachycardia. This phenomenon, which can also be reproduced experimentally after rapid electrical pacing of the heart is abruptly halted, is called overdrive suppression.

One explanation for overdrive suppression is based on the fact that the sodium pump is normally electrogenic and generates an outward (repolarizing) current when three sodium ions are pumped out of the cell in exchange for only two potassium ions (Chapter 9). This outward current is increased when the sodium pump is stimulated. As increased $[Na^+]_i$ is well known to stimulate the sodium pump, overdrive suppression can be explained by the increase in this outward current, which occurs when rapid stimulation frequencies lead to a transient increase in $[Na^+]_i$. This in turn slows pacemaker activity immediately following the termination of a tachycardia by reducing the net inward current which causes diastolic depolarization in the pacemaker cells. Gradual reduction in the outward current generated by the sodium pump as $[Na^+]_i$ returns to normal allows the net inward current normally generated in the pacemaker cells to effect a normal rate of diastolic depolarization.

Mechanisms Responsible for Supraventricular Tachycardias: Reciprocal Beating

The mechanism of origin of the paroxysmal supraventricular tachycardias, and whether they represent abnormally rapid pacemaker discharge or re-entrant arrhythmias, is not known in most cases. Several features of these arrhythmias (e.g., their abrupt onset and termination, and the relative insensitivity to the slowing

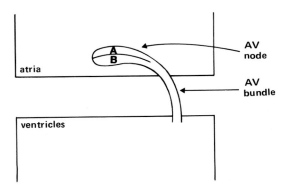

FIG. 18.4. Dual conduction pathways in the AV node. This diagram, based on experimental findings in animals, shows the existence of two parallel pathways in the AV node (A and B). These pathways can conduct impulses independently in either direction between the atria and ventricles.

effects of powerful vagal stimulation) suggest that they arise from re-entrant mechanisms. In some cases it has been possible to demonstrate with considerable assurance that these arrhythmias represent examples of *reciprocal beating*. This is a special form of re-entry involving the AV node which suggests the existence of "dual pathways" within this structure (Fig. 18.4). If one of the pathways is an abnormally depressed portion of the AV node that can conduct only very slowly in the retrograde direction (i.e., exhibits unidirectional, antegrade block), then an impulse conducted into the ventricles from the atria by way of the more rapidly conducting pathway (*A*, Fig. 18.4) reaches the ventricular end of the slowly conducting pathway (*B*, Fig. 18.4), when the latter is fully excitable. The impulse is then able to return to the atria by way of the depressed pathway in which it is slowly propagated. This re-entrant impulse therefore returns after a delay to the atrial end of the more rapidly conducting pathway. If the timing of this retrograde impulse is such that it arrives at the atrial end of the AV node before the next sinus impulse, the re-entrant wave of depolarization emerging from the slowly conducting pathway (*B*) can return to the ventricles by way of pathway *A*, giving rise to a *reciprocal beat* of the ventricles. Repetition of this re-entrant mechanism results in a reciprocal tachycardia, which has the characteristics of paroxysmal supraventricular tachycardia. This mechanism of reciprocal beating and the existence of dual pathways in the AV node have been documented in the hearts of experimental animals, where it is possible to obtain microelectrode recordings from multiple points in the AV node. The occurrence of a similar mechanism in man seems quite likely to produce some of the supraventricular tachycardias.

The ability of strong vagal stimulation to "break" paroxysmal supraventricular tachycardias while causing only minimal slowing prior to cessation of the

arrhythmia (Fig. 18.3) is not fully understood. In the case of a re-entrant pathway in the AV node, where conduction is depressed by vagal stimulation, the
depression caused by vagal stimulation can convert the unidirectional block
shown in Fig. 18.4 to complete block, so that the re-entrant pathway is interrupted. In the case of a re-entry pathway within the atrial myocardium, where
vagal stimulation speeds conduction (Chapter 19), the ability of interventions
such as carotid sinus pressure to stop an atrial tachycardia might be explained
by the phenomenon of inhibition. Under these conditions the interposition of
a wave of depolarization within the re-entry pathway, caused by more effective
conduction from a point of entry outside the loop (such as is shown in Fig. 17.15),
could block conduction in the loop. In this way accelerated conduction into the
re-entry pathway would terminate the re-entry mechanism and thus break the
tachycardia. This latter possibility, however, remains only speculative.

A special type of reciprocal beating has been shown to occur in pre-excitation.
Here the second pathway linking atria and ventricles (in addition to the normal
pathway in the AV node) is usually believed to be the bundle of Kent (Fig. 18.5).
In this situation an impulse entering the ventricles by way of the AV node may
be conducted back to the atria via the bundle of Kent and so re-enter the AV
node prior to the arrival of the next sinus impulse. Conversely, a reciprocal
rhythm can occur when the impulse reaches the ventricles via the accessory
pathway and returns to the atria by way of the AV node, although this is less
common. Either allows a reciprocal rhythm to be established. The likelihood of
such a mechanism, which is responsible for the tendency for patients with pre-
excitation to exhibit paroxysmal supraventricular tachycardia, has led to a number of attempts (some successful) to relieve this condition by surgical interruption
of the accessory AV conduction pathway.

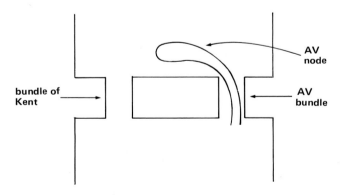

FIG. 18.5. Dual conduction pathways linking atria and ventricles. These pathways, the AV node
and bundle of Kent, represent two independent conduction pathways between the atria and
ventricles that are functionally similar to the dual pathways in the AV node, except that conduction in the bundle of Kent is usually rapid and transmits atrial impulses to an abnormal site in
the ventricles (i.e., one outside the Purkinje network).

Ventricular Tachycardia

A tachycardia in which the QRS complexes are widened (> 0.12 sec) and bear no fixed relationship to P waves is most often ventricular in origin (Fig. 18.6). The rates of ventricular tachycardias are similar to those of the paroxysmal supraventricular tachycardias, although the rhythm in ventricular tachycardia often shows slight irregularities, in contrast to the characteristically fixed rhythm in the paroxysmal supraventricular tachycardias. As the parasympathetic innervation of the ventricles is sparse, vagal stimulation is usually without effect on the rates of ventricular tachycardia; nor do interventions like carotid sinus pressure break these tachycardias. They are usually more ominous than the corresponding paroxysmal supraventricular tachycardias and can herald the advent of ventricular flutter or fibrillation (see below).

One important criterion for the diagnosis of ventricular tachycardia is the occurrence of a fusion beat (Chapter 17). In the ECG shown in Fig. 18.6, the QRS complex labeled V_F is less bizarre and its duration less prolonged than the other QRS complexes in this record. This beat is preceded by a P wave with a P-R interval of 0.16 sec and so can be presumed to represent a fusion beat that is initiated partly by the impulse arriving from the atria by way of the AV node and partly by the abnormal focus in the ventricles. The presence of a fusion beat, which is seen only occasionally in ventricular tachycardia, serves to differentiate this arrhythmia from a paroxysmal supraventricular tachycardia with persistent aberrant conduction or coexistent intraventricular block.

Ventricular tachycardias often occur in "runs," a phenomenon called *repetitive ventricular tachycardia.* One such brief burst of three beats of ventricular origin

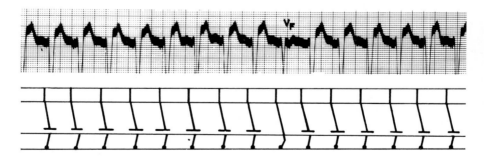

FIG. 18.6. Ventricular tachycardia. The dominant ventricular rhythm gives rise to prolonged QRS complexes (QRS duration = 0.16 sec) that occur at a rate of 115. P waves, which are inverted in lead III in this patient, bear no fixed relationship to the QRS complexes that follow (the apparent P-R interval is usually 0.08–0.15 sec), so the criteria for ventricular tachycardia are met. In the tenth beat (V_F) the P precedes the QRS complex by 0.16 sec and so is able to share in activation of the ventricles. The resulting QRS (V_F), which is narrower (duration = 0.11 sec) and more similar to the normal QRS complexes in an ECG taken prior to the onset of the tachycardia, represents a fusion beat. The presence of this fusion beat confirms the diagnosis of ventricular tachycardia, as fusion beats do not occur in supraventricular tachycardia with aberrant conduction. (ECG from Katz and Pick, 1956.)

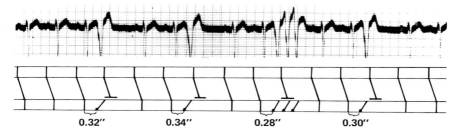

FIG. 18.7. Brief run of ventricular tachycardia caused by the occurrence of a ventricular premature systole during the vulnerable period. This record contains three single premature systoles (which produce the fourth and seventh QRS complexes, reading from the left; and the third QRS complex, reading from the right). These follow the preceding QRS complex by intervals of 0.32, 0.34, and 0.30 sec, respectively (numbers at bottom of the Lewis diagram). A fourth ventricular premature systole (the tenth, reading from the left), which appears 0.28 sec after the preceding QRS complex, occurs during the vulnerable period of the preceding ventricular beat and initiates a brief run of ventricular tachycardia. (ECG from Katz and Pick, 1956.)

is seen in the FCG in Fig. 18.7, which also shows frequent ventricular premature systoles.

The Vulnerable Period

Figure 18.7 illustrates the very important concept of the *vulnerable period of ventricular repolarization.* This concept refers to the frequent correlation between the ability of a ventricular premature systole to induce a run of ventricular tachycardia and the degree of its prematurity. Thus of the four ventricular premature systoles shown in Fig. 18.7, only the third initiates a brief run of ventricular tachycardia. Figure 18.7 demonstrates that this premature systole follows the onset of the QRS complex in the preceding sinus beat by 0.28 sec, whereas the other ventricular premature systoles, which do not initiate a burst of ventricular tachycardia, come 0.30–0.34 sec after the preceding sinus beat. The tendency of very early ventricular premature systoles to induce ventricular tachycardia is very well documented—so much so that the period of ventricular repolarization immediately following the peak of the T wave is called the *vulnerable period* (Fig. 18.8). Premature systoles that depolarize the ventricles during the vulnerable period tend to produce repetitive ventricular tachycardia or the much more serious ventricular fibrillation. Similarly, direct electrical stimulation of the ventricles (e.g., by an artificial pacemaker) is most likely to induce ventricular tachycardia or ventricular fibrillation when the stimulus falls near the peak of the T wave.

Recognition of the vulnerable period of ventricular repolarization, during which stimulation tends to produce ventricular arrhythmias, provided strong support for the view that ventricular premature systoles, as well as ventricular tachycardia and fibrillation, result from phenomena associated with re-entry. Early studies of the electrophysiology of the heart showed that electrical stimula-

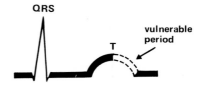

FIG. 18.8. ECG representation showing the vulnerable period *(unshaded)* during the middle and terminal phases of the T wave.

tion during the vulnerable period was most likely to produce runs of tachycardia. In contrast, stimulation of the ventricles earlier during the cardiac cycle failed to elicit any response, and electrical stimuli delivered later in the cardiac cycle produced only a single response to the stimulus. These phenomena can be explained in light of the mechanisms responsible for re-entry described in Chapter 17. Stimuli that reach the ventricles during the S-T segment find the ventricular myocardium wholly refractory and so are unable to elicit a propagated wave of depolarization. Stimuli arriving much later, after the end of the T wave, find the ventricles fully recovered and so initiate a single, well-organized wave of depolarization that is conducted rapidly throughout the ventricles. Stimuli delivered during the vulnerable period, however, reach the ventricles at a time when the gating mechanism controlling the fast inward current in some portions of the ventricular myocardium has recovered only partially. Therefore at this time the ability to respond with a full-sized action potential is depressed. Instead, the action potentials which arise during the vulnerable period propagate slowly and exhibit the characteristics of decremental conduction. The vulnerable period therefore represents that time when portions of the ventricles are most likely to exhibit slow conduction and unidirectional block, so that premature systoles and electrical impulses arriving during the vulnerable period are most likely to initiate re-entrant arrhythmias.

ATRIAL FLUTTER AND FIBRILLATION

Very rapid activation of the atria results in two characteristic arrhythmias: *atrial flutter,* in which the rate is rapid and the rhythm extremely regular; and *atrial fibrillation,* in which the atria are activated at an even more rapid rate but in which the rhythm is wholly irregular. These atrial arrhythmias can change from one to another, as is seen in "impure atrial flutter."

Atrial Flutter

Atrial flutter is like a rapid atrial tachycardia except that the rates are usually 250–350 and the electrocardiographic manifestations of atrial activity are not a series of discrete P waves but a sawtooth-like pattern called F waves (Fig. 18.9). As shown in Fig. 18.9, the QRS complexes are characteristically normal (unless there is aberrant conduction or coexistent bundle branch block), and there is usually 4:1 AV conduction (one QRS complex per four F waves). The result is

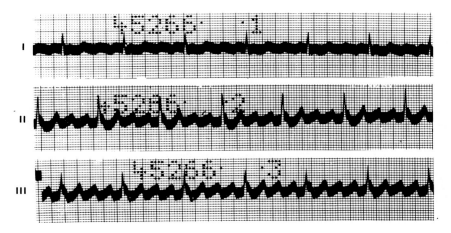

FIG. 18.9. Atrial flutter with 4 : 1 AV conduction. Atrial activity is manifest as sawtooth undulations in the baseline. The latter, which are regular at a rate of 250, represent F waves typical of atrial flutter. The ventricular rate is exactly one-fourth that of the atria, indicating that one of each four F waves traverses the AV node to activate the ventricles. (From Katz and Pick, 1956.)

regular ventricular beating at a rate of approximately 75. The failure of the AV node to conduct all of the atrial impulses into the ventricles demonstrates the "protective" role of the normally slow conduction in the AV node. Were the AV node to conduct all of the atrial impulses into the ventricles, the resulting ventricular rate of 300 would be severely disabling if not fatal. Thus the normal decremental conduction in the AV node protects the patient from the serious hemodynamic sequelae of a rapid ventricular rate.

The absence of 1:1 AV conduction in atrial flutter does *not* represent AV block, as this term should be used to describe conditions in which failure of AV conduction is due to an abnormal degree of block in the AV node. Instead, the 4:1 AV conduction commonly seen in atrial flutter is more correctly called *AV dissociation*. The term AV block should be reserved for those conditions in which failure of AV conduction is due to an abnormal degree of decremental conduction in the AV node (Chapter 16), whereas *AV dissociation* is a more general term that can be used for any condition in which not all atrial beats are conducted to the ventricles, whether due to the normal degree of block in the AV node (as in atrial flutter or rapid supraventricular tachycardias) or when the block is caused by an abnormal degree of decremental conduction in this structure (Chapter 16).

Carotid sinus pressure (vagal stimulation) characteristically has little or no effect on the atrial rate in atrial flutter, but this maneuver usually increases the degree of AV dissociation. In 2:1 atrial flutter, for example, where the atrial rate is typically 300 and the ventricular rate 150, the increased vagal activity caused by carotid sinus pressure characteristically exerts its major effect to depress AV conduction. The most common result is a sudden increase in the degree of AV dissociation, which causes an abrupt slowing of the ventricular rate to 75. For reasons that are not fully understood, but which may relate to the phenomenon of concealed conduction (see below), 3:1 AV conduction is rare in atrial flutter.

Atrial Fibrillation

Atrial fibrillation is much more common than atrial flutter, to which it is related. The atrial rates in atrial fibrillation are greater than 400, and the rhythm is completely irregular. As a result, the atria in this arrhythmia do not contract coherently but instead resemble a bag of worms so that the disorganized atrial contraction is ineffective in raising intra-atrial pressure. As is usually true in atrial flutter, the ventricular rates are much less than those in the atria; unlike atrial flutter, the ventricular rhythm in atrial fibrillation is usually grossly irregular. The ECG in atrial fibrillation is characterized by: (a) an absence of P waves, which are replaced by (b) undulations in the baseline that are irregular in amplitude and frequency (f waves), and (c) irregular beating of the ventricles (Fig. 18.10).

> The marked irregularity of ventricular beating in atrial fibrillation is generally stated to reflect the irregularity in the arrival of atrial impulses at the upper end of the AV node. Yet this explanation, which is usually accepted without further consideration, is often inadequate to explain the marked variations in R-R interval seen in some patients with atrial fibrillation. If the refractory period in the

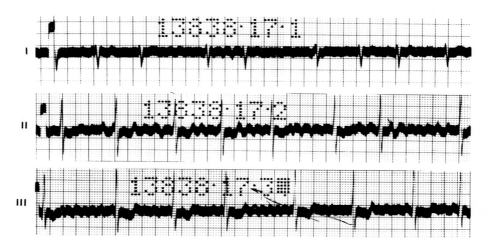

FIG. 18.10. Atrial fibrillation. Atrial activity is manifest as irregular undulations in the baseline. The intervals between these undulations vary between 0.13 and 0.17 sec, which corresponds to an atrial rate of 350–460. Ventricular beating is also grossly irregular, with R-R intervals of 0.56–1.16 sec, which corresponds to a ventricular rate of 52–106. The most likely explanation for 0.60-sec variations in the intervals between successive ventricular depolarizations, as opposed to only 0.04-sec variations in the intervals between atrial depolarizations, is concealed conduction of some of the atrial depolarizations within the AV node (Fig. 18.11). (From Katz and Pick, 1956.)

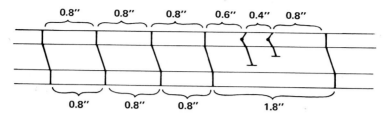

FIG. 18.11. Concealed conduction in the AV node. The arrival of a pair of atrial premature systoles (the fifth and sixth vertical lines in the upper space of this Lewis diagram) causes a 1.8-sec pause in ventricular beating (lower space). The AV node and ventricles, however, are clearly able to conduct at intervals of at least 0.8 sec, as demonstrated by normal conduction of sinus impulses at a rate of 75 in the initial portion of this diagram. The failure of the second atrial premature systole to activate the ventricles can be attributed to concealed conduction of the impulse arising from the first atrial premature systole within the AV node. This impulse fails to reach the ventricles, but by depolarizing the AV node renders the node unable to conduct the second atrial premature systole.

AV node were constant (e.g., 0.3 sec), refractoriness in the AV node would allow the ventricles to beat every 0.3 sec (200 times/minute) in response to impulses entering the AV node from the atria. Atrial frequencies in atrial fibrillation are usually much more than 300/minute, however, so that on a random basis an impulse should reach the upper end of the AV node every 0.2 sec. This means that, on the average, the interval between ventricular beats should be 0.5 sec, varying little because of the high frequency with which the atria are depolarized. Yet in the ECG shown in Fig. 18.10, R-R intervals are frequently as long as 1.2 sec, although the atrial rate is clearly greater than 300. An explanation must be found, therefore, to account for the fact that R-R intervals can exceed 1 sec even though the intervals between successive waves of atrial depolarization average 0.2 sec or less and the refractory period of the AV node cannot be more than 0.3–0.4 sec (as evidenced by R-R intervals less than 0.5 sec). It is therefore unlikely that these large variations in R-R intervals are due simply to marked variation in the interval between the arrival of successive atrial impulses at the upper end of the A-V node. A much more likely explanation is that the very long R-R intervals result from increased refractoriness in the AV node. This latter explanation, which is now believed to be correct, raises yet another question: What causes the very large variations in the length of the refractory period in the AV node? The answer lies in a phenomenon called "concealed conduction," in which atrial impulses can enter the AV node but cannot traverse it. The only effect of the penetration of the depolarization wave into the AV node, therefore, is to render it refractory to the impulse which follows.

Concealed Conduction

The phenomenon described in the preceding paragraph is diagrammed in Fig. 18.11, which illustrates a sinus rhythm at a basic rate of 75, i.e., an interval between successive beats of 0.8 sec. The arrival of a pair of atrial premature systoles coming at intervals of 0.6 and 0.4 sec, respectively, causes an interruption of ventricular beating because neither of these atrial premature systoles is conducted to the ventricles. The failure of the first premature systole to be conducted is readily understood because it arrives at the upper end of the AV node during the refractory period left behind by the preceding normal systole. The failure to conduct of the second atrial premature systole, which arrives at the AV node a full second after passage of the last normal systole, cannot be attributed to refractoriness in the AV node resulting from the preceding conducted impulse because the ability of the AV node to transmit impulses every 0.8 sec has already been demonstrated. Thus penetration of the wave of depolarization initiated by the first atrial premature systole into the AV node must have been responsible for failure of the second atrial premature systole to traverse the AV node. This allows us to conclude that the first atrial premature systole exhibits the phenomenon of concealed conduction. It is *conducted* into the AV node because of its effect to block the subsequent impulse; the conduction is *concealed* because the first atrial premature systole is not transmitted through the AV node and so does not initiate a QRS complex.

The concept of concealed conduction explains a number of phenomena besides the marked variability in ventricular rate in atrial fibrillation. A full discussion of these electrocardiographic phenomena is beyond the scope of this book. One example, however, is mentioned here because of the ease with which this phenomenon can be demonstrated. If a heart preparation (e.g., turtle heart) is impaled with fine copper wires and arranged so that electrical stimuli well above threshold can be administered by depressing a switch, then at slow frequencies of stimulation each depression of the switch is followed by a ventricular contraction. As the rate of stimulation is slowly increased, the heart initially contracts in response to each stimulus. At still higher rates the response becomes irregular owing to varying degrees of block around the wires; e.g., 2:1, 3:2, etc. block can be seen (the depressed tissue around the copper wires serving, like the AV node, as a region of decremental conduction). Further increases in stimulation frequency commonly (virtually always in the author's experience) lead to "standstill;" i.e., no contractions occur even though stimuli are rapidly arriving in the depressed areas. That this standstill is not due to irreversible damage to the heart is readily shown by abruptly stopping the stimulation for a few seconds, after which a single depression of the switch is followed by a contraction. Failure of conduction at high rates of stimulation is most easily explained if each stimulus produces only a local response in the depressed areas around the copper wires. Because of decremental conduction these local responses are not effective enough to be conducted into the remainder of the heart, although they are able to prevent the subsequent impulses from reaching the normal regions of the heart. In other words, the cardiac standstill can be attributed to repetitive concealed conduction.

Mechanism of Atrial Flutter and Fibrillation

In the older literature there is a now classic debate regarding the mechanism of atrial flutter and fibrillation. Electrophysiologists were, between the early 1930s and the 1950s, divided into two camps: On the one hand there were the proponents of the view that these arrhythmias arose from single or multiple *ectopic foci,* whereas others believed that atrial flutter and fibrillation were due to *circus movements* in the atria. These once mutually exclusive explanations now appear, however, to represent different ways of looking at the same phenomena.

The "ectopic focus" explanation of atrial flutter postulated that this arrhythmia arose from a single rapidly discharging focus in the atria, whereas atrial fibrillation was produced by multiple foci discharging at different rapid rates. The proponents of this explanation presented evidence that application of an irritant (e.g., aconitine) to a single point in the atria of the open-chested dog could produce rapid atrial beating that exhibited the electrocardiographic features of atrial flutter. Multiple points of irritation produced a more rapid, irregular arrhythmia that resembled atrial fibrillation. For this reason it was postulated that atrial flutter in man arose from a single ectopic focus, and that atrial fibrillation was due to multiple ectopic foci in the atria.

The proponents of the "circus movement" explanation for these atrial arrhythmias based their theory on an observation made by Mines during the early part of this century. Mines prepared a ring of excitable tissue and, after temporarily clamping one portion of the ring, delivered a stimulus to the excitable tissue away from the clamp (Fig. 18.12). The stimulation initiated a wave of depolarization that, in the example shown in Fig. 18.13, passed in a clockwise direction; it did not move in a counterclockwise direction because of the local block caused by the clamp. If the clamp was quickly removed prior to the arrival of the impulse at the site of local block via the clockwise direction, restoration of normal conductivity allowed the impulse to continue to travel around the ring of tissue. In this way a circus movement could be established that would continue to go around and around the ring of tissue virtually indefinitely (i.e., until the isolated preparation deteriorated). This experiment led to the view that atrial flutter resulted from a circus movement, like that shown in Fig. 18.13, which passed around the atria. The circus movement is one type of re-entry mechanism, so that its genesis in the heart can be understood in terms of the concepts

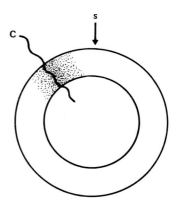

FIG. 18.12. Establishment of a circus movement in a ring of excitable tissue. If the tissue is lightly clamped (C) and then stimulated adjacent to the clamp (s), counterclockwise propagation of the impulse is blocked. Removal of the clamp prior to arrival of the impulse propagated in the clockwise direction at the site of block allows the impulse to continue to pass around the ring of tissue in a clockwise direction.

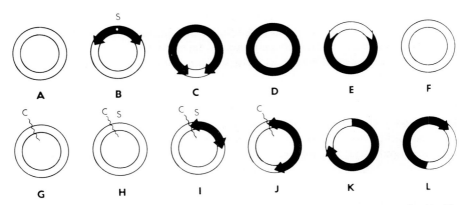

FIG. 18.13. Role of unidirectional block in establishing the circus movement described in Fig. 18.12. Application of a stimulus to a ring of excitable tissue *(unshaded area)* in the absence of block **(B)** initiates an impulse *(shaded area)* that depolarizes the entire ring **(D)**. Mutual cancellation of the impulses moving in opposite directions **(C)** allows the tissue to repolarize completely **(E, F)**. However, if unidirectional block is established by temporary clamping of the tissue (C in **H–J**), the impulse propagated in the clockwise direction can continue to travel around the ring **(K, L)**, thereby establishing a circus movement. (From Silber and Katz: *Heart Disease,* 1975. Macmillan, New York.)

presented in Chapter 17. A number of investigators provided evidence that circus movements could appear in the atria of experimental animals, and large circus movements were documented by slow-motion cinematography of fluttering atria in open-chested anesthetized dogs. The proponents of this theory argued that similar but multiple and disorganized circus movements could account for atrial fibrillation.

The response of these atrial arrhythmias (including atrial tachycardia) to certain physiological and pharmacological agents supported the circus movement theory (but did not rule out the ectopic focus theory). This evidence was based on the finding that circus movements are stopped both when conduction is accelerated and when the refractory period is prolonged. Accelerated conduction of the front of activation allows the wave of depolarization to "catch up" with the regions that have not yet recovered their excitability after prior passage of the wave front, while prolongation of refractoriness accomplishes the same thing by delaying the recovery of excitability (Fig. 18.14). By preventing the front of the wave of depolarization from reaching regions of excitable tissue, therefore, interventions that accelerate conduction or prolong the refractory period stop a circus movement. A useful analogy is to consider the impulse traveling around the circular pathway as a snake which, if its head catches up with its tail, bites itself and dies. According to this rather homely analogy, speeding the forward motion of the head of the snake or holding its tail in place longer terminates its movements. The ability of vagal stimulation—which speeds conduction in the atria (Chapter 19)—to interrupt atrial tachycardias was sometimes taken as evidence for the former type of interruption, while the frequently successful treatment of atrial tachycardias, flutter, and fibrillation with drugs like quinidine (Chapter 19), which prolong the refractory period, was cited as evidence for the latter means of terminating the postulated circus movement. This way of looking at these phenomena is still useful, although the current views concerning the genesis of re-entrant arrhythmias has been refined since these arguments held sway.

The controversy between the circus movement and ectopic focus explanations for atrial flutter and fibrillation has virtually disappeared, but not because either of these theories has proved to be correct or invalid. Instead, it has become apparent that the distinction between these mechanisms is much less obvious than was once believed. The blurring of the distinction between a circus movement and an ectopic focus is apparent if one considers the re-entry mechanisms described in Chapter 17. A circus movement such as that shown in Fig. 18.13 is but a special type of re-entry mechanism. Similarly, an ectopic focus can be produced by a re-entry mechanism in a tiny area of the myocardium, e.g., when an ectopic focus is induced by an irritant, and so can itself represent a miniature circus movement through a very small loop of depressed myocardial tissue.

An experiment that sheds a great deal of light on the mechanism of these arrhythmias was described in 1917 by Garrey. Basing his study on the observation that fibrillation was exceedingly difficult to produce in small hearts (e.g., that of the cat) but hard to avoid in large hearts (e.g., that of the cow), Garrey systematically examined the effect of myocardial mass on this arrhythmia. Taking a large heart, causing it to fibrillate, and then cutting it into smaller and smaller pieces, he found that as the mass of fibrillating tissue was reduced, the myocardium

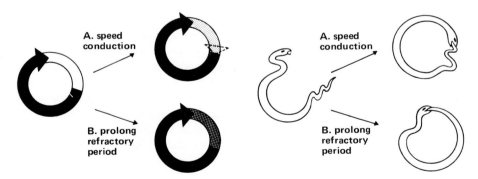

FIG. 18.14. Two ways in which a circus movement can be terminated. **Left:** The diagram at the left depicts a circus movement as shown in panel K of Fig. 18.13. If conduction is accelerated (A), the front of the impulse can extend ahead so as to reach the previously depolarized tissue during its refractory period, thereby terminating the circus movement. Prolongation of the refractory period (B) can also terminate the circus movement by causing the front of the impulse to reach tissue that is in a refractory state. **Right:** These two diagrams can be viewed in terms of a snake traveling in circles who can bite himself by reaching his fangs further ahead to catch his tail (A) or by slowing his tail so as to allow the fangs traveling at a constant speed to catch the tail (B).

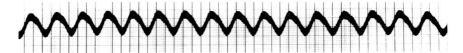

FIG. 18.15. Ventricular flutter. Electrical activity of the ventricles is manifest as a regular undulation in which prolonged QRS complexes cannot be distinguished from T waves. Atrial activity is not seen. (From Katz and Pick, 1956.)

tended to stop its fibrillation. As the mass of fibrillating tissue was made progressively smaller, each piece eventually ceased to fibrillate; instead, it began to beat synchronously or else stopped contracting altogether. For this and other reasons already discussed, it now appears likely that atrial and ventricular fibrillation commonly occur as the result of disorganization and "wandering" of fronts of depolarization within a large mass of myocardial tissue, especially when conduction is depressed. This observation explains the very high incidence of fibrillation in "giant" atria such as occur in patients with chronic mitral stenosis and insufficiency. Similarly, where conduction is depressed in normal-sized atria, the result is the same: Slowed conduction produces the same tendency for the front of depolarization to become disorganized, i.e., to find multiple re-entry pathways. In many cases of atrial flutter, a large circus movement can appear when large atrial size or slow conduction establishes a long pathway which permits the tail of the snake to slip ahead of its head, i.e., for a wave of depolarization to begin to go around and around the atria as a giant re-entry mechanism.

VENTRICULAR FLUTTER AND FIBRILLATION

Both flutter and fibrillation can occur in the ventricles. Unlike the corresponding atrial arrhythmias, which not infrequently persist for years and in the case of atrial fibrillation can last for a lifetime, persistent ventricular flutter and fibrillation are lethal arrhythmias. Both of these ventricular arrhythmias probably arise through re-entrant mechanisms of the sort discussed at many points in this chapter. The ECG in ventricular flutter (Fig. 18.15) often resembles a sine wave. This arrhythmia, which may result from a large circus movement traversing the ventricles, generally causes the pumping action of the ventricles to cease or at least to become severely impaired. In ventricular fibrillation, where the

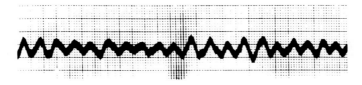

FIG. 18.16. Ventricular fibrillation. This lethal arrhythmia causes the chaotic, rapid undulations seen in this ECG. (From Katz and Pick, 1956.)

electrocardiographic appearance of the QRS complex is chaotic (Fig. 18.16), no effective ventricular contraction takes place. For this reason the hemodynamic consequences of ventricular fibrillation are the same as those of cardiac standstill (Chapter 16), i.e., cardiac arrest.

It is extremely important to understand not only the mechanisms which initiate and sustain ventricular flutter and fibrillation, but also to be able to recognize the abnormalities that herald these lethal arrhythmias. One example of a forerunner of ventricular fibrillation has already been discussed, i.e., an early premature ventricular systole which falls during the vulnerable period (Fig. 18.7). Several additional examples of electrocardiographic warnings that these arrhythmias may develop are described in Chapter 19. The early recognition of these electrocardiographic abnormalities and the pathological conditions or drugs which produce them is of critical importance clinically. The cardiac patient has already greatly benefited through institution of appropriate prophylactic therapy when such warning signs appear on the ECG. Even greater benefits can be expected from the rapidly growing knowledge of these abnormal mechanisms and the continuing development of improved means to prevent them.

BIBLIOGRAPHY

Garrey, W. E. (1914): The nature of fibrillary contraction of the heart.—Its relation to tissue mass and form. *Am. J. Physiol.,* 33:397–414.

Goldreyer, B. N., and Bigger, J. T., Jr. (1971): Site of reentry in a paroxysmal supraventricular tachycardia in man. *Circulation,* 43:15–26.

Langendorf, R. (1948): Concealed A-V conduction: The effect of blocked impulses on the formation and conduction of subsequent impulses. *Am. Heart J.,* 35:542.

See also references to Chapters 16 and 17.

19

Ionic and Pharmacological Actions on Cardiac Rate and Rhythm

The arrhythmias described in the preceding chapters arise from abnormal mechanisms of impulse formation and impulse conduction in the heart. The electrocardiographic manifestations of these arrhythmias were thus described in terms of abnormal slowing or acceleration of the sinus pacemaker, the emergence of pacemaker activity in abnormal regions of the heart, and disordered mechanisms of impulse conduction through the myocardium. Many of these abnormal mechanisms are re-examined in this chapter as they relate to the electrocardiographic features of the arrhythmias they produce and especially in terms of the way in which a number of important ionic and pharmacological agents act both to produce and alleviate these abnormalities. For this reason many of the phenomena described in the following pages are the same as those presented previously in other contexts. It is hoped this duplication of material will serve to reinforce the reader's understanding of the relationship between the cardiac action potential (Chapter 14), the arrhythmias (Chapters 16–18), and the actions of specific ions and pharmacological agents. The present chapter, in addition, provides a tentative description of the important clinical actions of the antiarrhythmic agents, although knowledge of the mechanism of action of these important drugs remains incomplete.

ELECTROLYTE ABNORMALITIES

The ECG is a sensitive indicator of abnormal serum electrolyte levels, especially altered potassium and calcium concentrations. The characteristic disturbances in cardiac rhythm and electrocardiographic contour that accompany elevation or reduction in serum concentrations of these ions reflect the effects of these abnormalities on the action potentials of the myocardial cells.

Hyperkalemia

Elevation of serum potassium influences both depolarization and repolarization in cardiac muscle, although the mechanisms responsible for these effects are quite different. The effects of hyperkalemia on the depolarization phase of the cardiac action potential are due primarily to the direct effect of elevated extracellular potassium concentration to lower resting potential (Chapter 14). Because

356 PHARMACOLOGICAL ACTIONS

resting potential reflects the $[K^+]_i/[K^+]_o$ ratio an elevated $[K^+]_o$ causes the cell to be partially depolarized during diastole. This partial depolarization inactivates the channels which normally allow sodium to enter the cell during the upstroke of the action potential (Chapter 14). The resulting decrease in the fast inward current reduces both the rate of rise and the amplitude of the cardiac action potential (Fig. 19.1). By the mechanism described in Chapter 16, these effects on depolarization can account for the ability of hyperkalemia to slow conduction velocity. The resulting appearance of decremental conduction is of considerable importance in the genesis of the serious and often lethal arrhythmias that accompany severe hyperkalemia (see below).

The effects of hyperkalemia on repolarization, unlike the effects on depolarization just discussed, are not attributable directly to the increased concentration of potassium outside the cell or to a reduction of membrane potential. One might predict that the decrease in the $[K^+]_i/[K^+]_o$ ratio would reduce the outward, repolarizing potassium currents. However, hyperkalemia *accelerates* repolarization and thereby shortens the plateau phase of the cardiac action potential (Fig. 19.1). This effect of high extracellular potassium can be attributed to an action of high $[K^+]_o$ that increases both the rate and the extent of opening of the channels which carry the repolarizing potassium current i_x.

> To understand the mechanism by which hyperkalemia shortens the duration of the cardiac action potential, it is necessary to recall the inward-going (anomalous) rectification that normally accounts for the long plateau phase (Chapter 14). The extent of this rectification process, in which membrane depolarization causes potassium permeability to fall, is reduced in hyperkalemia. As a result, the potassium channels that control the outward, repolarizing current i_x close to a lesser degree when $[K^+]_o$ is increased. The exact mechanism that produces this change and whether it is a direct action of the high extracellular potassium, an effect of the reduced action potential amplitude, or both is not fully understood. Regardless of the causative mechanism, the earlier opening of these potassium channels allows hyperkalemia to accelerate repolarization and thus to shorten the cardiac action potential.

The characteristic tall, peaked T waves seen in the ECG of patients with hyperkalemia (Fig. 19.2) can be attributed to the acceleration of repolarization described above. Similarly, shortening of the Q-T interval reflects abbreviation

FIG. 19.1. Effects of hyperkalemia on the cardiac action potential. Elevated serum potassium causes partial depolarization of the resting cell, which leads to slowing of the upstroke and reduction in the amplitude of the action potential. Repolarization is accelerated so the duration of the action potential is reduced.

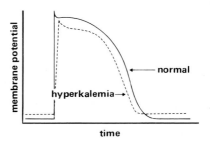

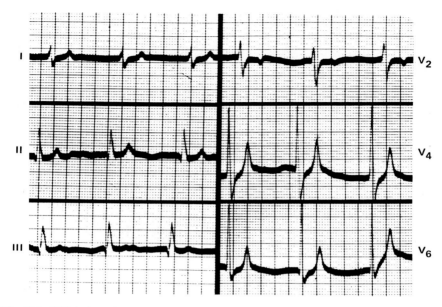

FIG. 19.2. ECG in hyperkalemia, showing tall, peaked T waves in leads V_4 and V_6, widening of the QRS complex, a slightly shortened Q-T interval, and absent P waves. (From Littman, 1972.)

of the action potential (Chapter 15). The widening of the QRS complex, which is 0.14 sec in Fig. 19.2, reflects slowed conduction that arises from the effects of hyperkalemia on the upstroke of the action potential. Reduction in both the rate of rise and the amplitude of the action potential (Fig. 19.1) prolongs the time required for the passage of the wave of depolarization through the ventricles— hence the prolongation of the time required for inscription of the QRS complex.

AV block, which can be caused by moderately severe hyperkalemia, leads to prolongation of the P-R interval. Intra-atrial block is also common. The slowing of conduction through the atria causes widened P waves that are also diminished in amplitude. SA block is also seen in hyperkalemic patients and is manifest by the absence of P waves, as in the ECG in Fig. 19.2. The disappearance of the P waves in the face of evidence of continuing SA nodal pacemaker activity is explained by evidence that conduction from the SA node to the AV node (by way of the SA ring bundles) can persist at a time when conduction of the impulse from the SA node into the atrial myocardium has failed. This phenomenon reflects a greater sensitivity of the atrial myocardium to the detrimental effects of hyperkalemia and might possibly be related to the normally brief duration of the atrial action potential, which would augment the inhibitory response to further shortening caused by hyperkalemia. The finding that impulses continue to travel from the SA node to the AV node when P waves are absent in the hyperkalemic heart indicates that conduction continues through the SA ring bundles (the preferential pathways which connect the SA and AV nodes) at a time when propagation of the impulse into the atrial myocardium is blocked. It is thus likely that in the ECG shown in Fig. 16.2 sinus rhythm is present, even though no P waves are seen.

Ventricular fibrillation can occur in severe hyperkalemia. This lethal arrhythmia is commonly heralded by ventricular premature systoles and bizarre abnormalities in ventricular rhythm. These arrhythmias are most likely the result of decremental conduction, which increases the propensity for development of re-entrant arrhythmias (Chapter 16). Abbreviation of the action potential, which shortens the refractory period, also tends to favor the development of re-entrant arrhythmias. For these reasons severe hyperkalemia represents a life-threatening abnormality in which electrocardiographic changes such as those shown in Fig. 19.2 provide a clear warning that treatment of the electrolyte disturbance must begin promptly to prevent sudden death.

Hypokalemia

Low serum potassium levels can have an anomalous effect on resting membrane potential in the heart. Reduction in $[K^+]_o$ would be predicted from the Nernst equation to cause an increase in the magnitude of the resting potential. The observed increase, however, is less than that predicted from the increase in the $[K^+]_i/[K^+]_o$ ratio, and when $[K^+]_o$ falls into a very low range (below approximately 3 mM) further lowering of serum potassium can cause a paradoxical decrease in resting potential (Fig. 14.4). This in turn is associated with a fall in potassium conductance. As a result of this fall in gK, potassium efflux is reduced, allowing a small "background" inward sodium current to cause partial depolarization of the membrane.

A second effect of lowered serum potassium is to prolong the cardiac action potential. This effect is opposite to the effects of hyperkalemia described above and can be attributed to an exaggeration of the normal inward-going (anomalous) rectification which inhibits the opening of the channels that control the outward (repolarizing) flux of potassium. This effect of hyperkalemia (Fig. 19.3) is of paramount importance in understanding the genesis of the arrhythmias seen when serum potassium levels become lowered (see below).

FIG. 19.3. Effects of hypokalemia on the cardiac action potential. Resting potential and the upstroke and height of the action potential are normal. The early portion of the plateau is reduced in amplitude by exaggeration of the inward-going rectification while the plateau is prolonged because of delayed opening of the potassium channels that carry outward, repolarizing currents.

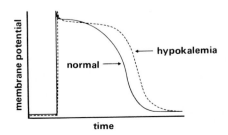

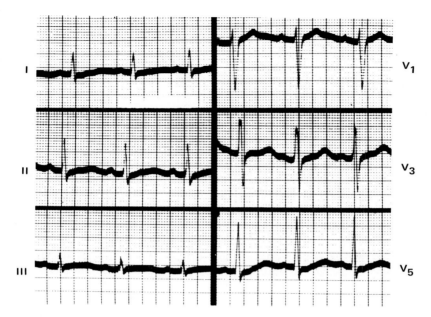

FIG. 19.4. ECG in hypokalemia, showing flat T waves, prominent U waves, a prolonged Q-T interval, and a prolonged P-R interval. (From Littman, 1972.)

The initial electrocardiographic manifestations of hypokalemia reflect the abnormalities of repolarization. The T waves become reduced in amplitude, and prominent U waves appear that often merge with the T wave (Fig. 19.4). The Q-T interval is prolonged, reflecting prolongation of the action potential (Fig. 19.3.)

Slowing of the rate of repolarization increases the propensity to the development of arrhythmias because a subsequent wave of excitation may arrive in some regions of the heart before the resting potential has returned to normal. Action potentials arising in these partially depolarized regions of the heart (Chapter 14) exhibit decremental conduction that is due to reduced opening of the fast sodium channels that decreases both the rate of rise and amplitude of the action potential. The resulting decremental conduction accounts for the widening of the QRS complex in severe hypokalemia and the tendency of patients with severe hypokalemia to develop ventricular fibrillation. Increased decremental conduction in the AV node also explains the prolonged P-R interval, which often leads to advanced AV block.

Hypercalcemia

Elevation of serum calcium characteristically shortens the duration of the cardiac action potential while increasing the extent of depolarization (Fig. 19.5). The latter effect, which shifts the plateau to a level of greater positivity, is readily

FIG. 19.5. Effects of hypercalcemia on the cardiac action potential. Elevated serum calcium increases the height of the plateau by enhancing the slow inward current. Shortening of the duration of the plateau is probably due to an effect of hypercalcemia to increase the postassium currents that normally cause the cell to repolarize.

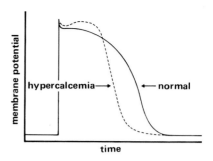

understood as being due to an increase in the slow inward current caused by the greater $[Ca^{2+}]_o/[Ca^{2+}]_i$ ratio. This increase in the slow inward current increases the depolarizing effect of calcium ions. The mechanism for the acceleration of repolarization (Fig. 19.5) is not well understood. It is likely that high $[Ca]_o$ increases the potassium conductances which cause repolarization.

The characteristic electrocardiographic manifestation of hypercalcemia is a shortened Q-T interval that can be attributed to the abbreviation of the action potential. Abnormalities also are seen in the S-T segment and T waves that arise from altered repolarization (Fig. 19.6).

Hypocalcemia

The effects of low serum calcium on the cardiac action potential are the opposite of those of hypercalcemia: The action potential is prolonged and its

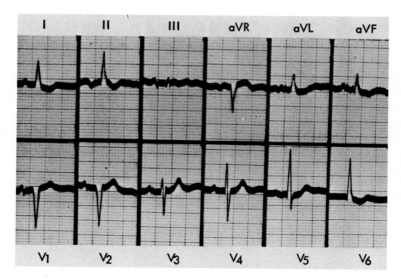

FIG. 19.6. ECG in hypercalcemia showing "sagging" S-T segments (leads I, aVL, and V_6) and a shortened Q-T interval. (From Littman, 1972.)

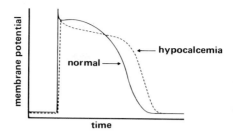

FIG. 19.7. Effects of hypocalcemia on the cardiac action potential. Lowered serum calcium slows the upstroke and decreases the amplitude of the action potential by reducing the opening of the fast sodium channels. This effect is probably due to an action of low serum calcium to enhance the voltage-dependent inactivation of the fast channels. Reduction in the height of the plateau reflects the lessening of the slow inward current caused by the reduced calcium concentration gradient across the sarcolemma, while prolongation of the action potential probably results from delayed appearance of the outward potassium currents that normally cause the cell to repolarize.

amplitude becomes reduced (Fig. 19.7). The reduced amplitude of the action potential plateau is due partly to the reduction of the slow inward current caused by the lesser concentration gradient for calcium. A decline in the rate of rise of the action potential is also sometimes caused by hypocalcemia. This latter effect has been attributed to an effect of lowered extracellular calcium on the relationship between resting potential and inactivation of the fast inward sodium current.

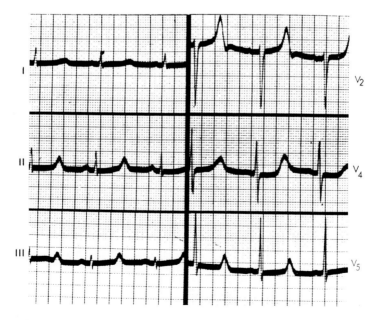

FIG. 19.8. ECG in hypocalcemia showing marked prolongation of the Q-T interval. (From Littman, 1972.)

Recall (Chapter 14) that depolarization of the cardiac cell membrane inactivates the opening of the sodium channels. The extent to which a degree of depolarization inactivates the fast inward current is modified by extracellular calcium. When $[Ca^{2+}]_o$ is low, the relationship between membrane voltage and inactivation of this sodium current is shifted so that the extent of inactivation is increased at any level of depolarization. When hypocalcemia is severe, the fast inward current is reduced even at normal levels of resting potential. This effect thus explains the action of low serum calcium concentration to reduce the rate of rise and extent of depolarization and so to increase the tendency to decremental conduction. The appearance of decremental conduction, together with the likelihood that the prolongation of the relative refractory period is not uniform, provides an explanation for the frequent occurrence of arrhythmias in patients with severe hypocalcemia.

The ECG in hypocalcemia is characterized by prolongation of the Q-T interval and S-T segment (Fig. 19.8), which reflect the increased duration of the plateau phase of the action potential.

AUTONOMIC NEUROTRANSMITTERS

Parasympathetic Neurotransmitters

Acetylcholine, the mediator of parasympathetic influences on the heart, has its greatest effects in the cells of the atria and the SA and AV nodes. Although effects of acetylcholine and stimulation of the parasympathetic nervous system have been detected also in the ventricular myocardium, they are of much less functional significance.

The effect of acetylcholine to slow the pacemaker activity of the SA node was already described in terms of sinus bradycardia in Chapter 16. This response is due to the general effect of acetylcholine to increase potassium conductances in the myocardium. In the SA node this effect is manifest as hyperpolarization and a slowing in the rate of the closure of the potassium channels which contribute to the spontaneous diastolic depolarization of the pacemaker cells (Fig. 19.9).

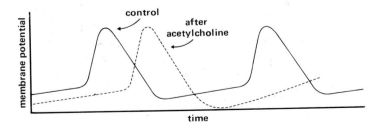

FIG. 19.9. Effects of acetylcholine, or vagal stimulation, on the SA node. Pacemaker activity is slowed because the resting potential is increased and the rate of diastolic depolarization is reduced.

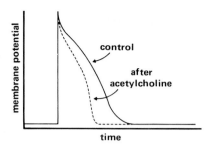

FIG. 19.10. Effects of acetylcholine, or vagal stimulation, on the atrial action potential. The duration of the action potential is shortened because the slow inward current is reduced and the outward, potassium currents that cause repolarization are increased.

Both of these actions tend to slow the spontaneous rate of pacemaker discharge.

The effects of acetylcholine on the atria, like those on the SA node, can be attributed to actions which promote opening of potassium channels. Most prominent of these effects is a dramatic shortening of atrial action potential duration (Fig. 19.10), which is attributable to an increase in the outward potassium currents that normally cause repolarization and to marked reduction of the slow inward current. The ability of acetylcholine to reduce contractility in the atria may result from this marked shortening of action potential duration and to reduction of the slow inward current. As discussed earlier in relation to the negative inotropic effect of high extracellular potassium, a reduction in the duration of the plateau of the action potential can reduce contractility both by shortening the active state and by reducing intracellular calcium stores when the slow inward current is abbreviated (Chapter 11).

The very marked shortening of action potential duration in the atria by acetylcholine may explain the tendency of vagal stimulation to induce and maintain atrial fibrillation. The direct relationship between shortened action potential duration, a shortened refractory period, and the establishment and maintenance of re-entrant arrhythmias (Chapter 18) is probably responsible for this effect of the parasympathetic neurotransmitter.

Under conditions where low resting potassium conductance causes membrane potential to be less than the potential predicted by the Nernst equation for potassium, the ability of acetylcholine to enhance potassium permeability leads to hyperpolarization. This hyperpolarizing effect allows acetylcholine and vagal stimulation to increase the rate of depolarization and the amplitude of the action potential owing to the voltage dependence of the opening of the sodium channels (Chapter 14).

Acetylcholine has a powerful effect to slow conduction in the AV node. The mechanisms responsible for this effect, however, remain incompletely understood because the small size of the AV nodal cells hampers precise measurements of changes in the ionic currents that are responsible for these effects. Acetylcholine appears to have little direct effect on action potential configuration in the cells of the lower (NH) region of the AV node, whereas in the cells of the AN and N regions (Fig. 14.15) the parasympathetic neurotransmitter shortens and reduces the amplitude of the action potential. These findings are in accord with evidence that the major effects of acetylcholine to slow AV conduction occur in the AN and N regions of the AV node. Other evidence suggests that transmission of the normal wave of depolarization through the AN region of the AV node, which is made up of small cells that have a low-amplitude, slowly rising action potential, is slowed by acetylcholine. Microelectrode recordings from cells in this region of extremely slow conduction demonstrate small "notches" on the upstroke of the action potential. These have been interpreted as evidence that the wave of depolarization is propagated through this region by the summation of several action potentials which arrive slightly out of synchrony. If this hypothesis is correct, then propagation of the impulse through the AV node would normally require that several cells together contribute to the depolarizing currents that activate the excitable tissue ahead. This process is similar to that of summation (Chapter 17; Fig. 17.14), which allows two or more subthreshold impulses to act together to provide an effective stimulus for impulse propagation. It is possible, therefore, that the major effects of acetylcholine to inhibit AV conduction are due to the reduction of action potential duration, which would tend to reduce the ability of impulses to summate. This view is supported by the finding that acetylcholine can increase the prominence and separation of the notches on the upstroke of the action potential in the AN region of the AV node (Fig. 19.11).

An alternative explanation for the ability of acetylcholine to slow AV conduction is that this neurotransmitter dissociates two ionic currents that contribute to the AV nodal action potential. According to this latter view, acetylcholine delays the onset of a slow depolarizing current, possibly carried by calcium, thus separating this inward current from a smaller initial rapid depolarizing current carried by sodium.

Very high concentrations of acetylcholine can shorten action potential duration in the cells of the His-Purkinje system and in the ventricles. These effects, which again can be attributed to an increase in potassium conductance, are probably of little physiological significance.

The effects of acetylcholine on the electrophysiological properties of the various regions of the heart are summarized in Table 19.1. The responses of the cells of the SA node and of the atrial myocardium can be attributed to the ability of the parasympathetic neurotransmitter to increase potassium permeability. The mech-

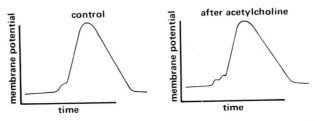

FIG. 19.11. Effects of acetylcholine, or vagal stimulation, on the AV node. Acetylcholine causes separation of notches on the upstroke of the action potential, which becomes reduced in amplitude.

TABLE 19.1. *Effects of acetylcholine on the electrophysiological properties of the heart*

Region	Physiological response	Effects on action potential
SA node	Slowing of pacemaker	Hyperpolarization [a] Slowed diastolic depolarization [a]
Atrial myocardium	Shortened refractory period (Depressed contractility)	Acceleration of depolarization [a] Reduced slow inward current
AV node	Slowed conduction	Reduced "summation" of impulses in AN region (Acceleration of repolarization and decreased amplitude) [b]
His-Purkinje system and ventricular myocardium	Little or none	Acceleration of repolarization only at extremely high concentrations [a]

[a] Probably due to increased potassium conductance.
[b] Possibly due to increased potassium conductance.

anism is less clearly defined in the case of the slowing of impulse conduction through the AV node. In this tissue as well, shortening of action potential duration may be due to an increased potassium conductance that accelerates repolarization.

Sympathetic Neurotransmitters

Norepinephrine, which is released from sympathetic nerve terminals in all regions of the heart, and *epinephrine,* which is released into the bloodstream along with norepinephrine from the adrenal glands, have similar actions on the myocardium. The effects of these catecholamines on the heart are more complex than those of acetylcholine and include enhanced contractility, accelerated conduction, increased heart rate, and shortening of action potential duration. The general mechanism by which these effects could be mediated by the cyclic AMP-protein kinase system was described in Chapter 9 and so is not repeated here. A role for cyclic AMP and membrane phosphorylation in producing the electrophysiological responses to catecholamines remains unclear. It now appears that cyclic AMP does participate in these responses, but evidence for membrane phosphorylation is still inconclusive.

The acceleration of pacemaker activity caused by catecholamines in the Purkinje fiber results from accelerated closure of the channels that control the outward potassium current (i_{K_2}). The resulting more rapid decrease in outward current flow accelerates diastolic depolarization by allowing the constant inward current that is carried by sodium or calcium ions to depolarize the cell more rapidly (Fig. 19.12). The increased rate of reduction in outward current caused by catecholamines results from a shift in the voltage dependence of the rate of closure of the potassium channel, which causes the membrane to repolarize more rapidly, especially when membrane potential is close to its fully repolarized level.

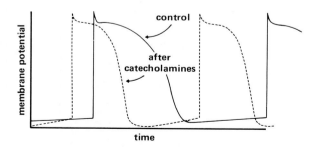

FIG. 19.12. Effects of catecholamines, or sympathetic stimulation, on the Purkinje fiber. Even though catecholamines cause hyperpolarization early in diastole, the rate of diastolic depolarization is increased sufficiently by accelerated closure of the potassium channel (i_{K_2}) to speed pacemaker activity. The action potential is shortened because the outward potassium currents that cause repolarization are increased by a shift in the voltage dependence of their opening.

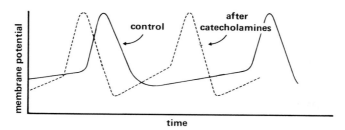

FIG. 19.13. Effects of catecholamines, or sympathetic stimulation, on the SA node. Even though there is hyperpolarization early in diastole, the rate of diastolic depolarization is increased sufficiently to accelerate pacemaker activity. In contrast to the response of the Purkinje fiber, accelerated diastolic depolarization in the SA node is due to an increased inward current, possibly one carried by calcium.

A more important effect of catecholamines on the rate of pacemaker discharge is that which occurs in the SA node where, as in the Purkinje fiber, the physiological response is an accelerated rate of firing. In both regions of the heart this response is brought about by an increased rate of diastolic depolarization (Fig. 19.13). There is reason to believe, however, that the mechanism which accelerates diastolic depolarization in the SA node may be significantly different from that described for the Purkinje fiber. In the SA node the outward potassium current whose decay is responsible for spontaneous diastolic depolarization may be i_x (Chapter 14), which, unlike i_{K_2} of the Purkinje fiber, is also involved in repolarization (Table 14.1). Studies of the effects of catecholamines to accelerate repolarization in the SA node suggest that these agents may increase an outward potassium current during diastole. For this reason another explanation for the accelerated rate of diastolic depolarization in the SA node must be sought. One such explanation is an effect of catecholamines to increase inward current flow during diastole. This latter explanation is based on the fact that an increased rate of opening of channels that carry inward current has the same effect of accelerating depolarization as an increased rate of closure of channels that carry outward current. It is thus possible that accelerated opening of the channels which control calcium flux into the myocardial cell might explain catecholamine-induced acceleration of pacemaker activity in the SA node. In view of the well-documented ability of catecholamines to increase inward calcium currents (see below), such an action could accelerate depolarization in the SA node if, as has been postulated, a diastolic component of this slow inward calcium current is present.

In addition to accelerating the rate of diastolic depolarization, catecholamines also cause hyperpolarization in pacemaker cells (Figs. 19.12 and 19.13). This effect, which woulld tend to slow pacemaker discharge, is much less than the effect to accelerate diastolic depolarization, so that the net response is an increased rate of pacemaker firing. The mechanism for the hyperpolarizing effect of catecholamines is not fully understood. It may result from the increased repolarizing potassium current (i_x), as was already discussed.

Another explanation for the hyperpolarizing effects of catecholamines stems from evidence that these agents may, at least at high concentrations, stimulate the Na-K-ATPase. As the sodium pump transports 3 moles of Na^+ out of the cell for each 2 moles of K^+ brought in, the pump is electrogenic; and because it produces a net outward current, it tends to promote hyperpolarization. This reported ability of catecholamines to stimulate the sodium pump, however, remains controversial.

The physiological significance of the action of catecholamines to shorten mechanical systole was described in Chapter 9. The ability of the heart to pump blood at the rapid rates that occur when catecholamine levels are high requires that there be sufficient time for diastolic filling and that the refractory period be shortened. Accelerated relaxation, and thus abbreviation of mechanical systole, is brought about by stimulation of the calcium pump of the sarcoplasmic reticulum and by a reduction in the Ca^{2+} affinity of troponin (Chapter 9). The ability of the heart to respond to the rapid rate of pacemaker discharge produced by catecholamines (i.e., abbreviation of electrical systole) is due partly to the interval-duration relationship (Chapter 14) and partly to a direct effect of these agents to promote repolarization. This latter effect is seen in the Purkinje fiber as an increase in the repolarizing potassium current (i_{x_1}). The resulting increased outward current more than balances the increased slow inward calcium current during the later part of the plateau (see below, and Chapters 9 and 14), so that the net effect of catecholamines in the Purkinje fiber is to shorten electrical as well as mechanical systole. In cells of the SA node and atrial myocardium as well, the outward potassium currents that promote repolarization (i_x) are increased by catecholamines. The resultant acceleration of repolarization allows for more rapid recovery of the ability of the sodium channels to reopen (Chapter 14). In this way the heart can respond electrically to the increased rate of pacemaker discharge brought about by the catecholamines.

The ability of catecholamines to increase the slow inward current carried by calcium ions has been mentioned at several points. The fact that this ionic current directly affects the mechanical performance of the heart (Chapter 9) as well as its electrical properties (Chapter 14) indicates the central importance of this response in the regulation of both electrical and mechanical functions in the heart.

Catecholamines have a well-documented and extremely important ability to provoke premature systoles and tachycardias. These effects are probably responsible for a number of cases of "sudden cardiac death," especially those provoked by sudden or severe physical and emotional stress. These arrhythmias arise in part because the catecholamines can cause different degress of action potential abbreviation in adjacent regions of the heart. The resulting inhomogeneities in repolarization are able to produce re-entrant arrhythmias by the mechanisms described in Chapter 17. In the diseased heart the shortening of action potential duration and refractory periods produced by these agents are especially nonuniform. The resulting marked inhomogeneities of repolarization are probably partly responsible for the well-known ability of catecholamines to provoke ar-

TABLE 19.2. *Effects of catecholamines on the electrophysiological properties of the heart*

Region	Physiological response	Effects on action potential
SA node	Acceleration of pacemaker Shortened refractory period	Accelerated diastolic depolarization [a] Accelerated repolarization [b] (Hyperpolarization [b])
Atrial myocardium	Shortened refractory period (Enhanced contractility [a])	Accelerated repolarization [b]
AV node	Accelerated conduction	Increased amplitude [a] Increased rate of depolarization [a]
His-Purkinje system	Promotion of pacemaker activity Shortened refractory period	Accelerated diastolic depolarization [c] Accelerated repolarization [b] (Hyperpolarization)
Ventricular myocardium	Shortened refractory period (Enhanced contractility [a])	Accelerated repolarization [b] (Hyperpolarization) [b]

[a] Possibly or probably due to increased calcium conductance.
[b] Probably due to increased potassium conductance.
[c] Probably due to accelerated decrease in i_{K_2}.

rhythmias in patients with pre-existing heart disease. An additional mechanism by which catecholamines can induce arrhythmias is attributable to the increased slow inward current which increases the propensity toward the generation of slowly propagated action potentials in partially depolarized regions of the heart, thereby setting the stage for re-entrant arrhythmias (Chapter 17).

Catecholamines increase the rate of rise and amplitude of the action potential in the AV node and so accelerate conduction velocity. The mechanism for this effect remains uncertain, but one attractive hypothesis is that the increased conduction velocity is due to the catecholamine-induced increase in the slow inward current. This hypothesis fits well with other evidence that depolarization in the AV node is due largely to inward calcium currents (rather than sodium currents) and the lack of comparable effects of catecholamines on the upstroke of the action potential in the atria and ventricles, where action potentials are initiated by inward sodium currents. If the ability of catecholamines to increase the opening of calcium channels explains the increased rate of rise and amplitude of the AV nodal action potential, this mechanism may account for the important action of these agents to increase AV conduction and thus to reduce the extent of AV block in patients with heart disease.

The effects of catecholamines on the electrophysiological properties of various regions of the heart are summarized in Table 19.2. Unlike the responses to acetylcholine, most of which appear to reflect a single general mechanism (increased potassium permeability), those due to catecholamines appear to be more complex.

CARDIAC GLYCOSIDES

The actions of cardiac glycosides on myocardial contractibility have been discussed in terms of the well-documented ability of these agents to inhibit the sodium pump. The way in which sodium pump inhibition can also account for many of the electrophysiological effects of cardiac glycosides are described at this point. It is important, however, to note that cardiac glycosides also have an important reflex effect in the intact animal and man. This reflex action is mediated by increased parasympathetic tone, so that in the intact animal and in man a large part of the electrophysiological response to the administration of cardiac glycosides is indirect and can be attributed to the actions of acetylcholine described earlier in this chapter. These reflex effects are not discussed further at this point; only the direct electrophysiological effects of the cardiac glycosides on the heart are considered here.

The action of cardiac glycosides to inhibit the sodium pump can explain the direct actions of high concentrations of this class of drugs on resting potential. The fact that the sodium pump is electrogenic and generates a small outward current may partly explain the depolarizing effects of toxic doses of the cardiac glycosides. The replacement of intracellular potassium with sodium, however, probably causes the major portion of the depolarizing effect seen in cardiac glycoside toxicity as resting potential falls when the $[K^+]_i/[K^+]_o$ ratio is decreased (Chapter 14). The decreased resting potential inhibits the opening of the sodium channels and thereby reduces both the rate of rise and the amplitude of the action potential (Chapter 14). Cardiac glycosides also may increase the resistance of the intercalated disc and thereby slow conduction. The resulting increase in the tendency for decremental conduction (Chapter 17) probably plays a major role in the tendency of patients receiving cardiac glycosides to develop cardiac arrhythmias.

The ability of cardiac glycosides to provoke premature systoles and tachycardias may be due not only to the tendency toward the development of re-entrant arrhythmias described above but also to abnormal pacemaker activity in cells of the ventricular conduction system. The ability of cardiac glycosides to promote pacemaker activity in the Purkinje fibers, and thus to cause ventricular premature systoles and tachycardias, is well documented. Recent evidence indicates that this effect is not due solely to accelerated closing of potassium channels (i.e., the normal mechanism of pacemaker acceleration) but also to an action to open calcium channels during diastole. This latter effect allows calcium to carry a positive charge into the cell during diastole, thereby causing membrane depolarization and abnormally active pacemaker activity. Cardiac glycosides may also increase the systolic calcium influx that is associated with the slow inward current during the plateau phase of the cardiac action potential.

The interaction between serum potassium level and the effects of cardiac glycosides on the cardiac cell are of considerable clinical significance. The well-established and extremely important ability of lowered serum potassium to exacerbate cardiac glycoside toxicity and of elevated serum potassium to reduce the toxic manifestations in patients who have received excessive doses of the cardiac glycosides probably result from the well-documented interactions between potassium and the cardiac glycosides on the breakdown of the phosphorylated sodium pump enzyme (Chapter 9).

The major effects of cardiac glycosides on electrocardiographic contour are a shortening of the Q-T interval and abnormalities in the S-T segment and T waves (Fig. 19.14). These findings suggest that the cardiac glycosides affect the repolarization process, although electrophysiological evidence for these actions is contradictory. Prolongation as well as abbreviation of the cardiac action potential have been reported, and the effects of cardiac glycosides on the ionic currents responsible for repolarization remain incompletely understood.

Cardiac glycosides have been suggested to decrease the outward potassium current (i_{K_2}), which is responsible for the pacemaker activity of Purkinje fibers. This effect has been attributed to an action of increased intracellular sodium concentration, which is caused by inhibition of the sodium pump. This finding suggests that partial membrane depolarization, which increases the tendency for ventricular arrhythmias to develop in hearts exposed to cardiac glycosides, is due not only to a decrease in the potassium gradient across the sarcolemma but also to an effect of increased $[Na^+]_i$ to inhibit the outward movement of potas-

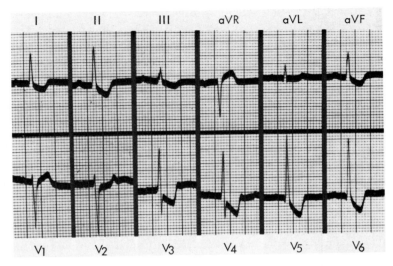

FIG. 19.14. Effects of cardiac glycosides on the ECG showing "sagging" S-T segments (leads I, II, aVF, V₅, and V₆), T wave abnormalities, and shortening of the Q-T interval. The P-R interval is 0.20 sec, the upper limit of normal. (From Littman, 1972.)

sium. Inhibition of the electrogenic sodium pump, an alternative or possibly an additional explanation for the action of cardiac glycosides to inhibit outward currents, was already mentioned in relation to the depolarizing effects of these drugs.

The inhibition of the small outward current generated by the sodium pump would have its greatest effect on membrane potential when membrane resistance is high, especially toward the end of the plateau of the cardiac action potential. Some evidence suggests that the sodum pump is active throughout the cardiac cycle and that the inhibition of this electrogenic pump by cardiac glycosides may reduce outward currents during repolarization. These studies have been interpreted to mean that the "background"outward current (i_{K_1}) is not due to potassium efflux through a channel such as that described in Chapter 14, but instead that this current is produced by the sodium pump.

ANTIARRHYTHMIC DRUGS

Utilization of the rapidly growing knowledge of the ionic basis of cardiac action potential for the benefit of the patient with heart disease represents one of the most important challenges to the modern cardiologist. At the present time, however, this field of research is in a confused state, although one must remember that this confusion has resulted from an explosion of knowledge at all levels of study regarding this very important problem. New data and concepts are appearing so rapidly in clinical as well as experimental studies that it has not yet been possible to organize the findings in a clear, unambiguous manner.

The modern cardiologist who wishes to use an antiarrthymic drug must be aware of a number of clinical, physiological, and biophysical observations. The *clinical* data are often based on clinical impressions, i.e., observations which may not have been proved by meticulously controlled double-blind studies but which nevertheless are of considerable value. For example, it is commonly taught that quinidine is a better agent in the treatment of atrial fibrillation than is procainamide, although one is hard pressed to find statistically validated proof for this observation, which is generally accepted as being correct. From a *physiological* standpoint, antiarrhythmic drugs are often analyzed in terms of their ability to speed or slow conduction, or to shorten or lengthen the refractory period. These physiological observations are for the large part related to the findings discussed in Chapter 18 in terms of the "snake analogy." Very recently antiarrhythmic agents have been examined from a *biophysical* point of view, i.e., the way in which they modify time dependency, voltage dependency, or other characteristics of the ionic currents and the gating mechanisms by which they are controlled. This plethora of data has not yet been fully organized, so that the following pages represent but one way of looking at these often confusing, but very important findings.

Difficulties arise in attempting to understand the mechanisms of antiarrhythmic drug action for several reasons. In the first place there are many types of data that must be encompassed in any systematic presentation of this field. In addition, re-entrant arrhythmias can be terminated by agents that either prolong or shorten the refractory period in areas of decremental conduction, as well as by measures that either depress or improve conduction (Chapter 18). Thus each of the clinically used antiarrhythmic agents may have multiple actions on the cardiac action potential and its underlying ionic properties, and so the present confusion regarding the mechanism of action of these agents is understandable.

Classification of Antiarrhythmic Agents

A number of classifications of antiarrhythmic drugs have been proposed, but there is no agreement whatsoever between leading investigators in this field as to which if any of the current classifications is most suitable. For this reason the classification adopted here (Table 19.3) is very general and almost inevitably will have to be revised as knowledge in this field grows.

TABLE 19.3. *Tentative classification of the antiarrhythmic agents*

Agents used to treat bradycardias
    Sympathetic agonists (e.g., ephedrine)
    Parasympathetic antagonists (e.g., atropine)

Agents used to treat tachycardias
    Membrane-stabilizing agents
        Class 1 agents (e.g., quinidine, procainamide)
        Class 2 agents (e.g., lidocaine, diphenylhydantoin)
    β-Blocking agents (e.g., propranolol)
    Calcium influx inhibitors (e.g., Verapamil)

Agents Used to Treat Bradycardia

Slowing of the rate of ventricular beating, when chronic, can cause signs and symptoms of heart failure (Chapter 21); when it is abrupt in onset it may lead to sudden death due either to ventricular standstill or the appearance of ventricular fibrillation. The latter can arise as a complication of the depressed conduction in the ventricles and "awakening" of latent abnormal pacemakers which appear in the heart when extreme bradycardia causes blood pressure to fall. These dangerous bradycardias are usually due to AV block, but a minority of cases arise from the sick sinus syndrome (Chapter 16).

Prior to the introduction of safe and effective electrical pacemakers, these bradycardias were treated, and efforts were made to prevent them, by administering agents whose actions mimicked those of the sympathetic transmitters, and by anticholinergic drugs. These forms of treatment, whose effect on the heart was already described, are often effective. Drug therapy for the bradycardias has proved to be unreliable and is often accompanied by serious side effects, so that in current clinical practice these agents are generally used only to maintain the patient's cardiac rate until an electrical pacemaker can be inserted or, if the bradycardia is transient or due to a reversible cause, until the arrhythmia has disappeared.

Agents Used to Treat Premature Systoles and Tachycardias

The difficulties in classifying the important therapeutic agents used for premature systoles and tachycardias have already been alluded to. Because these abnormalities can arise from both accelerated pacemaker activity (diastolic depolarization) and re-entry, and because either improvement or further depression of membrane function in re-entrant pathways can terminate these arrhythmias, the formulation of a rational basis to classify these agents on clinical or even physiological grounds is difficult. An ideal scheme by which the synergistic, parallel, and antagonistic actions of these agents can be understood probably must await the time when we have additional knowledge concerning how each of these drugs acts on specific ionic conductances in the various regions of the heart. As this information appears to lie several years in the future, only a general classification has been adopted here (Table 19.3). It is likely that a number of agents whose actions differ in significant details have been grouped together under the broad heading "membrane-stabilizing agents." Two other classes of antiarrhythmic drugs, the β-blocking agents and calcium influx inhibitors, are also described, although these agents often exhibit membrane-stabilizing types of action.

Membrane-stabilizing agents.

The category "membrane-stabilizing agents" includes a large number of antiarrhythmic agents whose effects are sometimes referred to as "local anesthetic actions." Some of these drugs, notably diphenylhydantoin, may also act partly through reflexes initiated by drug actions in the central nervous system, leading for example to depression of sympathetic tone. This class of therapeutic agents, however, appears to have a common general action on the heart—a membrane-stabilizing or local anesthetic effect, which reflects the ability of these agents to reduce passive ion fluxes across the cardiac sarcolemma.

Actions on pacemaker activity. The membrane-stabilizing agents slow pacemaker activity, both in the SA node and in abnormal sites of pacemaker activity. The mechanisms by which these effects are brought about are largely unknown. In the case of the SA node, their ability to slow diastolic depolarization may arise from slowing of a time-dependent increase in calcium conductance (Chapter 14). The ability of these agents to slow pacemaker activity in other regions of the heart in which diastolic depolarization is brought about by a decline in potassium conductance suggests that membrane-stabilizing agents also reduce maximal potassium conductance or slow the rate of closure of the potassium channels.

Actions on action potential upstroke velocity and conduction velocity. A controversy exists regarding the ability of different membrane-stabilizing agents to slow the upstroke velocity (phase 0) of the action potential. Quinidine and procainamide have been found by virtually all investigators to slow upstroke velocity and are sometimes called class 1 agents. Lidocaine and diphenylhydantoin, on the other hand, have been reported by some but not all investigators to have little or no action to slow upstroke velocity at low, therapeutic concentrations, and so have been designated class 2 agents. It is agreed, however, that high concentrations of class 2 agents, like class 1 agents, slow the upstroke velocity.

One explanation of the controversies regarding the membrane-stabilizing agents with class 1 and class 2 actions also illustrates the problems in evaluating the mode of action of these agents on the basis of currently available data. If, for example, the class 2 agents are, as some investigators have suggested, more effective than class 1 agents in slowing pacemaker activity, the resulting decrease in heart rate would prolong diastole. As a result, membrane potential would have more time to return to a fully repolarized state, allowing for greater recovery of the fast inward current, which is both time- and voltage-dependent (Chapter 14). These effects of slowing the heart rate would therefore increase indirectly the extent of opening of the fast sodium channels and thus tend to mask a direct effect of the class 2 agents to slow upstroke velocity.

Consideration of the way in which the membrane-stabilizing agents could act to slow upstroke velocity provides yet another possible explanation for the differences between class 1 and class 2 agents. Recovery of the ability of the membrane to open its sodium channels, and thus to initiate the fast inward current that produces the upstroke of the action potential, is both time- and voltage-dependent (Chapter 14). It is thus possible that class 1 and class 2 agents might have different relative degrees of action on these two parameters. There is in fact some evidence that this view may be correct. Lidocaine, a class 2 agent, reduces upstroke velocity by slowing the time-dependent recovery of the ability of the sodium channels to reopen but has little effect on the myocardial cell after it is fully repolarized. For this reason, lidocaine would be expected to have little or no effect on upstroke velocity at slow or even normal heart rates. In contrast, quinidine, a class 1 agent, has little effect on the time-dependent recovery of the fast inward current, but instead slows upstroke velocity at all levels of resting potential. In other words, quinidine inhibits upstroke velocity by its action to block a given fraction of the fast channels at any level of membrane potential. If these data can be generalized to other class 1 and class 2 agents, it might be predicted that the former would be most useful in preventing tachycardias in patients whose heart rates are normal, whereas the class 2 agents would be most useful in treating the established tachycardias, where their action to delay the time-dependent recovery of the fast inward current would be most pronounced. The validity of this hypothesis, which is suggested by some clinical observations, must be tested by additional experimentation.

The actions of the membrane-stabilizing agents on conduction velocity can be predicted to a large extent from their effects on the fast inward current (Chapter 16). For this reason class 1 agents, which appear to have a greater ability to decrease upstroke velocity, would be expected to have a greater tendency to slow conduction than the class 2 agents. This slowing of impulse conduction tends to abolish re-entrant arrhythmias (Chapter 18).

The direct actions of the membrane-stabilizing agents to inhibit the opening of the fast sodium channels also promotes decremental conduction and thus *increases* the tendency to develop re-entrant arrhythmias. This effect, which accounts for the ability of high doses of the membrane-stabilizing agents to cause arrhythmias that are sometimes fatal, illustrates how a single drug can exhibit both antiarrhythmic and arrhythmogenic actions. Furthermore, it is apparent that a single action, in this case to depress upstroke velocity and thus to promote decremental conduction, can have both beneficial and detrimental effects.

Actions on action potential duration. As was true for their effects on upstroke velocity, the membrane-stabilizing agents appear to have two types of action on the duration of the cardiac action potential. Class 1 agents have been found in virtually all studies to prolong the action potential while low concentrations of class 2 agents have been reported in some but not all studies to cause abbreviation of the action potential. The discrepancies between the conclusions reached in different studies with the class 2 drugs may arise from differences in the tissues studied (see below). The ability of high concentrations of these drugs, especially those of class 1, to prolong the action potential accounts for the marked prolongation of the Q-T interval seen when an agent like quinidine is administered in toxic doses (Fig. 19.15).

Actions on refractory period. Remember that the duration of the refractory period in the heart is determined both by time- and voltage-dependent properties of the recovery of the fast sodium channels. While all the membrane-stabilizing agents can prolong the refractory period, it has already been pointed out that at least one of the class 1 agents (quinidine) does so by inhibiting this recovery process such that there is less recovery of the ability of the sodium channels to

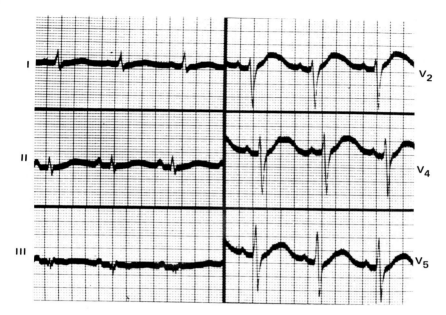

I   V₂

II V₄

III V₅

FIG. 19.15. Effects of quinidine on the ECG showing slight widening of the QRS complex, marked prolongation of the Q-T interval, and prominent U waves. (From Littman, 1972.)

reopen at any given membrane voltage. In the case of lidocaine, a class 2 agent, the refractory period is prolonged mainly by inhibition of the time-dependent recovery of these channels.

It has recently become apparent that differences in the responses of various tissues to the membrane-stabilizing agents may explain not only some of the discrepancies in published data regarding their effects on various electrophysiological parameters but also some of their antiarrhythmic actions. In the partially ischemic heart, for example, lidocaine prolongs the refractory period in the ischemic regions to a greater extent than it does in the normally perfused areas. Because abbreviation of the action potential appears to be one of the underlying causes of premature systoles and tachycardias in patients with ischemic heart disease (Chapters 17 and 22), any agent that has a disproportionate effect of prolonging action potential duration in ischemic tissue can reduce the resulting inhomogeneities in repolarization and so can prevent and treat such arrhythmias.

β-Blocking agents.

The use of β-blocking agents (e.g., propranolol) to prevent and treat premature systoles and tachycardias can be understood in terms of their ability to reverse the arrhythmogenic effects of the catecholamines described earlier in this chapter. The mechanism responsible for these antiarrhythmic actions lies in the ability of the β-blocking agents to inhibit the binding of catecholamines to β-receptors, thereby reducing the influence of the sympathetic neurotransmitters on the heart.

Most of the β-blocking agents also have membrane-stabilizing effects, although the latter usually appear at higher serum levels than are needed to cause the β-blocking effects. Efforts are now being made to develop "pure" β-blocking agents which lack membrane-stabilizing effects. Agents like Practolol and Sotanol have an increased ratio between the β-blocking and local anesthetic actions. There remains some disagreement, however, as to whether these newer agents lack membrane-stabilizing effects when administered in effective antiarrhythmic doses.

Calcium influx inhibitors.

The recent recognition of the role of slow potentials (Chapter 17) in causing cardiac arrhythmias has led to the search for agents with primary effects to inhibit the depolarizing currents that arise when calcium enters the cell by way of the slow channel. A new class of agents (of which Verapamil can be considered a prototype) has been developed whose actions appear to be primary in inhibiting this calcium current.

Verapamil depresses the slow inward current but has less effect on the fast inward current carried by sodium ions. The depression of the slow inward current caused by calcium-influx inhibitors can be partially overcome by increasing extracellular calcium concentration, so that Verapamil may act to block a portion of the slow channels that allow calcium entry during the plateau of the action potential.

The ability of calcium influx inhibitors to reduce the depolarizing effects of the slow inward current may be responsible for many of their antiarrhythmic actions. These effects would be especially important in depressed areas of the heart where re-entrant arrhythmias are initiated and sustained by "slow potentials" (Chapters 17 and 22). The interruption of re-entrant pathways that would result from inhibited conduction of slow potentials may account for the reported antiarrhythmic effects of these agents in ischemic heart disease, where sizable areas of the heart are partially depolarized (Chapter 22) and so may be activated only by slow potentials.

Because of the ability of the calcium-influx inhibitors to reduce calcium-dependent depolarizing currents, these agents would also be expected to slow pacemaker activity in the SA node and to depress conduction in the AV node (Chapter 14). Both of these effects have been found. In most cases the slowing of the sinus pacemaker represents a "side effect" of this class of drugs, while inhibition of AV conduction can have both beneficial and detrimental effects. The tendency of Verapamil to depress conduction in the AN and N regions of the AV node can give rise to the often undesirable development, or worsening, of AV block. On the other hand, the depression of AV nodal conduction may abolish re-entrant tachycardias due to reciprocal rhythm in some patients (Chapter 18). Recently Verapamil was found to prolong the refractory period in the AV node. This effect, like that of depressing AV nodal conduction, allows the calcium-influx inhibitors to reduce the tendency for the development and maintenance of re-entrant tachycardias in this structure that arise from reciprocal beating (Chapter 18).

There is evidence that the calcium-influx inhibitors, like the β-blocking agents, also have actions similar to those of the membrane-stabilizing agents. For this reason a part of their antiarrhythmic actions may arise from the mechanisms described earlier in this chapter. In view of their actions to reduce the inward movement of calcium, it should be recognized that these agents also decrease myocardial contractility.

Knowledge of the mechanism of action of antiarrhythmic drugs is incomplete. Yet rapid progress now being made in this important area, based on the growth of knowledge regarding the ionic basis of the normal cardiac action potential (Chapter 14), holds considerable promise for managing the cardiac patient. Precise knowledge of the mechanisms by which the antiarrhythmic agents act to modify physiological and biophysical aspects of cardiac excitability, coupled with an understanding of the way in which disease processes influence these same parameters, promises a new era in the prevention and treatment of cardiac arrhythmias.

BIBLIOGRAPHY

Bassett, A. L., and Hoffman, B. F. (1971): Antiarrhythmic drugs: Electrophysiological actions. *Annu. Rev. Pharmacol.,* 11:143–170.

Chen, C-M, Gettes, L. S., and Katzung, B. G. (1975): Effect of lidocaine and quinidine on steady-state characteristics and recovery kinetics of $(dV/dt)_{max}$ in guinea pig ventricular myocardium. *Circ. Res.,* 37:20–29.

Cranefield, P. (1975): *The Conduction of the Cardiac Impulse. The Slow Response and Cardiac Arrhythmias.* Futura Publishing Co., Mount Kisco, N. Y.

Dreifus, L. S., and Likoff, W. editors (1966): *Mechanisms and Therapy of Cardiac Arrhythmias.* Grune & Stratton, New York.

Dreifus, L. S., Likoff, W., and Moyer, J. H., editors (1973): *Cardiac Arrhythmias.* Grune & Stratton, New York.

Gettes, L. S. (1975): Electrophysiologic basis of arrhythmias and acute myocardial ischemia. In: *Modern Trends in Cardiology,* Vol. 3, edited by M. F. Oliver, pp. 219–246. Butterworths, London.

Giles, W., and Noble, S. J. (1976): Changes in membrane currents in bullfrog atrium produced by acetylcholine. *J. Physiol. (Lond.),* 261:103–123.

Kupersmith, J., Antman, E. M., and Hoffman, B. F. (1975): In vivo electrophysiological effects of lidocaine in canine acute myocardial infarction. *Circ. Res.,* 36:84–91.

Littman, D. (1972): *Textbook of Electrocardiology.* Harper & Row, New York.

Rosen, M. R., and Hoffman, B. F. (1973): Mechanisms of action of antiarrhythmic drugs. *Circ. Res.,* 32:1–8.

Vaughan Williams, E. M. (1970): Classification of antiarrhythmic drugs. In: *Symposium on Cardiac Arrhythmias,* edited by E. Sandoe, E. Flensted-Jensen, and K. H. Olesen, pp. 449–472. Astra, Sweden.

20

Valvular Heart Disease

Diseases of the valves of the heart in which the valves become insufficient (leaky) or their orifices become stenotic (narrowed) cause predictable abnormalities in the pressures and flows within specific chambers of the heart and in the circulation as a whole. The latter effects, which tend to reduce the pumping ability of the heart, are discussed in Chapter 21. Here we discuss some of the more common clinical abnormalities of valve function and their effects on intracardiac pressures.

As was true for the arrhythmias, the descriptions here are not intended to be a complete and systematic review of the subject of valvular heart disease, nor do they represent thorough coverage of these conditions as they are encountered by the clinical cardiologist. Instead, the descriptions are provided to help the reader understand the way in which valvular stenosis and insufficiency alter the normal pressure and flow patterns in the heart and circulation.

The reader is encouraged to review the material at the end of Chapter 1 before reading further in this chapter. For those who wish to obtain a more exhaustive discussion of these topics, reference should be made to one of the textbooks of clinical cardiology that are cited at the end of this chapter.

INTRODUCTION

Valvular heart disease is due in most cases either to rheumatic fever or congenital abnormalities. In the case of rheumatic fever, the immune responses of the body to streptococcal infection can lead to both acute and chronic inflammation of the heart valves, and thus to the development of valvular stenosis and insufficiency. The mitral and aortic valves are most commonly affected by these processes; tricuspid valve involvement is uncommon, and rheumatic pulmonic valve disease is rare. Multiple valve involvement in rheumatic heart disease is frequently encountered but for the sake of clarity is not described further in this text. Any of the heart valves may be abnormal due to a congenital anomaly, and multiple valve involvement is also common in congenital heart disease although the patterns of multiple valve involvement are quite different from those seen in rheumatic valvular diseases. Defects in the interatrial and interventricular septum, which also occur in congenital heart disease, commonly complicate abnormalities of the cardiac valves by allowing shunting of blood between the various chambers of the heart. Valvular heart disease, usually aortic and mitral insufficiency, can complicate a variety of systemic diseases. Infection of the heart valves often causes valvular insufficiency, while traumatic valve rupture is much rarer.

The following descriptions center around four abnormalities of the valves on the left side of the heart: mitral stenosis and insufficiency, and aortic stenosis and insufficiency. Similar abnormalities affecting the tricuspid and pulmonic valves on the right side of the heart also occur, but their effects on right ventricular and atrial pressure are similar to those produced by the corresponding valve abnormalities on the left side of the heart. The focus here is not on a clinical description of these conditions but on the way in which valvular function abnormalities cause predictable changes in the pressures within the heart and great vessels, thereby altering the hemodynamic features of cardiac pumping.

MITRAL STENOSIS

Narrowing of the mitral valve impairs emptying of the left atrium into the left ventricle during diastole. The primary effects of mitral stenosis therefore are a rise in left atrial pressure and a fall in cardiac output. The latter can be attributed to the lowering of left ventricular end-diastolic volume as a result of reduced filling of this chamber from the left atrium. Left ventricular systolic and aortic pressures are not reduced, except in *very* severe mitral stenosis (Chapter 21).

Mitral stenosis produces characteristic abnormalities in the heart sounds, as well as readily identifiable murmurs. The latter arise from the turbulence caused when blood flows rapidly through the narrowed mitral orifice, so that the timing of the murmurs coincides with the cardiac cycle phases during which a pressure gradient exists across the open mitral valve. In addition, the deformity of the mitral valve in most cases of rheumatic mitral stenosis increases the amplitude of the first heart sound (S_1), which is associated with mitral valve closure, and also causes the mitral valve opening to become audible. The latter phenomena arise because fusion of the mitral commissures, which produces the stenosis, also causes the valve to resemble a sail. Hence the increased amplitude of S_1 can be likened to the filling of a sail when a sailboat "jibes" (the wind direction from the stern shifting from port to starboard, or vice versa. Closure of the deformed, stenotic mitral valve when left ventricular pressure rises causes a loud sound, much like that heard when the wind suddenly fills a sail from behind. Similarly, mitral valve opening in patients with mitral stenosis often causes a snapping sound, the *opening snap* (OS), which is similar to the sound made by a sail in a boat "coming about" (the wind direction from the bow shifting from port to starboard or vice versa in a sailboat facing a strong wind).

It is a curious custom in clinical cardiology to devote the greatest care in evaluating the intensity and acoustic characteristics of murmurs and abnormal sounds, whereas from a pathophysiological standpoint it is their *timing* that provides the most information about the degree and often also the nature of the underlying hemodynamic abnormality. Although the abnormalities in the heart sounds and murmurs are qualitatively similar, regardless of the degree of severity of the mitral stenosis, several quantitative differences, especially in timing, are of considerable importance clinically. The different physical findings associated with mitral stenosis of different degrees of severity illustrate clearly the value of the "Wiggers diagram" (Fig. 1.16) in clinical cardiology. The following discussion treats mild, moderate, and severe mitral stenosis in separate sections.

Mild Mitral Stenosis

The abnormalities in intracardiac pressure that result from mild mitral stenosis are shown in Fig. 20.1. During atrial systole, when left atrial pressure rises, the stenotic mitral valve fails to transmit sufficient blood to the left ventricle, so that left atrial pressure becomes abnormally elevated and comes to exceed that in the left ventricle. In other words, an abnormal pressure gradient develops across the mitral valve. The left atrial pressure remains slightly elevated during ventricular systole, when the mitral valve is closed, because further emptying of the atrium cannot take place (Fig. 20.1). As left ventricular pressure declines during isovolumic relaxation, the elevated left atrial pressure causes the mitral valve to open earlier during the cardiac cycle than is normal. This is apparent in Fig. 20.1 as a slight leftward shift at the point at which left ventricular pressure falls below that in the left atrium. The narrowed mitral valve causes an abnormal pressure gradient to reappear during the rapid filling phase of early diastole. This is demonstrated by the fact that the left atrial pressure falls more slowly than usual, remaining higher than the left ventricular pressure until, toward the end of the rapid filling phase, the pressures equalize (Fig. 20.1).

Two murmurs characteristically appear in mild mitral stenosis (Fig. 20.1). Both coincide with the phases of the cardiac cycle during which an abnormal pressure gradient exists across the mitral valve: atrial systole and rapid filling. The former gives rise to a *presystolic murmur,* while the murmur that coincides with the rapid filling phase of diastole produces a *middiastolic murmur* that is usually "rumbling" in character. The duration of the latter is brief in mild mitral stenosis because the left atrial and ventricular pressures equilibrate relatively quickly.

Several important changes in the heart sounds are caused by mitral stenosis. An atrial sound is not heard in this condition because mitral valve narrowing prevents sudden emptying of the left atrium. Similarly, the stenotic mitral valve slows blood flow into the left ventricle so that a third heart sound (III) cannot be produced. Indeed, an audible third heart sound, which signifies rapid ventricular filling, denies the existence of mitral stenosis. Instead of the third sound, which is broad and low-pitched, and heard normally 0.13–0.15 sec after the second heart sound (II), the patient with mitral stenosis has a higher-pitched opening snap (OS), which comes earlier in the cardiac cycle. In mild mitral stenosis it follows the second heart sound by an interval of approximately 0.10–0.12 sec.

Moderate Mitral Stenosis

As in mild mitral stenosis, the left atrial pressure in moderate mitral stenosis is abnormally elevated during those phases of the cardiac cycle when blood flows

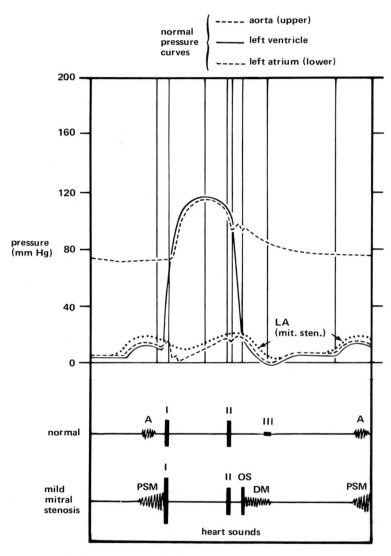

FIG. 20.1. Mild mitral stenosis. Left atrial pressure is elevated (·····), causing an abnormal diastolic pressure gradient across the mitral valve, especially marked during atrial systole and the rapid filling phase of the cardiac cycle. Resulting turbulent blood flow causes a presystolic (PSM) and a diastolic (DM) murmur. Mitral valve opening and closing become audible and cause an opening snap (OS) and an accentuated first sound (I).

across the mitral valve, i.e., atrial systole and rapid filling. In addition to greater elevation of left atrial pressure during these two phases of the cardiac cycle, increased severity of mitral stenosis prolongs the period when the abnormal pressure gradient exists between left atrium and ventricle during rapid ventricular filling (Fig. 20.2). This causes the middiastolic murmur of mitral stenosis to

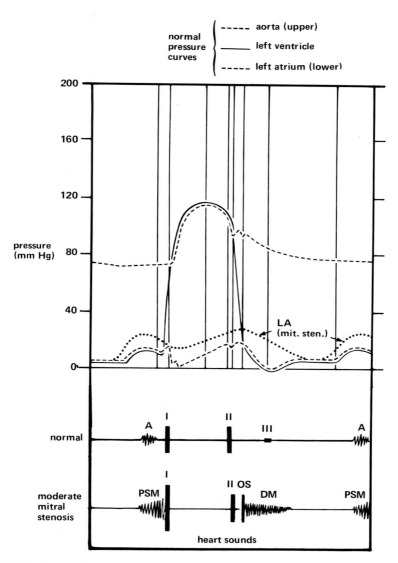

FIG. 20.2. Moderate mitral stenosis. Left atrial pressure is higher (·····) than in mild mitral stenosis (Fig. 20.1) so the presystolic murmur (PSM) is louder. The longer time needed for left atrial and left ventricular pressures to equilibrate at the beginning of diastole prolongs the diastolic murmur (DM). Mitral valve opening occurs sooner after the second sound when left atrial pressure becomes more elevated, so the II-OS interval is shorter than in mild mitral stenosis.

become prolonged as the stenosis becomes more severe. Greater elevation of left atrial pressure also causes the opening snap to occur sooner after the second heart sound. This is apparent in Fig. 20.2 where the point at which left ventricular pressure falls below that in the left atrium is seen to be shifted not only upward (to a higher level) but also to the left, i.e., to an earlier time after the second heart sound than in Fig. 20.1. As mitral stenosis worsens from mild to moderate, therefore, the II-OS interval is shortened to 0.08–0.10 sec.

Severe Mitral Stenosis (With Atrial Fibrillation)

The hemodynamics of severe mitral stenosis as shown in Fig. 20.3 depict not only the effects of severe narrowing of the mitral valve orifice but also those of *atrial fibrillation.* The latter, which is a common complication in patients with severe mitral stenosis, can be understood in light of the atrial dilatation that develops when emptying of the left atrium is impeded by a narrowed mitral valve orifice. The consequent enlargement of the left atrium, which develops because the atrium both dilates (owing to the elevation of left atrial pressure) and hypertrophies (owing to the chronic hemodynamic overloading; Chapter 21) predisposes to the development of re-entrant arrhythmias (Chapter 17). Loss of the atrial "primer" pump causes left atrial pressure to be elevated throughout the cardiac cycle (Fig. 12.11) and so contributes to the clinical disability in these patients. The loss of atrial systole of course is accompanied by disappearance of the presystolic murmur.

The existence of severe mitral stenosis is also reflected in the finding that the middiastolic murmur becomes so prolonged it lasts throughout almost all of diastole. The great length of this murmur reflects the very slow fall of left atrial diastolic pressure and its failure to equilibrate with that in the left ventricle (Fig. 20.3). The interval between the second heart sound and the opening snap becomes shortened still further in severe mitral stenosis as mitral valve opening occurs at a very high left ventricular pressure. The II-OS interval in severe mitral stenosis is 0.05–0.07 sec.

> Although an opening snap is depicted in Fig. 20.1–20.3, this sound is not always heard in patients with mitral stenosis. When present the opening snap provides evidence that the mitral valve is flexible; therefore its absence implies that the stenotic valve has become either fibrotic or calcified. For this reason the presence or absence of the opening snap provides an indication about the *anatomical* severity of the mitral stenosis but does not directly indicate its *hemodynamic* severity (the degree of obstruction of the mitral valve orifice). As would be expected, loss of the opening snap is accompanied by diminution of the intensity of the first heart sound.

MITRAL INSUFFICIENCY

Failure of the mitral valve to close tightly causes blood to leak from the left ventricle back to the left atrium during those phases of the cardiac cycle when left ventricular pressure exceeds that in the left atrium. This abnormal regurgitant flow therefore occurs throughout ventricular systole, beginning almost at the onset of isovolumic contraction and ending only toward the end of isovolumic relaxation. The abnormal flow of blood from ventricle to atrium causes left atrial

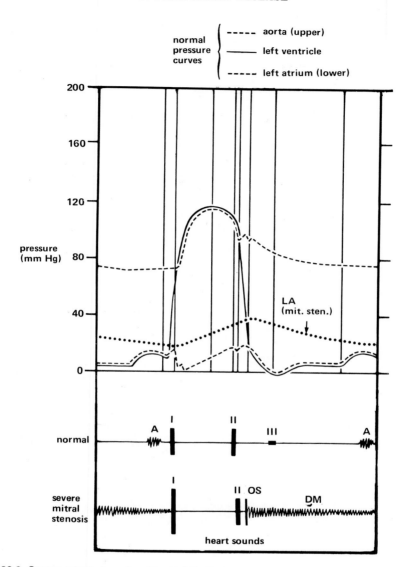

FIG. 20.3. Severe mitral stenosis with atrial fibrillation. Left atrial pressure is elevated further (·····) by extreme narrowing of the mitral valve. Loss of atrial systole leads to disappearance of the presystolic murmur. As there is a significant pressure gradient across the mitral valve throughout almost all of diastole, the diastolic murmur (DM) fills this phase of the cardiac cycle. The very high left atrial pressure reached at the end of ventricular systole causes the mitral valve to open early during the phase of isovolumic relaxation, causing a very short II-OS interval.

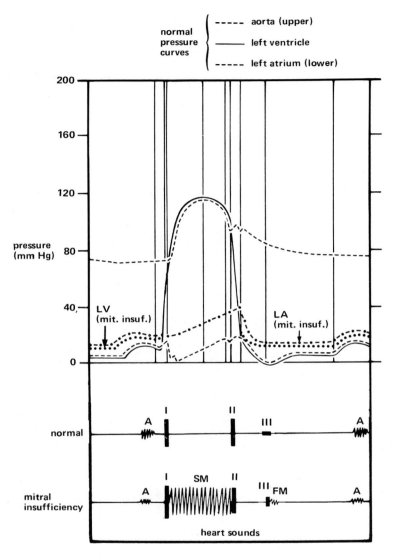

FIG. 20.4. Mitral insufficiency. Regurgitation of blood across the mitral valve during ventricular systole causes left atrial pressure (·–··–··) to rise sharply and produces a murmur (SM) that lasts throughout systole. The regurgitant blood in the left atrium contributes to an increased return to the left ventricle during diastole and so elevates left ventricular diastolic pressure (·····). The high left atrial pressure at the onset of diastole increases the rapid filling rate, which accentuates the third heart sound (III) and causes a short flow murmur (FM).

pressure to rise throughout ventricular systole (Fig. 20.4). It can easily be appreciated that diversion of a portion of the left ventricular output in an abnormal direction, into the left atrium, tends to reduce cardiac output. While the regulatory mechanisms in the systemic circulation maintain mean aortic pressure at or very near a normal level, cardiac output is progressively diminished as mitral insufficiency increases in severity.

The regurgitant flow in rheumatic mitral insufficiency characteristically causes considerable turbulence and so is associated with a pansystolic (holosystolic) murmur, these names implying that the murmur lasts throughout ventricular systole as shown in Fig. 20.4. This regurgitant blood flow must be returned to the left ventricle during diastole, where it is added to the normal forward stroke volume that has also entered the left atrium from the lungs during the cardiac cycle. As a result of this increase in left ventricular filling, mitral insufficiency causes a "volume overload" in which each left ventricular contraction pumps the forward stroke volume into the aorta and, in addition, an abnormal regurgitant volume back into the left atrium.

There are other conditions besides rheumatic heart disease that can give rise to mitral insufficiency. One of these is *Barlow's syndrome* in which a midsystolic "click" is followed by a murmur late in systole. This abnormality is often caused by a "floppy" mitral valve in which the fibrous and elastic tissue of the valve degenerates. In these cases the click represents a sudden abnormal valve opening during midsystole, when left ventricular pressure is at its highest, while the late onset of the murmur occurs because the insufficiency is not present prior to this time. Another cause of mitral regurgitation is papillary muscle insufficiency in which loss of contractility of one or more of the papillary muscles—often caused by ischemic heart disease (Chapter 22)—causes the mitral valve to lose its support and so to become leaky. When mild, papillary muscle insufficiency can produce a crescendo (increasing in intensity) murmur that begins in midsystole. When severe, papillary muscle insufficiency usually causes a pansystolic murmur. In some cases of very severe mitral insufficiency, as when a papillary muscle ruptures—due, for example, to myocardial infarction (Chapter 22)—the systolic murmur may be very faint as the wide open mitral valve orifice may fail to generate enough turbulence to produce a loud noise even though the regurgitant flow is grossly increased. This finding illustrates the point that the intensity of a murmur is only a rough guide to the severity of the underlying hemodynamic abnormality.

It can be appreciated that because both the forward stroke volume and the abnormal (backward) regurgitant volume must be pumped with each left ventricular contraction, the diastolic filling of the ventricle is increased in mitral insufficiency. This has two major consequences. First, the left ventricle becomes dilated by the abnormal preload, so that end-diastolic left ventricular and left atrial pressures rise (Fig. 20.4). Second, the torrential flow of blood across the mitral valve during early diastole, which must occur to allow both the forward stroke volume and the regurgitant volume to enter the left ventricle, accentuates the third heart sound. (Remember that this sound is produced by rapid ventricular filling.) The torrential flow across the mitral valve also causes a short diastolic murmur. The latter, often attributed somewhat misleadingly to "relative mitral stenosis," arises because an increased flow of blood passes through a normal (or nearly normal) size mitral valve orifice. A better name for this short diastolic murmur is "flow murmur."

> Mitral flow murmurs are associated with a number of conditions, in addition to mitral insufficiency, that increase mitral blood flow. These include ventricular septal defect and patent ductus arteriosus. Flow murmurs are also heard over the tricuspid valve in conditions like tricuspid insufficiency and atrial septal defect, where blood flow from the right atrium to the right ventricle is increased.

Although mitral flow murmurs occur during diastole, they are usually distinguished easily from the diastolic murmurs of mitral stenosis by their brevity. Thus even though an abnormally large volume of blood flows across the mitral valve early during diastole, the normal valve orifice is able to transmit this increased volume of blood at a rate sufficiently rapid for left atrial and ventricular pressures to equilibrate quickly. Mitral flow murmurs therefore are brief in duration.

Unlike mitral stenosis, which places no abnormal load on the left ventricle, mitral insufficiency leads to both dilatation and hypertrophy of the left ventricle. Dilatation is an inevitable consequence of mitral insufficiency as a large end-diastolic volume is needed to accommodate the abnormally large volume of blood that must be pumped during each cardiac cycle (see above). Dilatation also reflects the operation of the Frank-Starling relationship, which helps the ventricle to meet this demand for increased stroke work. The stimulus that leads to left ventricular hypertrophy—which represents an increased left ventricular mass caused by the individual muscle fibers enlarging in order to provide additional contractile elements to meet the augmented work load—is not well understood. Possible causal mechanisms of initiating cardiac hypertrophy include the increased wall tension (which occurs even when left ventricular systolic pressure is normal, due to the operation of the law of Laplace; Chapter 12), stretching of the muscle fibers, and relative myocardial hypoxia or energy lack due to the increased work load. Whatever the initiating factor or factors, hypertrophy allows the increased demands for left ventricular work to be distributed among a greater number of contractile elements and so reduces the load on each (Eq. 12.4).

AORTIC STENOSIS

Unlike diseases of the mitral valve, which alter the relationship between left atrial and left ventricular pressures, diseases of the aortic valve directly alter the relationship between pressures and flows in the aorta and left ventricle. Changes in left atrial pressure accompany these abnormalities but are secondary to the overloading of the left ventricle.

The direct effects of aortic stenosis are related to the impediment to blood flow across the aortic valve. One might expect to see both a rise in left ventricular pressure and a fall in aortic pressure in this condition, but the compensatory mechanisms that control the pressures in the systemic arterial circulation tend to maintain mean aortic pressure at or near a normal level (Chapter 21). For this reason the most prominent hemodynamic abnormalities in aortic stenosis are a rise in left ventricular pressure caused by a large pressure gradient across the aortic valve during the phases of ejection (Fig. 20.5) and a fall in cardiac output.

Although mean aortic pressure is maintained by adjustments of the cardiovascular system in patients with aortic stenosis, slowing of ejection causes a modest fall in aortic pulse pressure. This is associated with reduction in the rate at which aortic pressure rises (Fig. 20.5). The resulting slowly rising, low-amplitude aortic pulse (called an anacrotic pulse) is characteristic of aortic stenosis. This abnormality can be appreciated by carefully palpating the pulse in such patients.

Aortic stenosis is characterized by a systolic murmur that increases in intensity during early systole as ejection rate increases, then decreases during late systole as ejection slows. The resulting "ejection murmur" is typically diamond-shaped (Fig. 20.5). The ejection murmur of aortic stenosis is therefore usually easy to distinguish from the pansystolic murmur of mitral insufficiency. (Aortic ejection murmurs also are usually heard at different locations over the chest, are transmitted in different directions, and are harsher in tone than mitral pansystolic murmurs.)

The characteristic diamond shape of the aortic ejection murmur can be understood if it is remembered that aortic and left ventricular pressures are identical at both the beginning and end of ventricular ejection. At these times there is no pressure gradient across the stenotic aortic valve and thus no turbulence of flow. The aortic valve gradient becomes maximal during midsystole when the pressure in the left ventricle reaches its peak (Fig. 20.5), so that the murmur is loudest at this time. In contrast, the abnormal flow of blood across the mitral valve in mitral insufficiency takes place between a high-pressure chamber (the left ventricle) and a low-pressure chamber (the left atrium), so there is a large pressure gradient from the end of the brief phase of isovolumic contraction to the beginning of isovolumic relaxation. For this reason the mitral pansystolic murmur lasts longer than the aortic ejection murmur and is more nearly constant in amplitude throughout systole.

Aortic stenosis causes a "pressure overload" on the left ventricle; i.e., left ventricular systolic pressure must increase in order to force blood through the narrowed aortic valve into the aorta. The resulting increase in left ventricular systolic pressure increases ventricular wall tension, so more tension must be developed by each muscle fiber in the walls of the left ventricle. One might expect the increased left ventricular work load to be overcome partly through dilatation of this chamber, so increased left ventricular volume could, through operation of the Frank-Starling relationship, increase the ability of the heart to meet the overload. There are many theoretical disadvantages to this compensatory mechanism, as is apparent from the considerations discussed in Chapter 12. Because the elevation of left ventricular pressure in aortic stenosis causes the tension on the muscle fibers of the left ventricle to increase, the efficiency of left ventricular

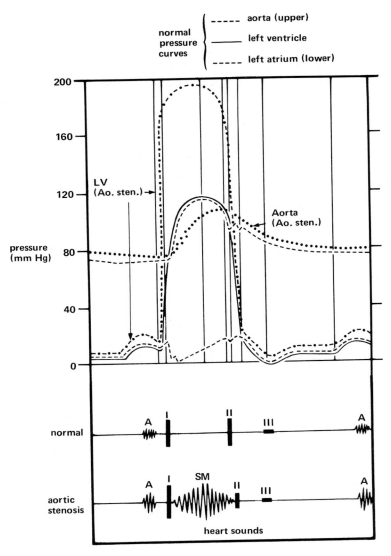

normal
pressure
curves
{
    ----- aorta (upper)
    ——— left ventricle
    ----- left atrium (lower)
}

FIG. 20.5. Aortic stenosis. Obstruction to blood flow across the aortic valve causes an abnormal systolic pressure gradient and marked elevation of left ventricular systolic pressure (·—·—·). Mean aortic pressure in aortic stenosis is essentially normal, but the aortic pulse pressure is reduced and the upstroke of the aortic pressure curve (·····) is slowed (anacrotic pulse). Blood flow across the stenotic aortic valve causes a systolic ejection murmur (SM), and the atrial sound (A) is often accentuated when the left atrium contracts against the "stiff," hypertrophied left ventricle. (The abnormal left atrial pressure curve is not shown here, as left atrial diastolic pressure is only slightly higher than that in the left ventricle.) The amplitude of the aortic second sound is often reduced by the aortic valve abnormality.

contraction is reduced. Were the left ventricle to undergo dilatation, the consequences of the law of Laplace would increase wall tension to still higher levels, thereby causing a further loss of muscular efficiency. It is probably for these reasons—although how this is achieved remains a mystery—that the left ventricle in aortic stenosis is characterized not by dilatation but by hypertrophy. As a result of this hypertrophy, left ventricular wall thickness is increased while cavity size remains virtually normal. Hypertrophy also allows the abnormally high pressure to be developed by a greater number of myofibrils, thereby reducing the load on each. The law of Laplace [Eq. (12.4)] states that wall tension increases with increasing left ventricular pressure and radius but decreases as the walls of the left ventricle become thickened. These considerations probably account for the common finding that in severe aortic stenosis prior to the onset of left heart failure (Chapter 21) the compensatory mechanisms available to the heart cause such massive hypertrophy of the walls of the left ventricle that left ventricular volume is increased very little if at all.

One consequence of the compensatory mechanism just described is that left ventricular stroke volume tends to become fixed. This occurs because the ability of the left ventricle to accommodate an increased end-diastolic volume becomes impaired as the hypertrophied muscle becomes noncompliant (stiff). At the same time, the ability of the ventricle to reduce its end-systolic volume (as, for example, when contractility is increased; Chapter 13) is lessened by the pressure overload and by the massively thickened left ventricular walls. For these reasons patients with severe aortic stenosis often experience a fall in systemic arterial blood pressure when muscular exercise causes peripheral vasodilation. Thus an inability of the left ventricle to increase its stroke volume in order to fill the systemic arterial circulation under these circumstances often causes the patient to faint (syncope).

Marked dilation of the left ventricle in patients with aortic stenosis is seen only when the compensatory mechanisms described in the preceding paragraphs become exhausted. This can occur when the aortic valve orifice becomes severely narrowed, when myocardial damage develops in patients with a longstanding pressure overload (Chapter 21), or when both are present. The relatively late occurrence of dilation in the pressure-overloaded left ventricle, which in aortic stenosis is an ominous sign that heralds a fatal outcome within months or a few years, contrasts with the left ventricular dilation that *inevitably* accompanies the diastolic overloading caused by mitral (see above) or aortic (see below) insufficiency. In the latter conditions the left ventricular cavity must dilate in order to accommodate the regurgitant volume of blood that has to be pumped, in addition to the forward stroke volume, with each beat. For this reason, *although both volume and pressure overloads lead to left ventricular hypertrophy, only the former requires that left ventricular end-diastolic volume be increased.*

The fact that aortic stenosis is accompanied by an increase in left ventricular wall thickness (and when the condition is longstanding, by fibrosis of its walls) contributes to the rise in left atrial systolic pressure usually seen in aortic stenosis.

Elevation of left atrial systolic pressure, which is accompanied by a corresponding increase in left ventricular pressure during the phase of atrial systole (Fig. 20.5), occurs because the ability of the ventricle to accept blood pumped to it from the atrium is reduced by the decreased compliance of the left ventricle. The increased "stiffness" of the chronically hypertrophied left ventricle causes the energy transmitted to it during left atrial systole to appear as an abnormal rise in pressure rather than as increased left ventricular filling. A loud atrial sound (A, Fig. 20.5) is commonly produced by these hemodynamic phenomena.

Slowing of the upstroke of the aortic systolic pressure pulse (Fig. 20.5) is a characteristic finding in patients with aortic stenosis. The narrowed aortic valve delays the passage of blood from the left ventricle to the aorta and so causes a slowly rising central aortic pulse that can be readily appreciated when the carotid or brachial arteries are palpated. This abnormality in the aortic pulse is virtually diagnostic of aortic stenosis, and the degree of slowing of the upstroke provides a better indication of the severity of this condition than does the intensity of the systolic murmur. (Indeed, in *very* severe aortic stenosis stroke volume can fall to such an extent that the turbulence produced by the narrowed valve causes virtually no murmur. Under these conditions, however, the pulse remains slowly rising.)

AORTIC INSUFFICIENCY

When the aortic valve becomes incompetent (leaky), blood can flow backward from the aorta to the left ventricle during ventricular diastole. This abnormal flow of blood across the aortic valve occurs mainly during early diastole, when the pressure gradient between the aorta and left ventricle is maximal (Fig. 20.6). This regurgitant flow produces a high-pitched decrescendo (i.e., decreasing in intensity) *early diastolic murmur* that begins immediately after the aortic second heart sound (Fig. 20.6). The latter is often reduced in amplitude by the same deformity of the aortic valve leaflets that produces the valve insufficiency.

The arterial pulse pressure in aortic insufficiency is widened. Systolic pressure in the aorta is elevated because both the stroke volume and the rate of ejection by the left ventricle are increased (see below), while the aortic diastolic pressure is reduced due to regurgitation of blood across the aortic valve during diastole. The lowered aortic diastolic pressure allows left ventricular ejection to begin somewhat earlier than usual, thereby shortening the phase of isovolumic contraction. The rapid, early ejection of blood into the aorta at a reduced aortic pressure is probably responsible for the finding that the peak of aortic pressure occurs earlier during the ejection phase than normal, and is followed by a "systolic collapse" in which aortic pressure begins to fall rapidly later during systole. These abnormalities give rise to a characteristic "collapsing" pulse, which is readily appreciated by palpating the carotid or brachial arteries of patients with aortic insufficiency. When this lesion is severe, an extremely rapid upstroke of the arterial pulse is followed by an abrupt decline in pressure, producing a "water

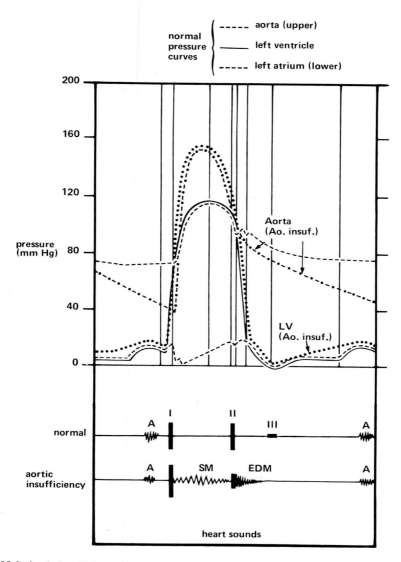

FIG. 20.6. Aortic insufficiency. Regurgitation of blood through the aortic valve during diastole produces an early diastolic murmur (EDM) and causes aortic pressure (·-·-·-·) to fall throughout diastole. Aortic and left ventricular (·····) pressures are increased during systole because an abnormally increased stroke volume must be ejected by the left ventricle. The increased flow rate across the aortic valve during ejection often causes a soft systolic ejection murmur (SM). Left ventricular and left atrial diastolic pressures are also increased by the augmented diastolic filling of the left ventricle caused by the regurgitation of blood from the aorta.

hammer pulse." (The pulse feels like an old-fashioned water hammer toy—a hollow, evacuated tube half-filled with water in which, when the tube is tipped from end to end, the column of water drops abruptly through the vacuum to strike the bottom of the tube with a sharp blow like a hammer.)

Aortic insufficiency represents a volume overload on the left ventricle because with each cardiac cycle the left ventricle must pump not only the blood that enters from the left atrium as the normal stroke volume but also the abnormal flow of blood that has entered from the aorta. This increased stroke volume, while passing through the deformed aortic valve, commonly causes a turbulence that produces an aortic ejection murmur (Fig. 20.6). This murmur can be extremely loud, even in the absence of coexistent aortic stenosis, but should not interfere with making a correct diagnosis of aortic insufficiency because of both the decrescendo early diastolic murmur and especially the characteristic collapsing pulse of aortic insufficiency. The latter, like the slowly rising pulse of aortic stenosis, is thus a better index to the severity of the aortic insufficiency than are the characteristics of the early diastolic murmur.

SUMMARY

The four simple lesions described in this chapter were selected because they illustrate the way in which knowledge of the Wiggers diagram can aid in evaluating and analyzing the clinical manifestations of valvular heart disease. In this introductory text, it is not necessary to extend this list of examples or to add further classes of abnormalities such as those caused by the shunting of blood between various chambers of the heart, or between the heart and great vessels that occur in congenital heart disease. It should be emphasized, however, that the Wiggers diagram is even more useful for understanding the signs and symptoms of the more complex forms of heart disease than it is for the simple abnormalities discussed in this chapter. Without a full understanding of the normal physiology of the heart, the signs and symptoms of heart disease represent merely dull lists of facts to be memorized, whereas application of the principles of cardiac physiology to the clinical problems posed by patients with heart disease can be intellectually rewarding and, more importantly, a critical guide to the correct diagnosis and proper treatment of these patients. Furthermore, by careful physical examination at the bedside, the physician can gain a surprisingly precise knowledge of both the nature of the hemodynamic lesion and its severity.

BIBLIOGRAPHY

Hurst, J. W., Logue, R. B., Schlant, R. A., and Wenger, N. K., editors (1974): *The Heart, Arteries and Veins.* McGraw-Hill, New York.
Leon, D. F., and Shaver, J. A. (1975): *Physiologic Principles of Heart Sounds and Murmurs.* AHA Monograph No. 46. American Heart Association, New York.
Wood, P. (1954): An appreciation of mitral stenosis. *Br. Med. J.,* 1:1051–1063, 1113–1124. [A true classic!]
Wood, P. (1956): *Diseases of the Heart and Circulation.* Lippincott, Philadelphia.
Silber, E. N., and Katz, L. N. (1975): *Heart Disease.* Macmillan, New York.

21

Heart Failure

The heart transfers blood coming to the ventricles from the low-pressure reservoirs of the systemic and pulmonary veins into regions of high pressure in the pulmonary artery and aorta by its pumping action (Fig. 21.1). When cardiac performance is impaired, therefore, the consequences can be twofold: (a) failure to empty the venous reservoirs, and (b) reduced delivery of blood under pressure into the pulmonary artery and aorta. This rather simplified view of cardiac function and its modification by heart failure permits the major signs and symptoms of this condition to be understood.

When the heart fails, four primary changes can occur: systemic venous pressure and pulmonary venous pressure can rise, and the ejection of blood into the pulmonary artery and aorta can be reduced (Table 21.1). If the right ventricular pump alone were to fail, the resulting "right heart failure" would cause systemic venous pressure to rise and the ejection of blood into the pulmonary artery to decrease. In the case of pure "left heart failure," pulmonary venous pressure would rise and ejection of blood into the aorta would decrease. Neither right nor left heart failure can occur in a pure form, however, because the ventricles are arranged in series within the circulation. For this reason a decrease in right ventricular function not only leads to a rise in systemic venous pressure but because of the reduced right ventricular output the work of the left ventricle also decreases (Fig. 21.2). In the case of left ventricular failure, right ventricular function is lessened by the fall in left ventricular output; in addition, the right ventricle encounters an abnormal pressure load produced by the elevated pulmonary venous pressure, which is transmitted through the lungs to increase pulmonary arterial pressure (Fig. 21.3). For this reason, although right or left heart failure can predominate in a given patient, in all cases the circulation as a whole, including the dynamics of function in the opposite ventricle, becomes disordered.

The fact that blood moves in a circle also tends to diminish the heuristic value of a once prevalent concept that a dichotomy existed between "forward failure" and "backward failure." Backward failure describes those signs and symptoms due to the rise in pulmonary and systemic venous pressure that results from failure of the ventricles to empty the veins (Fig. 21.4). When they are due to heart failure (as distinct from certain forms of circulatory failure; see below), they are regularly accompanied by a fall in cardiac output and thus some of the clinical features of forward failure.

A reduction in the ability of the ventricles to deliver blood under pressure into the arterial systems (forward failure) is almost always manifest initially by a fall

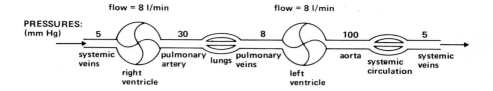

THE NORMAL CIRCULATION

FIG. 21.1. The normal circulation. Reading from left to right, the systemic veins empty into the right ventricle, which pumps blood through the pulmonary artery to the lungs. Blood returns via the pulmonary veins to the left ventricle from which it is pumped into the systemic circulation via the aorta. Efflux from the systemic circulation returns to the right ventricle via the systemic veins. As the blood moves continuously in a circle, the outputs of the two ventricles are equal, the normal cardiac output *(above)* being approximately 8 liters/min. Normal mean pressures are approximately 5 mm Hg in the systemic veins, 30 mm Hg in the pulmonary artery, 8 mm Hg in the pulmonary veins, and 100 mm Hg in the aorta.

in cardiac output. If forward failure existed in a "pure" state, uncomplicated by other cardiovascular adjustments, then regardless of the ventricle primarily involved the condition would cause a decrease in cardiac output (Fig. 21.5). A decline in ventricular work can of course also lead to a reduction in ejection pressure (Chapter 11), so that one might expect blood pressure, as well as cardiac output, to be reduced in forward failure. A decline in arterial pressure, however, is a very late sign in the evolution of the clinical picture of heart failure because virtually all of the compensatory mechanisms available to the heart and circulatory system operate to maintain perfusion pressure (instead of cardiac output) as near normal as is feasible. In this way these circulatory adjustments provide pressure for the maintenance of blood flow to vital organs.

As encountered in clinical practice, heart failure assumes various characteristics, depending on both the cause of the disorder in cardiac function and on the compensatory mechanisms which operate in the individual patient. Most commonly, heart failure is caused by decreased left ventricular performance such as occurs in valvular heart diseases like aortic stenosis, chronic overloading caused by arterial hypertension, and myocardial disease such as that caused by ischemic heart disease. In these conditions the predominant alterations in circulatory

TABLE 21.1. *Primary changes in heart failure*

Site of failure	Backward failure	Forward failure
Right heart failure	Increased systemic venous pressure	Reduced ejection into pulmonary artery
Left heart failure	Increased pulmonary venous pressure	Reduced ejection into aorta

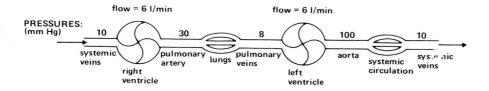

RIGHT HEART FAILURE

FIG. 21.2. "Right heart failure." Impaired pumping by the right ventricle causes the output of both ventricles to be reduced so that cardiac output falls, e.g., to 6 liters/min. Systemic venous pressure rises (e.g., to 10 mm Hg) because right ventricular end-diastolic pressure is increased, but circulatory reflexes tend to maintain mean pulmonary artery pressure and left ventricular end-diastolic pressure at virtually normal levels.

function include a rise in pulmonary venous pressure and a fall in cardiac output. These are complicated by a greater or lesser degree of pulmonary arterial hypertension, which by impairing right ventricular output leads to increased systemic venous pressure. Only in very severe cases is there a significant fall in systemic arterial pressure. A moderately severe example of this condition is shown in Fig. 21.6.

SIGNS AND SYMPTOMS OF HEART FAILURE

The clinical picture of heart failure consists of *signs*, which are objective manifestations of depressed cardiac performance, and *symptoms*, which are abnormalities perceived by the patient. The most important signs of heart failure are usually produced when reduced pumping by the right heart causes systemic venous pressure to rise. The major symptoms of heart failure, on the other hand,

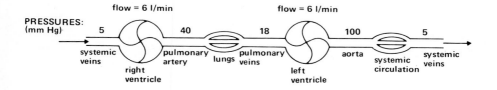

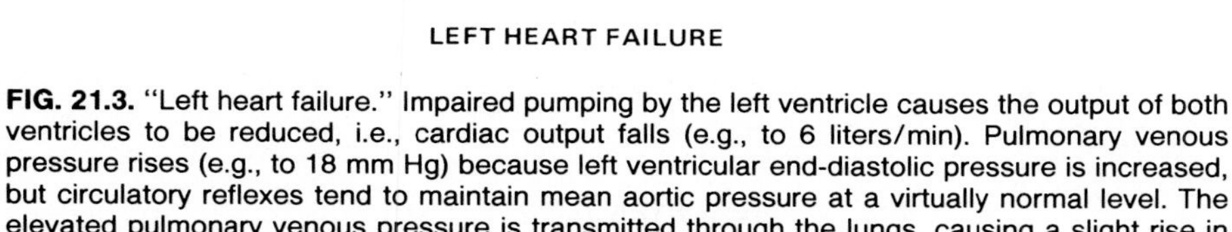

LEFT HEART FAILURE

FIG. 21.3. "Left heart failure." Impaired pumping by the left ventricle causes the output of both ventricles to be reduced, i.e., cardiac output falls (e.g., to 6 liters/min). Pulmonary venous pressure rises (e.g., to 18 mm Hg) because left ventricular end-diastolic pressure is increased, but circulatory reflexes tend to maintain mean aortic pressure at a virtually normal level. The elevated pulmonary venous pressure is transmitted through the lungs, causing a slight rise in mean pulmonary artery pressure, e.g., to 40 mm Hg.

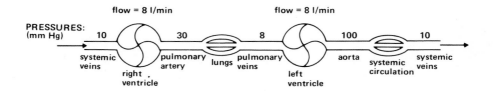

A. "BACKWARD FAILURE" OF THE RIGHT HEART

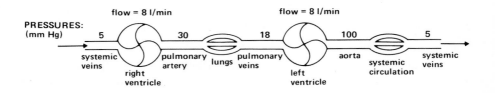

B. "BACKWARD FAILURE" OF THE LEFT HEART

FIG. 21.4. "Backward failure." "Pure" backward failure of the right heart (A) would increase systemic venous pressure (e.g., to 10 mm Hg) without causing other abnormalities. "Pure" backward failure of the left heart (B) would increase pulmonary venous pressure (e.g., to 18 mm Hg) without causing other abnormalities.

are due mainly to the elevated pulmonary venous pressure and fall in cardiac output that result from impaired pumping by the left heart.

The manifestations of severe heart failure are recognized as a syndrome called *congestive heart failure.* This syndrome, or constellation of signs and symptoms, is the most common but not the only way in which impairment of cardiac performance appears in clinical practice. The patient with congestive heart failure is characteristically troubled by symptoms of weakness, fatigue, and shortness of breath. The latter is usually called dyspnea (difficulty in breathing). Examination of such patients typically reveals a small rapid pulse, an enlarged heart,

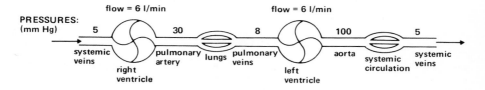

"FORWARD FAILURE"

FIG. 21.5. "Forward failure." "Pure" forward failure of either ventricle would reduce cardiac output (e.g., to 6 liters/min) without causing other abnormalities.

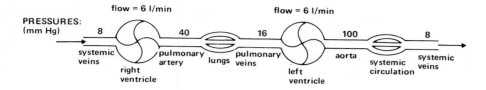

PRESSURES:
(mm Hg)

flow = 6 l/min   flow = 6 l/min

8   40   16   100   8

systemic veins   pulmonary artery   lungs   pulmonary veins   aorta   systemic circulation   systemic veins

right ventricle   left ventricle

CLINICAL HEART FAILURE

FIG. 21.6. Clinical heart failure. As encountered in most patients, heart failure is due to impaired pumping of the left ventricle. When moderately severe, heart failure is accompanied by a fall in cardiac output (e.g., to 6 liters/min), significant elevation of pulmonary venous pressure (e.g., to 16 mm Hg), modest elevation of mean pulmonary artery (e.g., to 40 mm Hg), and systemic venous (e.g., to 8 mm Hg) pressures, with no significant abnormality in mean aortic pressure.

elevated systemic venous pressure, and an enlarged liver; there is often fluid (edema) in the dependent parts of the body, the abdominal cavity (ascites), and the pleural space which surrounds the lungs (pleural effusion). When a stethoscope is applied to the chest of such patients, bubbling sounds (rales) are commonly heard during respiration. The latter sign signifies the presence of fluid that has entered the air passages of the lungs from the pulmonary capillaries because of the elevated pulmonary venous pressure. Although this clinical picture is not produced only by heart failure, and heart failure does not invariably give rise to all of these signs and symptoms, the following paragraphs focus on the way in which impairment of the pumping action of the heart produces the typical signs and symptoms described above.

The signs and symptoms of heart failure are characteristically exacerbated by physical or emotional stress. The degree of such stress needed for their provocation depends on the extent to which cardiac performance is impaired. When cardiac function is only mildly disordered, these manifestations are absent under ordinary conditions, appearing only during extreme stress. As the pumping action of the heart becomes progressively more severely impaired, the degree of stress needed to provoke them becomes less until, when cardiac function is severely impaired, this picture becomes manifest even at rest. For this reason the amount of physical exertion needed to provoke the clinical features of heart failure serves as a very useful index as to the severity, although not necessarily the nature, of the underlying heart disease. This generalization does not always hold, however, as some of the features of congestive heart failure are more readily provoked than others, and a number of complicating factors, notably salt and water retention by the kidney, can modify this relationship. For example, the way in which circulatory reflexes and other compensatory mechanisms adjust for the decline in cardiac performance varies greatly from one individual to another, and effective therapy reduces the signs and symptoms produced by a given degree of impaired cardiac function.

Certain of the key features of the clinical picture of heart failure are discussed here in terms of the mechanisms responsible for their production. This section does not, however, attempt to provide a comprehensive description of the clinical features of heart failure; for this the reader is referred to the many textbooks of clinical medicine and cardiology. The present discussion is intended only to illustrate the way in which disorders in the physiology and biophysics of the pumping action of the heart affect the cardiac patient, much as Chapters 15–18 attempted to illustrate the effects of disordered electrophysiological behavior on the ECG and on cardiac rate and rhythm.

Failure To Empty the Systemic Venous Reservoir

One of the major consequences of impairment of the pumping action of the right ventricle is reduced emptying of the reservoirs of blood in the great veins: the superior and inferior venae cavae. The cause of this failure to relieve the "back pressure" on the heart is readily apparent in Fig. 13.15, which shows the "family" of Starling curves. When the heart shifts to a lower Starling curve, as happens when right ventricular contractility is depressed (Fig. 21.7A) or when a hemodynamic overload causes the right ventricular myocardium to expend additional energy to eject blood normally (Fig. 21.7B), a greater filling pressure (end-diastolic pressure) is needed to achieve a given level of external work. In the absence of compensatory responses within the circulation, impairment of the pumping ability of the right ventricle causes right ventricular end-diastolic pressure to increase until the end-diastolic volumes reach levels that provide for an adequate right ventricular work output.

A reduction in right ventricular contractility is an unusual cause for impaired emptying of the systemic venous reservoir. Instead, the requirement for abnormally high levels of ventricular work is the more common cause of elevated systemic venous pressure in heart failure. Such increases in right ventricular work can occur when the pulmonary valve orifice is abnormally narrowed (pulmonic stenosis) or when there is regurgitation (insufficiency) of the tricuspid valve. Most commonly, the abnormally high levels of right ventricular work which lead to elevated systemic venous pressure in heart failure are caused by disorders of left ventricular function that lead to elevated pulmonary venous pressure and an increased resistance to blood flow through the lungs. A description of the mechanisms by which elevated pulmonary venous pressure leads to increased pulmonary artery resistance is beyond the scope of this text, but it should be noted that chronic left ventricular failure commonly leads to changes (both physiological and anatomical) in the small vessels of the lung that increase the resistance to blood flow through the lungs and thereby elevate pulmonary arterial pressure. For this reason the rise in right ventricular end-diastolic pressure that is characteristic of heart failure is usually not due to depressed right ventricular contractility (Fig. 21.7A) but is a part of the compensatory response by which the right ventricle overcomes an abnormally increased hemodynamic load (Fig. 21.7B) that is engendered by left ventricular disease.

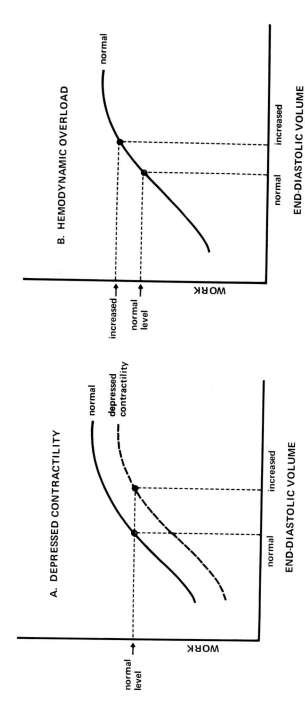

FIG. 21.7. Ventricular end-diastolic volume is increased at normal levels of cardiac work when contractility is impaired **(A)**, at increased work levels when contractility is normal **(B)**, or as the result of a combination of these situations. When end-diastolic volume increases because of depressed contractility, cardiac performance has shifted to a lower Starling curve **(A)**. When end-diastolic volume increases because of hemodynamic overload at a constant level of contractility, ventricular function has shifted along a normal Starling curve **(B)**. In most clinical cases of longstanding hemodynamic overloading, both contribute to the rise in end-diastolic volume because cardiac work increases and myocardial contractility is reduced.

When the work of the right ventricle is increased, its end-diastolic pressure also increases. This elevated "filling pressure" is transmitted throughout the systemic venous circulation and so is responsible for the distended neck veins and enlarged liver that are characteristic of the clinical syndrome of heart failure. Transmission of the increased hydrostatic pressure further "upstream" into the systemic capillaries increases intracapillary pressure, which in turn forces fluid from the capillaries into the surrounding tissues, causing edema, ascites, and pleural effusion.

Failure To Empty the Pulmonary Venous Reservoir

The mechanisms by which impaired pumping of the left ventricle causes an increased left ventricular end-diastolic pressure are the same as those described in relation to the right ventricle (Fig. 21.7). In contrast to the right ventricle, however, primary disorders of contractility comprise a more common cause of elevated filling pressures in the left ventricle (see below). In addition, ischemic heart disease represents a major cause for impaired left ventricular contractility (Chapter 22). Increased left ventricular work can also be responsible for the elevation of pulmonary venous pressure, as is the case in systemic hypertension or abnormalities such as aortic stenosis and insufficiency of the aortic or mitral valves (Chapter 20).

Increased left ventricular end-diastolic pressure increases left atrial and pulmonary venous pressures and so causes distention of the left atrium and pulmonary veins. The latter abnormalities are apparent on radiographic examination of the chest but only rarely give rise to recognizable signs. On the other hand, increased pressure in the pulmonary venous circulation causes dyspnea, a subjective sensation of difficulty in breathing related to transmission of the elevated left ventricular diastolic pressure "upstream" into the pulmonary capillaries. Here increased capillary pressure forces fluid into the walls and eventually the cavities of the alveoli, thereby impairing gas exchange by the lungs. In its milder form increased pulmonary capillary pressure and transudation of fluid into the alveoli are associated with dyspnea, although the way in which these abnormalities lead to the subjective awareness of breathing difficulty is still not fully understood.

When pulmonary capillary pressure is markedly elevated, pulmonary edema ensues. This condition, which occurs when an elevated pulmonary capillary pressure forces large amounts of fluid into the alveoli, is characterized by severe dyspnea accompanied in its late stages by the appearance of frothy fluid from the lungs in the mouth and nose of the patient. Ultimately pulmonary edema may be fatal, as the patient can literally drown in this fluid. These features of failure of pumping by the left ventricle can be understood as being caused directly by the elevated diastolic pressure in the left ventricle, which can result from impaired left ventricular contractility (Fig. 21.7A) and an increased work load on this ventricle (Fig. 21.7B), as well as from mitral stenosis (Chapter 20).

Cardiomegaly

Enlargement of the heart (cardiomegaly), which constitutes one of the important signs of heart failure, is readily understood in the light of the foregoing discussion. An increased end-diastolic volume is either or both ventricles, which accompanies hemodynamic overloading or impaired cardiac performance, as described above, leads directly to cardiomegaly. Cardiomegaly can be detected by physical examination and by a chest radiograph. This sign is an important feature in the clinical picture of heart failure, whether due to impaired myocardial contractility, an abnormal increase in the demands on the myocardium, or both.

Decreased Cardiac Work

The minute work of the heart can be estimated from the product $BP \times CO$ (Eq. 13.6). As mentioned earlier in this chapter, the initial effect of a decrease in cardiac work by the failing heart usually manifests almost entirely as a reduction in cardiac output. Blood pressure remains at or near its normal level in all but the most severe forms of heart failure, although pulse pressure (the difference between systolic and diastolic blood pressures) tends to fall because of the reduced stroke volume. A significant fall in mean blood pressure in a patient with heart failure is usually a terminal event in the evolution of this condition and generally heralds the impending death of the patient. The clinical finding that mean blood pressure is maintained at or near normal levels in patients in whom impaired cardiac performance can reduce cardiac output to one-third of normal or less reflects the fact that many vital organs cease to function if blood pressure falls. For example, a fall in mean blood pressure from its normal level of 90–100 to 70–80 mm Hg causes confusion and impaired consciousness owing to impaired blood flow to the brain. The same or a slightly greater reduction in mean blood pressure causes severe damage to the kidneys. For this reason the resistance vessels in various regions of the systemic circulation compensate for the reduced cardiac performance in heart failure by restricting blood flow to other, less critical organs (e.g., the skin and skeletal muscles) so as to maintain blood pressure at levels that ensure adequate perfusion of vital organs like the brain, kidneys, and the heart itself.

Reduction of blood flow to the muscles is largely responsible for the symptoms of weakness and fatigue associated with heart failure. When the impairment of cardiac pumping is mild, these symptoms appear only during exercise. Measurement of cardiac output in such patients shows that while resting cardiac output may be only slightly reduced the ability to increase cardiac output during exercise is much less than normal, as is the ability to increase the maximal level of total energy expenditure by the body during exercise. Reduced blood flow to the skin in heart failure causes the common finding of cool extremities.

The preceding descriptions represent only a partial list of the signs and symptoms of heart failure. They should, however, provide an indication as to the way in which these and other signs and symptoms encountered in patients with heart failure can be related to the disordered pumping action of the heart and ultimately to the derangements in the normal physiology and biophysics of the heart described in the earlier chapters of this book.

CAUSES OF HEART FAILURE

A large number of abnormalities can cause the signs and symptoms of heart failure described above. For this reason heart failure is not a distinct pathophysiological entity, but instead represents only one stage in the progressive deterioration of cardiac function caused by primary disorders of myocardial function (i.e., intrinsic myocardial disease) or by chronic overloading of the myocardium. With the exception of the cardiomyopathies, which are poorly understood disorders involving primarily a loss of contractility within the heart muscle itself (see below), the constellation of signs and symptoms generally recognized as heart failure appears when the myocardium is no longer able to overcome a sustained hemodynamic overload. Such conditions of cardiac overloading can occur when one or more of the heart valves become stenotic (narrowed) or insufficient (leaky), or when there is abnormal shunting of blood between the chambers of the heart. Heart failure can also develop in systemic and pulmonary hypertension, where resistance to blood flow is abnormally increased in the systemic or pulmonary circulations, or in the face of other conditions that lead to chronic and excessive demands on the myocardium. Similarly, when a significant fraction of the heart muscle is damaged because of ischemic heart disease, heart failure becomes apparent when the nonischemic regions of the heart become unable to carry out the pumping action of the heart adequately.

Circulatory Failure, Heart Failure, Myocardial Failure

It is important, both clinically and conceptually, to distinguish between circulatory failure, heart failure, and myocardial failure, three settings in which the signs and symptoms of heart failure can appear. In *circulatory failure* the clinical picture of heart failure can appear even though the capacity for cardiac function is normal or very nearly so. One can easily appreciate that infusion of large quantities of salt and water into the veins would eventually cause the pressures in the systemic and pulmonary veins to rise in any individual, thereby producing many but not all of the signs and symptoms of heart failure. Indeed, the unwary physician can be misled by the findings in some patients in whom large amounts of fluid are retained due, for example, to diseases of the liver or kidney. The resulting edema, ascites, and pleural effusion, which are often associated with dyspnea, may be erroneously attributed to heart failure. Although the circulation in such patients is clearly abnormal, the forms of circulatory failure described above must be distinguished from that of *heart failure,* in which similar signs and symptoms of circulatory failure arise from an abnormality in the pumping action of the heart. In other words, while heart failure typically produces the signs and symptoms of congestive heart failure, not all patients with this syndrome are suffering from disordered cardiac function.

Even more difficult than the distinction between circulatory failure due to noncardiac causes and that resulting from heart failure is evaluation of the role of *myocardial failure* in producing the clinical syndrome of heart failure. Heart failure can occur in the absence of abnormalities in the contractile properties of the heart muscle. In traumatic rupture of the aortic valve, such as may occur during an automobile accident, the clinical picture of heart failure, which develops suddenly, can hardly be attributed to an abnormality of myocardial performance in the patient in whom, minutes before an accident, cardiac function was normal. In clinical practice, however, it is extremely difficult to define the role of myocardial failure in producing the signs and symptoms in most cases of heart failure. Thus acute mitral insufficiency due to a ruptured leaflet of the mitral valve may be confused with a fulminating cardiomyopathy in which the rapid onset of myocardial weakness can produce a significant degree of mitral insufficiency. In most patients with cardiomyopathy, evidence can be obtained to rule out causes for congestive heart failure other than myocardial failure. Yet in patients with heart failure secondary to chronic valvular or other structural heart disease, the clinical picture is generally clouded by the coexistence of some degree of myocardial failure. These complicating disorders of myocardial function themselves, in addition to representing a major cause of clinical disability, may also prevent recovery after the primary defects are successfully repaired surgically.

It is now well established that any condition which causes sustained hyperfunction by the myocardium can lead to a decline in myocardial contractility. As a result, contractile function becomes significantly impaired in patients in whom the myocardium is subjected to longstanding hemodynamic overloading, as well as in cases of primary myocardial disease (i.e., the cardiomyopathies).

Cardiomyopathies

One of the open frontiers in cardiology is the systematic study of the diseases of cardiac muscle that produce the cardiomyopathies. Both the disorders that cause the myocardial weakness, which is the hallmark of the cardiomyopathies, and the mechanism by which these diseases lead to impaired myocardial contractility are very poorly understood.

A number of etiological classifications of the cardiomyopathies can be found in the literature and in standard clinical textbooks. While these differ in many important details, almost all include a list of the sort given in Table 21.2. Little or nothing can be gained within the context of our objectives by further discussion of these many and, for the large part, poorly understood causes of cardiomyopathy. It suffices to emphasize that the causation of these devastating and often fatal disorders of cardiac function continues to represent one of the major challenges to the student of cardiac function.

TABLE 21.2. *Causes of the cardiomyopathies*

Inflammatory diseases
  Due to infectious agents
  Associated with systemic diseases
  Unknown

Noninflammatory diseases
  Associated with metabolic or hormonal disorders
  Associated with hereditary disorders
  Due to physical or chemical agents
  Due to infiltration of myocardium with nonmuscle cells
  Unknown

In addition to the etiological classifications, the cardiomyopathies can be subdivided in terms of their clinical features. Goodwin described two clinical classes: *congestive cardiomyopathy,* in which the primary abnormality is ventricular dilation due to loss of contractility, and *hypertrophic cardiomyopathy,* in which the abnormality is primarily ventricular hypertrophy that is inappropriate (i.e., there is no hemodynamic overload to account for this response). The latter conditions, which are commonly familial, include idiopathic hypertrophic subaortic stenosis in which septal hypertrophy obstructs left ventricular outflow, thereby causing a picture that is similar in some ways to valvular aortic stenosis (Chapter 20). It is probably useful to consider also a third class—*restrictive cardiomyopathy*—as primary endocardial thickening or infiltrative diseases of the myocardium can produce a distinctive clinical syndrome. Although useful in aiding the physician in prognostication and choice of therapy, this clinical classification provides little direct understanding of the abnormal mechanisms which underline these conditions.

Sparse as the knowledge of the causes of cardiomyopathy is, our understanding of the mechanisms by which the different etiological factors give rise to the clinically evident myocardial dysfunction is even less adequate. In the case of certain infections and toxic etiologies, the mechanism leading to cardiac failure is probably simple cell destruction. Because the myocardium heals poorly and the adult heart lacks the ability to regenerate new myocardial cells, severe cellular damage leads to necrosis and eventually to replacement of contractile tissue by fibrous tissue. Simple death of myocardial cells, however, appears to give rise to a minority of the cases of cardiomyopathy seen in clinical practice. In many if not most such patients, the primary causes appear to lie in disorders of one or more of the processes (described in the earlier chapters of this book) which underlie normal cardiac function.

Advances in our understanding of these disease processes is now limited primarily by the inability of investigators to obtain cardiac tissue samples for detailed study, although recent progress in achieving safe methods for cardiac biopsy offers considerable promise that these disorders can soon come under rational study. The difficulty in defining meaningful hypotheses concerning possible mechanisms for the loss of myocardial function has now been overcome, as must be apparent to those who have read the first 13 chapters of this volume. Indeed, the problem is now that there are *too many* useful hypotheses to test, so that the investigator presented with a few milligrams of myocardial tissue from a patient suffering from one of the poorly understood forms of this condition (e.g., a hereditary cardiomyopathy) would be hard pressed to know where to begin a systematic study. Each of the growing number of well-characterized reactions involved in cardiac muscle contraction and its control (Chapters 5–11) represents a possible site for pathological change that could impair myocardial contractility. Abnormalities of any of the contractile proteins or in any of a number of calcium transport processes could give rise to the reduced myocardial contractility that characterizes the cardiomyopathies. If one adds to this growing list the many reactions involved in energy production (Chapters 3 and 4), the search for the basic defect in various forms of cardiomyopathy resembles the proverbial search for a needle in a haystack. Characterization of the pathophysiology of the cardiomyopathies is therefore now hindered as much by the large number of possible causal mechanisms as by a lack of hypotheses worthy of detailed investigation.

Progress in understanding this important group of diseases will probably remain slow until means to define specific functional defects can be found that do not require the removal of relatively large samples of cardiac muscle. Unfortunately, the early promise of cardiac mechanics in narrowing the search for specific abnormalities in various forms of cardiomyopathy has not fulfilled initial expectations. Other approaches to the definition of specific functional abnormalities in the intact myocardium are appearing, however. These approaches, which stem from the apparent safety of cardiac biopsy and from careful analysis of direct measurements, offer hope for a better understanding of pathogenesis and thus for prevention and cure of some forms of cardiomyopathy. Further refinements in existing methodology, possibly aided by new concepts coming from unexpected directions, offer promise that knowledge of the causes, and thus means to prevent and treat the cardiomyopathies, are within the grasp of the dedicated scholars in this field.

MYOCARDIAL FAILURE DUE TO LONGSTANDING OVERLOADING OF THE HEART [1]

The most common cause of depressed myocardial function is sustained hemodynamic overloading of the heart. Whether due to systemic or pulmonary hypertension, valvular heart disease, or loss of functional myocardial tissue (as in ischemic heart disease), chronic overloading of cardiac muscle calls into play a number of mechanisms that compensate for the increased expenditure of mechanical energy. To meet the increased rate of utilization of mechanical energy, the rate of production of chemical energy by the myocardium also must be increased. Yet the energy-generating capacity of the myocardium is limited,

---

[1] This section follows closely an article by the author: Congestive heart failure: Role of altered cellular control. *New England Journal of Medicine,* 293:1184–1191, 1975.

and there is little high-energy phosphate reserve, even when circulatory hemody-namics are normal. For this reason a rebudgeting of the energy-producing and energy-consuming reactions is a part of the compensatory mechanisms that evolve in the chronically overloaded heart. The myocardial response to a sustained hemodynamic overloading therefore represents a complex and as yet incompletely understood intermingling of adjustments that enhance the ability of the heart to pump blood and energy-sparing mechanisms that tend to depress cardiac performance. These regulatory mechanisms have been the subject of the earlier chapters of this book, and the interested reader is referred to Chapters 3 and 4 for a discussion of the mechanisms by which an increased rate of energy expenditure by the myocardium accelerates the rate of ATP generation from carbohydrate and fat metabolism in order to match the increased rate of ATP utilization.

The chronically overloaded myocardium appears to be reasonably successful in maintaining normal high-energy phosphate levels within the cells. It is unlikely that longstanding overloading reduces ATP or phosphocreatine concentrations to levels so low that substrate lack would directly affect the important energy-consuming reactions of the heart. Indeed it now appears to be very unlikely that the tissue levels of high-energy phosphate compounds play any physiological role in regulating energy-consuming reactions. [This is, of course, in marked contrast to the ability of energy-producing metabolic reactions to respond to slight changes in levels of ATP, ADP, AMP, P_i, and phosphocreatine (Chapters 3 and 4).] Insensitivity of known energy-consuming reactions to changing ATP levels in the physiological millimolar range is reflected in the low K_m values for ATP of the ion pumps and contractile proteins, which are less than 0.1 mM. This low K_m means that the substrate-binding sites of these effector mechanisms would remain more than 90% saturated, even if ATP levels were to decline to 20% of normal. Such a fall in ATP levels probably occurs only in the dying or, more likely, the virtually dead myocardial cell.

These conclusions must not be interpreted to mean that the myocardial weakness caused by a longstanding hemodynamic overload is not attributable to a fall in high-energy phosphate levels. What is meant is that high-energy phosphate lack does not impair contractility by depriving energy-consuming reactions of their substrate. New biochemical data from the author's laboratory and recent studies of ion fluxes across living membranes indicate that changes in ATP concentration at levels well above the K_m for sites that use ATP as substrate are able to modulate ion fluxes. These recent studies point to a novel way in which changing levels of ATP (and ADP) can alter both the electrical and mechanical properties of the myocardium.

Hypertrophy represents a major response of the heart to chronically increased hemodynamic demands. Up to a point, the increased mass of cardiac muscle is beneficial to both the myocardium and the circulation. The distribution of the increased demand for mechanical work among a large number of contractile elements reduces the energy expenditure of each, as well as providing for more effective cardiac pumping (Chapter 20). Hypertrophy, however, is not an unmixed blessing, for the new growth of cardiac muscular tissue does not result from an increased number of normal myocardial cells. Instead, because the muscle cells of the adult heart have little or no ability to divide, each cell becomes larger. This results in an increase in muscle mass but, for reasons not yet fully understood, a decrease in the strength of each contractile unit. Therefore although the total capacity for cardiac work is increased by hypertrophy, the newly formed myocardial tissue is not normal muscle.

Meerson's Three Stages of the Cardiac Response to Hemodynamic Overloading

A very useful description of the sequential changes that occur after the myocardium is overloaded was first published during the early 1960s by Meerson, who studied the response of experimental animals' hearts following the production of aortic stenosis. This description is valuable in that it aids in understanding the evolution of the cardiac response to a hemodynamic overload; but of even greater importance is evidence that after such an overload occurs the evolution of the myocardial response follows a pattern which, although it can proceed at different rates in individuals, offers the potential for defining the state of the myocardium in a given individual. Understanding this evolution therefore may allow future surgeons to choose the optimal time for such interventions as heart valve replacement. This is of considerable practical importance, for when a prosthetic valve is inserted earlier than necessary the patient is subject, for a needless period, to the risks that inevitably complicate this therapy (e.g., infection, thromboembolism); and if the operation is deferred too long, successful valve replacement can fail to benefit the patient because irreversible myocardial damage becomes so severe that correction of the hemodynamic abnormality does not restore health.

The three stages of myocardial response to a sudden and severe overload (Table 21.3) are: the first short-term stage of damage, the second long-term stage of relatively constant hyperfunction, and the third long-term stage of exhaustion and fibrosis. The first stage is a period during which the myocardium comes to compensate for the increased load; the second represents that period during which increased myocardial function allows a return toward normal circulatory dynamics; and the third stage gradually evolves when the myocardium becomes irreversibly damaged so that its function decreases and the clinical symptoms return.

In most clinical cases of valvular heart disease and hypertension, the first stage is not clearly seen, as the onset of the overload itself is gradual. In some patients (e.g., following rupture of a leaflet of the mitral valve or one of its supporting chordae tendinae) this first stage usually lasts a few days or weeks. The clinical picture is that of acute left heart failure, described earlier, associated with dilatation of the left ventricle and edema of its walls. The excessive energy demands cause a fall in substrate and high-energy phosphate (especially phosphocreatine)

TABLE 21.3. *Meerson's three stages of cardiac response to hemodynamic overloading of the left ventricle*

First short-term stages of damage
   Clinical: Left heart failure, pulmonary congestion.
   Pathological: Dilatation of the left ventricle.
   Histological: Swelling and separation of the myofibrils.
   Biochemical: Glycogen and ATP levels decreased, phosphocreatine level markedly decreased, lactate production slightly increased. Protein synthesis, RNA, and mitochondrial mass (especially the inner membranes) increased.

Second long-term stage of relatively constant hyperfunction
   Clinical: Relief of symptoms.
   Pathological: Hypertrophy.
   Histological: Increased size of cardiac fibers, minimal fibrosis.
   Biochemical: Glycogen, ATP, phosphocreatine levels normal. Lactate production increased. Protein synthesis, RNA level normal, DNA level decreased. Myofibrillar mass increased relative to that of the mitochondrial mass.

Third long-term stage of exhaustion and fibrosis
   Clinical: Reappearance of heart failure.
   Pathological: Fibrous replacement of muscular tissue.
   Histological: Disproportionate appearance of connective tissue, fatty dystrophy; muscle cell nuclei become pyknotic.
   Biochemical: As in second stage, except decline in protein synthesis and marked decline in DNA levels.

levels, while a slight increase in lactate production indicates that the heart has become abnormally dependent on anaerobic energy production. This is not unexpected in light of the effects of high-energy phosphate depletion described in Chapter 3. This first stage is also characterized by an increased protein synthesis rate, as well as an increase in RNA content and mitochondrial mass, all of which represent the start of the transition to the second stage.

The second stage occurs when hypertrophy increases the number of active muscular units in the heart, thereby leading to relief of symptoms. The return of protein synthesis rates and RNA levels to normal levels indicates the end of the stage of rapid muscle growth. Although glycogen and high-energy phosphate levels return toward normal, the hypertrophied myocardium is *not* normal muscle. An increased myofibrillar mass relative to that of the mitochondria and abnormally high rates of lactate production indicate that energy consumption during contraction is outstripping energy production. The fall in DNA content may arise from a preponderant increase in myofilaments, but the appearance of fibrosis heralds the transition to the third and irreversible stage.

The final stage in the overloaded heart occurs when muscle cells die and are replaced by connective tissue. The time required for this transition is highly variable and reflects individual variations within the myocardium and an often continuing progression of the underlying hemodynamic disorder. The process of fibrous replacement, which is essentially one of scarring, is irreversible because the adult myocardium has little or no ability to regenerate new cells. Loss of functioning myocardial cells causes a return of the signs and symptoms of heart failure. When correction of the underlying hemodynamic overload is impossible, this third stage progresses until the death of the patient.

The importance of Meerson's concepts cannot be overemphasized. Although the histological and biochemical features of these three stages are described only incompletely in Table 21.3 (and are not fully known), their characterization in the cardiac patient offers considerable promise to the cardiologist and cardiac surgeon who must select the appropriate time to perform a very serious operation. With the possibility of obtaining and studying cardiac biopsies from these patients in terms of this evolutionary process, the risks of this procedure may be more than balanced by the potential benefit to the patient.

Biochemical Defect in the Chronically Overloaded Heart

The recognition that chronic overloading of the heart leads to a fall in myocardial contractility was followed by a search for a "biochemical defect" in these hearts. This approach led investigators to attempt to identify, in newly discovered biochemical and biophysical reactions, abnormalities that could explain the impaired contractility seen in heart failure. Recognition of the role of oxidative phosphorylation in the generation of chemical energy for cardiac contraction, for example, was quickly followed by the search for a possible depression of energy production in mitochondria isolated from failing hearts. Similarly, the ability to measure the molecular weight of the myosin molecule led to studies of the physicochemical properties of myosin isolated from failing hearts. In both of these examples, as in many other studies of specific components and reaction mechanisms in the cardiac contractile process, early findings indicated the existence of significant abnormalities. Subsequent investigations, however, have contradicted or at least modified the initial interpretations that a biochemical defect which caused myocardial contractility to decline in the chronically overloaded heart had been identified. Much confusion has arisen and continues to arise because serious experimental problems are encountered in studies of enzymes and subcellular fractions derived from cardiac muscle. The extreme lability of these biological materials is not always appreciated, and on many occasions methodological pitfalls are overlooked by investigators whose interests are primarily cardiological rather than biochemical. Most of these errors have been corrected, however, and we are left with a number of suggested alterations of individual cellular functions that may explain, at least in part, the reduced contractility seen in the chronically stressed myocardium.

Abnormalities in the Contractile Proteins: Primary Changes

Over the years a great many changes have been suggested to occur in the contractile proteins of the failing myocardium. At the present time, one abnormality in these proteins appears likely to be significant in permitting the heart to adapt to a chronic hemodynamic overloading: a fall in myosin ATPase activity.

The ATPase activity of myosin isolated from animals with experimentally induced congestive heart failure has been found by a number of investigators to be abnormally low. This change, which is similar to that found experimentally in the hearts of older animals and in the presence of some endocrinopathies, would reduce myocardial contractility by lessening shortening velocity, especially at lighter loads (Chapter 11). In addition to this deleterious effect, which in the intact heart would decrease the rate of ejection of blood, a reduction in myosin ATPase activity can increase the mechanical efficiency in the heart that is contracting with high wall tension. The latter interpretation is based on comparisons between "fast" and "slow" skeletal muscles in which the slow muscles have been found to use less ATP than the fast ones when shortening against heavy loads (Chapter 2). Slowing of contraction in the chronically overloaded heart may therefore represent an adaptation to an abnormally sustained demand for tension output and the accompanying high rate of energy expenditure.

> There is some evidence that during the early stages of the response of the heart to a hemodynamic overload (Meerson's first and second stages) myosin ATPase activity may be increased. This finding has not been confirmed in all laboratories, however, and so must remain tentative pending further study. The significance of this finding, if correct, lies in the similarity to the situation in the hearts of animals subjected to intense physical training. Here, exercise leads to an increased myosin ATPase activity, so that this proposed initial response in the overloaded heart may represent a "physiological," rather than a "pathological" adjustment.

Hypertrophy of the pressure-overloaded heart is associated in its later stages with an increased myofibrillar mass at the expense of that of the mitochondria (Table 21.3). This adds another factor to the precarious balance between energy production and energy utilization. By reducing the number of energy-producing structures and increasing the proportion of the cell occupied by the energy-consuming contractile proteins, this change in the composition of the hypertrophied, overloaded heart accentuates the tendency to deplete energy reserves. Synthesis of a myosin molecule with low intrinsic ATPase activity thus has some value in that this change can be expected to increase the amount of mechanical energy derived from each mole of ATP utilized, albeit at the expense of a decrease in the maximum rate at which blood can be ejected. In this way, although activity is slowed, the energy demands for contraction are more easily met.

Abnormalities in the Contractile Proteins: Secondary Changes

Potassium loss.

The pioneering work of A. Szent-Györgyi showed that high potassium ion concentration depresses the activity of contractile proteins studied *in vitro*. These observations, which reflect a primary action of increasing ionic strength to reduce the interaction between actin and myosin, were later correlated with changes in potassium fluxes that occur when cardiac muscle is subjected to various iono-tropic interventions. Although there is a positive correlation between loss of potassium and enhanced myocardial contractility, a number of recent studies indicate that this relationship is indirect (Chapter 11). Furthermore, because total potassium loss is quite small and represents mainly exchange of intracellular potassium for sodium derived from the extracellular fluid, the ionic strength within the myocardium changes very little if at all. For these reasons changes in intracellular potassium ion concentration probably have little direct influence on the contractile proteins of the intact heart and so probably do not contribute to a fall in myocardial contractility in the chronically overloaded heart.

ATP Depletion.

The key role of ATP in providing chemical energy for the contractile process suggests that ATP lack might directly impair myocardial performance in the overloaded heart. While many of the changes in the myocardial cell that occur in response to chronic hemodynamic overloading probably are due ultimately to an imbalance between energy production and energy utilization, a *direct* effect of ATP depletion on the contractile proteins is unlikely to depress myocardial contractility (see above). Furthermore, in addition to its role of supplying energy for contraction, ATP has a second major effect on the contractile proteins. This is its "plasticizing" effect, which requires even higher levels of the nucleotide than are needed to fuel contraction (Chapter 6). Recall that the plasticizing effect of ATP is essential for muscle to relax, so that severe reduction of the ATP levels at the level of the contractile proteins causes muscle to develop rigor. Loss of this plasticizing effect in the heart is probably lethal in that rigor prevents the heart from filling during diastole. For this reason ATP lack seems unlikely to be directly responsible for the loss of contractility seen in the early stages of congestive heart failure. It should be emphasized that this conclusion does *not* mean that ATP deficiency does not set into motion other changes in the regula-tion of myocardial function that depress contractility when energy demands are chronically increased in the myocardium.

Acidosis.

When the demands for mechanical energy expenditure in the heart become excessive, the myocardium increases its dependence on the pathways of anaerobic glycolysis (Chapter 3 and Table 21.3). Under these conditions hydrogen ion is liberated when glucose and glycogen are metabolized to lactate. The resulting tendency toward intracellular acidosis may impair contractility in the overloaded heart because reduced pH has a marked negative inotropic effect (Chapter 11).

Abnormalities in the Sarcoplasmic Reticulum: Primary Changes

There is considerable evidence from both morphological and biochemical stud-ies that the sarcoplasmic reticulum is abnormal in the heart subjected to longstanding and severe hemodynamic overloading. The significance of these abnormalities, which have been found in studies of calcium transport into sarcoplasmic reticulum preparations studied *in vitro,* remains to be established. Although there is considerable indirect evidence that both the extent and rate of calcium release by the sarcoplasmic reticulum are impaired in congestive heart failure, failure of relaxation is not a prominent feature of this syndrome. As it is not now possible to study the calcium release process by purified sarcoplasmic reticulum *in vitro,* the functional significance of impaired calcium transport into the sarcoplasmic reticulum can be related only indirectly to abnormalities in cardiac function. It is possible, for example, that a reduced rate of calcium transport may lead to decreased stores of calcium at the site in the failing myocardium from which calcium is released for binding to troponin C.

The tendency to develop mechanical alternans in the chronically overloaded heart may reflect impaired calcium transport within the sarcoplasmic reticulum. This phenomenon, in which stronger beats alternate with weaker beats, is sometimes seen in severe heart failure, and transient mechanical alternans is not infrequently observed after premature systoles in such hearts. In the latter case maximum ventricular pressure in a series of beats after a premature systole resembles a damped oscillation in which the forceful postextrasystolic beat is followed by a weak beat, then a beat that is abnormally forceful although less so than the first postextrasystolic beat, then a somewhat less impaired beat, etc., until contractile tension returns to a steady state. While this behavior may in part reflect variations in ventricular filling (due to operation of the Frank-Starling relationship), it is possible that the weak contractions may also be due to the retention of calcium at a site in the sarcoplasmic reticulum where it is unable to be released to the contractile proteins. Such a cause for the alternating weak beats, which is analogous to the mechanism believed to be responsible for the negative staircase (Chapter 11), could result from abnormally slow recovery of the ability of calcium channels in the sarcoplasmic reticulum to open or from a reduced rate of calcium translocation within the sarcoplasmic reticulum. Direct evidence for the existence of such abnormalities remains to be obtained, however.

Abnormalities of the Sarcoplasmic Reticulum: Secondary Changes

The possibility that the properties of the sarcoplasmic reticulum are altered by other, primary, changes in the intracellular milieu of the chronically overloaded heart remains largely unexplored. Two examples of such possible alterations in intracellular environment are mentioned at this point to illustrate the type of abnormality that could contribute to the decline in myocardial contractility seen in the chronically overloaded myocardium.

Acidosis.

Because the pH optimum for calcium transport by the cardiac sarcoplasmic reticulum *in vitro* is between 7 and 8, intracellular acidosis could, by inhibiting calcium uptake, impair filling of intracellular calcium stores. A shift to anaerobic pathways of ATP production in the overloaded myocardium may lead to intracellular acidosis (See above). If this fall in pH were sufficient to slow the rate of calcium transport into the sarcoplasmic reticulum, a reduced calcium store in this membrane system might cause a loss of myocardial contractility.

ATP depletion.

The existence of an imbalance between energy production and utilization in the chronically overloaded heart raises the possibility that ATP lack might be responsible for the impairment of one or another of the membrane ion pumps. While this possibility cannot be excluded, the relatively slight decline in cellular ATP levels and the low requirements for ATP by these pumps do not support this hypothesis (see above). In the case of the calcium pump of the sarcoplasmic reticulum, for example, the K_m for ATP is less than 0.1 mM, whereas average cellular ATP levels, even in the failing heart, are much higher. However, compartmentalization of ATP within the cell might allow a localized decline in ATP concentration to impair one or more of the ion pumps that control myocardial contractility.

Abnormalities of the Sarcolemma

A possible role for sarcolemmal abnormalities in the pathogenesis of myocardial weakness seen in the chronically overloaded heart has not been carefully explored. The effects of hemodynamic overload on the slow inward current and on the sodium-calcium exchange mechanism (Chapter 11) have not been studied systematically. There is some evidence that the sodium pump is impaired under these conditions. Recent work cited on page 410 suggests that a modest fall in cellular ATP levels can modify ion fluxes across this membrane.

Abnormalities in Catecholamine Metabolism

It is now well documented that catecholamine metabolism may be abnormal in patients with heart failure. The uptake of catecholamines is reduced in the chronically overloaded heart, and a decrease in adenylate cyclase activity has been found in some but not all studies of these hearts. If the response to catecholamines is blunted when the heart is subjected to longstanding hemodynamic overloading, the resulting impairment of the ability of the heart to increase its metabolic and contractile activity would be in accord with other evidence already cited that the failing heart is unable to meet the increased demands of the circulation in such states as exercise and emotional stress.

Functional Significance of Reduced Contractility in Heart Failure

Alterations in the control systems of the myocardial cell could cause myocardial weakness and thus may be involved in the pathogenesis of some of the primary cardiomyopathies. In the myocardial weakness that develops secondarily in the chronically overloaded myocardium, however, the functional significance of such abnormalities is much less clear. There is no doubt that a lower level of myocardial contractility would increase the clinical disability in patients with longstanding hemodynamic overloading, such as is seen in hypertension, aortic stenosis, mitral insufficiency, etc. Similarly, loss of contractility in nonischemic regions of the heart would reduce the functional capacity of the hearts of patients with severe ischemic heart disease. Yet it cannot be assumed that loss of contractility is not entirely without beneficial effects.

Although a decrease in myocardial contractility would reduce the heart's capacity to perform mechanical work, such abnormalities would also attenuate the most "expensive" of the energy-consuming reactions of the heart. By reducing contractile activity to a "maintenance" level, this type of abnormality would tend to reserve chemical energy for synthetic and reparative processes, thereby delaying the onset of Meerson's third stage of exhaustion and fibrosis. Furthermore, the loss of myocardial contractile function could help avoid severe ATP depletion, which in skeletal muscle leads to a state of rigor that can be reversed only by restoration of high levels of ATP. In the heart, moreover, rigor is probably irreversible because intramyocardial tension, which impedes nutrient coronary flow, would be increased at the same time that the ability of the heart to generate aortic pressure, the motive force for coronary flow, is reduced. It is possible in this way that by producing small areas of rigor, severe ATP depletion may be partly responsible for the patchy necrosis and fibrosis seen in the hearts of patients with longstanding hemodynamic overloading. For this reason depression of myocardial contractility in the chronically overloaded heart might prolong life in patients with heart failure due to chronic hemodynamic overloading, even though survival is achieved at the expense of exacerbated clinical manifestations of congestive heart failure.

BIBLIOGRAPHY

DiPolo, R. (1976): The influence of nucleotides on calcium fluxes. *Fed. Proc.,* 35:2579–2582.
Goodwin, J. F. (1970): Congestive and obstructive cardiomyopathies. *Lancet,* 1:731–739.
Meerson, F. Z. (1969): The myocardium in hyperfunction, hypertrophy and heart failure. A. H. A. Monograph No. 26. American Heart Association, New York.
Rabinowitz, M. (1974): Overview on pathogenesis of cardiac hypertrophy. *Circ. Res. (Suppl. II),* 35:II-3–II-11.
See also the textbooks of cardiology cited at the end of Chapter 20.

22

The Ischemic Heart

Ischemic heart disease is one of a number of names given to the clinical syndrome produced when blood flow to a region of the heart is reduced. Other names for this condition include coronary heart disease and arteriosclerotic heart disease, the latter term arising from one of the designations (arteriosclerosis) given to the process that most commonly gives rise to this form of heart disease.

Little more than a generation ago, ischemic heart disease was accepted simply as a manifestation of old age. The increasing frequency with which this disease now appears in the Western world, and the steady increase in the number of young men and women whom it kills belies this view. Recognition of ischemic heart disease as a manifestation of disordered myocardial cellular function constitutes a necessary first step in a now impressive effort directed to its control and, more importantly, its prevention.

A description of the pathophysiology of the disorders which cause narrowing of the coronary arteries, as well as the abnormalities in lipid metabolism, blood coagulation, blood flow patterns, and coronary arterial structure with which these processes are associated, is beyond the scope of this text. Needless to say it is at this level—an understanding of the processes that operate in the arterial wall, causing coronary blood flow to be reduced—that progress in the prevention of ischemic heart disease holds greatest promise. It is appropriate at this point, however, to discuss at some length the two major sequelae of ischemic heart disease. These are a decline in myocardial contractility and disorders of cardiac rate and rhythm. Each of these is responsible for approximately half of the deaths due to ischemic heart disease in the United States.

The following discussion focuses on the mechanisms that contribute to the loss of contractility and the arrhythmias associated with ischemic heart disease. In no way should this discussion be viewed as a comprehensive survey of these conditions from the standpoint of the clinical cardiologist. These descriptions are intended only to provide the reader with some insight as to the way in which disorders of cardiac cellular function described in this text can become manifest in the cardiac patient.

LOSS OF MYOCARDIAL CONTRACTILE FUNCTION

Patients with ischemic heart disease who suffer from "pump failure" (i.e., a decline in contractile function) can be grouped into two categories: those who die during the acute phase that occurs soon after coronary flow to a region of the heart (almost always the left ventricle) is interrupted, and those in whom death occurs after a more or less prolonged period of congestive heart failure. The sequence of changes in the heart and circulation that accompany the latter situation were touched on in Chapter 21. After an initial loss of functional myocardial tissue places an abnormal burden on the remaining regions of the left ventricle, the overload can be tolerated for a greater or lesser period of time. So little normal myocardium remains in some patients that ischemic heart disease causes either acute or chronic heart failure. In such patients the loss of functional myocardium is great enough to lead to severe impairment of cardiac pumping. The clinical manifestations of this form of heart failure, which results from a loss of functioning myocardial tissue, were described in Chapter 21. The chronic heart failure that results from ischemic heart disease can be understood as being due to the death of large numbers of myocardial cells that were deprived of their blood supply. However, the initial response of the myocardium to ischemia, in which contractility is rapidly lost in cells that are still viable, is much less well understood. For this reason the remainder of this section is devoted to the mechanisms responsible for early pump failure of the ischemic heart.

EARLY PUMP FAILURE OF THE ISCHEMIC HEART [1]

When coronary arterial flow to a portion of the heart is interrupted, the ischemic regions lose their ability to contract almost immediately. Complete interruption of coronary flow to a segment of the canine heart is followed within a few seconds by abbreviation of cardiac systole and then by loss of contractility. As a result, after less than a minute the ischemic portion of the ventricle bulges outward during systole. These phenomena do not mean that the ischemic myocardium has completely lost its ability to develop tension. Instead, a marked diminution in contractility causes the tension generated by the ischemic portion of the ventricle to be unable to overcome the intraventricular pressure generated by the normally perfused myocardium.

To understand the early pump failure of the ischemic myocardium, the mechanisms that can cause the rapid decline in myocardial contractility after interruption in coronary blood flow must be defined. In this analysis of the myocardial response to ischemia it is useful to refer to the "four causes" defined by Aristotle. The *efficient cause* is the producing agency or the factor that sets into motion the processes that, in the specific case of the early pump failure of the ischemic heart, ultimately lead to the loss of contractility in the ischemic myocardium. The *formal* and *material causes* are, in this situation, the form and matter of the mechanical deterioration, while the *final cause* of the rapid decline in contractile function represents the end these phenomena may serve in the ischemic myocardium.

---

[1] This section follows closely an article by the author: Effects of ischemia on the contractile process of heart muscle. *American Journal of Cardiology,* 32:456–460, 1973.

Efficient Cause of Impaired Contractility

The rapid decline in myocardial contractility that occurs after coronary arterial occlusion could be due to one or both of two types of efficient causes: the lack of a substrate or substrates normally supplied by the coronary circulation, and the accumulation of one or more metabolites.

The substrate whose lack is felt most promptly by the ischemic myocardium is almost certainly oxygen. Within a minute after the blood supply to the heart is interrupted, intramyocardial oxygen tension falls to extremely low levels. This state of myocardial anoxia develops because the heart has virtually no stores of oxygen. In contrast, considerable quantities of glycogen persist long after the ischemic myocardium has ceased its effective contraction, and the myocardial content of fats actually increases when blood supply is interrupted. The view that oxygen is the critical substrate whose lack may be responsible for the early pump failure of the ischemic heart is supported further by the finding that anoxia, like ischemia, causes a precipitous decline in cardiac contractile function. However, the similarity between the effects of anoxia in the perfused myocardium and those of ischemia do not provide conclusive evidence that the accumulation of metabolites has no role in the mechanical deterioration after coronary occlusion (see below).

The precipitous decline in myocardial contractility that follows interruption of coronary blood flow is accompanied by an increased rate of glycolysis, in which glycogen breakdown is associated with increased cellular levels of cyclic AMP and the conversion of phosphorylase from the inactive b form to the more active a form. Of greater importance in accelerating glycolysis is release of the inhibitory effects of ATP and glucose-6-phosphate, which in the normal heart maintain phosphorylase b activity at a low level. This occurs when cessation of oxidative metabolism causes ATP levels to decline along with glucose-6-phosphate levels, while at the same time AMP and inorganic phosphate levels rise. The latter also contribute to the acceleration of glycogenolysis in the ischemic heart as both of these substances increase phosphorylase b activity (Chapter 3).

Glucose flux through the glycolytic pathways is increased in the ischemic heart as the result of stimulation of the reaction catalyzed by phosphofructokinase. As is the case for phosphorylase b (see above), the activity of this enzyme is enhanced when oxidative ATP production ceases. Stimulation of phosphofructokinase in the ischemic heart is effected by increased cellular levels of ADP, AMP, and P_i, which activate this enzyme, and by reduced concentrations of ATP and phosphocreatine, both of which are inhibitory at normal cellular levels. The increased rate of glycolysis in the ischemic heart is only transient, however. Eventual cessation of anaerobic ATP production is probably due to the accumulation of NADH and lack of NAD, which cause the glycolytic pathway to be inhibited at the step where glyceraldehyde-3-phosphate is reduced (Fig. 3.1). In addition, the increased rate of lactate production is accompanied by the accumulation of hydrogen ions, so that the rapid development of acidosis inhibits the step in the glycolytic pathway that is catalyzed by phosphofructokinase. The interested reader may wish to review Chapters 3 and 4 in order to re-examine these key regulatory steps and to evaluate the role of the general features of enzyme control summarized in Table 4.4 as they operate in the ischemic heart.

While oxygen lack and the accompanying cessation of aerobic ATP production are probably key initial steps in the efficient causation of the early pump failure that follows interruption of coronary arterial blood flow, the response of the heart to anoxia differs from that to ischemia. When a region of the heart is perfused with blood that contains no oxygen, the initial fall in myocardial contractility is generally similar to that seen in the ischemic myocardium, which receives no blood flow. In the case of myocardial anoxia, however, the glycolytic rate remains elevated. This persistence of active glycolysis in the perfused, anoxic heart is probably due to the washout of both hydrogen ions and lactate, which is not possible in the ischemic heart. As the anoxic heart remains perfused, the removal of hydrogen ions can partially release the inhibition of phosphofructokinase that is caused by acidosis. Washout of lactate in the perfused, anoxic heart facilitates pyruvate reduction and thereby allows partial renewal of the supply of oxidized NAD. In spite of these differences, which tend to maintain glycolytic energy production at a higher level in the anoxic than in the ischemic heart, it remains likely that the initial fall in contractility in both conditions is due in large part to oxygen lack and its sequelae.

Although oxygen is almost certainly the major substrate whose lack sets into motion the series of events that leads first to reduced myocardial contractility and ultimately to cell death, the nature of the other substrates available to the myocardium appears able to modify the response to ischemia. These effects would be especially important in regions of partial ischemia, where a reduced capacity for aerobic energy production could support marginal levels of function and viability. In such areas of partial ischemia, increased levels of carbohydrate substrates in the arterial blood could sustain both function and viability by providing additional substrate for anaerobic glycolysis. Fatty acids, on the other hand, may be detrimental, as high concentrations of these substrates have an "oxygen-wasting" effect that arises from their ability to increase oxygen consumption without a corresponding increase in the rate of ATP production.

The concept of areas of partial ischemia is extremely important in understanding some of the complications of ischemic heart disease. It is likely, for example, that both the chest pain (angina pectoris) and the arrhythmias associated with ischemic heart disease arise in partially ischemic regions of the myocardium. Once cell death occurs, the ability to initiate pain and generate arrhythmias is probably lost, although the accompanying loss of functioning myocardium clearly contributes to the overall contractile function of the heart.

Cell death (necrosis) generally occurs after 40–60 min of total myocardial ischemia. The mechanism of this ischemic cell death is probably related to a breakdown in membrane function caused when ATP concentrations fall below levels that are needed to maintain key ion pumps (approximately 0.1 mM). There is evidence that excessive entry of calcium is of major importance in this process. In addition, low ATP concentrations can lead to the formation of rigor bonds between the contractile proteins (Chapter 7). It now appears that reperfusion of ischemic areas of the heart after 30–60 min of ischemia can cause an almost "explosive" cell death, possibly because the sarcolemma of the ischemic cells has been sufficiently damaged to be unable to maintain the normally low intracellular levels of Ca^{2+}. For this reason reperfusion of ischemic areas of the heart—as might occur when emergency coronary bypass surgery is carried out more than an hour after the onset of symptoms of myocardial infarction—may actually hasten cell death in some regions of the heart.

The possibility that loss of potassium from the ischemic myocardium might contribute to the efficient cause of the fall in myocardial contractility was suggested many years ago when changes in potassium concentration in the extra- and intracellular spaces were believed to play a primary role in the regulation of myocardial contractility (Chapter 11). With the recognition that potassium plays only a minor role in regulating myocardial contractility, and that loss of cell potassium is accompanied by a gain of cell sodium, the view that potassium loss causes the early pump failure of the ischemic heart has been considerably weakened. Indeed exchange of intracellular potassium for extracellular sodium might be expected to cause an increase in contractility (Chapter 11). The finding that resting membrane potential remains virtually unchanged in the period immediately following myocardial anoxia when contractility declines markedly provides further evidence that significant changes in extracellular potassium concentration are not responsible for the immediate loss of contractility in the ischemic heart. In contrast, several lines of evidence suggest that changes in calcium fluxes between intra- and extracellular spaces may account, in part at least, for the loss of contractility in the ischemic heart. These changes are described in the subsequent section on formal and material causes.

In addition to substrate lack and metabolite accumulation, the loss of contractile function that occurs soon after a portion of the heart is made ischemic could be attributable to a fall in ATP concentration [2] that results from the interruption of aerobic energy production. Direct measurements show a significant decline in cellular ATP content[2] soon after coronary artery blood flow has been interrupted, but this decrease usually reaches levels not less than 50% of normal at a time when contractility has fallen to extremely low levels. The ATP content in biopsy samples from such hearts would, if ATP were distributed uniformly throughout the tissue water, represent average ATP concentrations in the millimolar range. Such concentrations are well above those needed to saturate the ATP-binding sites of myosin and the known ATP-utilizing ion pumps. These findings do not,

---

[2] It is important to distinguish between *concentration*, which is the amount of a substance per unit volume in a defined region of the myocardial cell, and *content*, which describes the amount of substance present per unit weight of a tissue sample. Metabolic reactions depend on substrate and metabolite concentrations in those areas where the reactions take place. Changes in these concentrations may often differ considerably from those occurring in overall substrate and metabolite content due to the distribution of these substances in "compartments" within the myocardial cell.

however, rule out the possibility that ATP depletion might serve as the efficient cause of the pump failure that accompanies myocardial ischemia. There is no assurance, for example, that the ATP content of a biopsy specimen provides an accurate index of ATP concentration in a small intracellular compartment that contains an ATP-utilizing system. Furthermore, it cannot be assumed that these measurements of ATP content are valid measurements of the ability of the energy-producing mechanisms in the heart to deliver high-energy phosphate to systems that utilize ATP. This view is supported by the very marked fall in phosphocreatine content, which far exceeds the decrease in ATP content. Because ATP and phosphocreatine should be in equilibrium, the proportionately much greater fall in the latter indicates that a part of the cellular ATP pool is in a "compartment" that is not in equilibrium with the phosphocreatine pool. Slight changes in ATP concentration may, through amplification mechanisms such as that described for phosphofructokinase in Chapter 3, influence certain key regulatory steps in the regulation of myocardial contractility. It is, however, very unlikely that a fall in ATP concentration acts directly on the contractile proteins or ion pumps in a manner that causes myocardial weaknesses because the initial response of these systems to ATP lack would be the development of rigor (Table 22.1) instead of the failure to contract seen in the ischemic heart.

At this time oxygen lack appears to be the efficient cause of the early pump failure of the ischemic heart. The mechanisms that link this initial step to a series of changes that leads eventually to myocardial weakness, however, remain largely speculative. ATP lack is probably not *directly* responsible for loss of myocardial

TABLE 22.1. *Effects of ATP lack on energy-consuming reactions associated with regulation of myocardial contractility*

Process	Immediate consequence	Mechanical effect
Actin-myosin interaction	Loss of "plasticizing" effect; failure of thick and thin filaments to dissociate	Rigor
Calcium pump of the sarcoplasmic reticulum	Reduction of calcium transport during diastole; failure to remove calcium from contractile proteins	Inhibition of relaxation; contracture
Sodium pump	Reduction of sodium efflux; increased intracellular sodium	Increased sodium efflux by Na-Ca exchange; reduction of Ca efflux; contracture
Sarcolemmal calcium pump (hypothetical)	Reduction of calcium efflux	Increased intra-cellular calcium; contracture
Mitrochondrial calcium pump	Reduction of calcium transport into mitochondria	Increased calcium levels in the cytosol; contracture

contractility, although a fall in ATP concentration is partly responsible for a transient acceleration of glycolysis that leads to lactate and hydrogen ion accumulation in the ischemic myocardium. Both cellular acidosis and alterations in ATP-dependent regulatory processes (see, for example, page 410) may participate in the sequence of steps which leads eventually to the loss of contractility, but it remains to be shown how ATP lack at the level of the major energy-utilizing systems could itself cause the mechanical abnormalities seen in the ischemic myocardium.

Formal and Material Causes of Impaired Contractility

In contrast to the efforts to define the efficient cause of the early pump failure of the ischemic heart, where tenable hypotheses are scanty and causal relationships poorly defined, a number of reasonable hypotheses can explain the direct (i.e., formal and material) causation of this loss of myocardial contractility. To appreciate how this effect can be brought about, it must be remembered that the phasic control of myocardial contractility is effected mainly by changes in the amount of calcium made available to, and bound to, the contractile proteins of the heart. The formal and material causes of the myocardial weakness in the ischemic heart therefore can involve any mechanism that either reduces the amount of calcium released during excitation-contraction coupling or prevents calcium from being bound to troponin, the calcium receptor of the contractile proteins.

Changes in the Cardiac Action Potential

Although prolonged myocardial ischemia eventually leads to failure of the action potential to propagate, the early and rapid deterioration of contractility in the ischemic heart is associated with only minor changes in action potential configuration. These latter abnormalities are primarily an abbreviation of the action potential caused by shortening of the plateau (phase 2). Preservation of normal resting potential indicates that the potassium-dependent properties of the membrane are not markedly altered, and the lack of major changes in the upstroke velocity and amplitude of the action potential provides evidence that the sodium-dependent properties of the membrane, which are responsible for the early fast inward current, also remain essentially normal during the initial phases of myocardial ischemia. However, the shortening of the action potential plateau indicates that ischemia significantly modifies the ionic processes responsible for the slow inward current that is largely responsible for this phase of the cardiac action potential. Because this slow inward current is carried largely by calcium, slight modifications of the plateau can have profound effects on contractility. In this way the early pump failure of the ischemic heart may reflect a reduction in the inward movement of calcium during the plateau of the action potential, so that ischemia-induced abbreviation of the action potential and a reduction in calcium influx can represent formal and material causes for the early pump failure of the ischemic myocardium. In the anoxic, perfused heart, however, profound loss of contractility is seen even if the shortening of the action potential plateau is prevented by high glucose concentration in the oxygen-free perfusate.

The mechanism responsible for the reduction in action potential duration and in the slow inward current in the ischemic heart remains poorly understood. Similar effects are sometimes but not always seen in the anoxic heart, and various inhibitors of oxidative phosphorylation can inhibit the opening of the slow channel. While the efficient cause of these changes in membrane permeability is not fully understood, one such cause might be the rapid accumulation of lactate that occurs when the heart comes to rely on anaerobic glycolysis as a major source of ATP. Alternatively, changes in ATP and ADP concentrations might directly influence the slow channel.

Changes in the Cardiac Sarcoplasmic Reticulum

Sarcoplasmic reticulum vesicles isolated from ischemic hearts show no irreversible abnormalities of calcium transport *in vitro*. This finding, however, does not rule out changes produced by abnormal conditions that may exist in the environment around the sarcoplasmic reticulum in the intact, ischemic heart. Examination of the transport processes believed to be responsible for calcium uptake by the sarcoplasmic reticulum (Chapter 9) provides some indication that calcium may be held more tightly within these membranes in the ischemic heart because lowering the pH may increase the affinity of these membranes for calcium. In other studies, however, the pH optimum for calcium transport by cardiac sarcoplasmic reticulum was 7.5–8.0 so that the acidotic state in the ischemic heart would be predicted to decrease calcium flux into this structure. The significance of these findings, and their relevance to the situation in the living heart during ischemia, however, remain uncertain. The slowing of calcium transport that would result from acidosis may explain the reduced rate of relaxation seen at certain phases in the response of the intact myocardium to ischemia and thus may provide an explanation for a transient reduction in cardiac compliance sometimes seen in patients with ischemic heart disease. The significance of this abnormality as a cause for the decrease in myocardial contractility, however, is less apparent.

Changes in the Cardiac Contractile Proteins

As with the sarcoplasmic reticulum, no irreversible changes in the properties of the contractile proteins isolated from acutely ischemic myocardial tissue have been found. This evidence, obtained in studies of purified actomyosins examined under controlled conditions *in vitro,* does not rule out changes in contractile protein interactions caused by abnormalities in the intracellular environment that occur in the ischemic myocardium. One such abnormality is the state of acidosis discussed above, which develops rapidly when coronary arterial blood flow to the heart is interrupted. Acidosis has a well-known negative inotropic action (Chapter 11), and studies of actomyosin *in vitro* show that reduced pH increases the calcium requirement for activation of both ATPase activity and tension development. This effect is currently believed to result from a competition between hydrogen and calcium ions for binding to the calcium binding site on troponin C as acidosis modifies the Ca^{2+} dependence of the interactions between the contractile proteins studied *in vitro*. Much higher levels of Ca^{2+} are thus needed to produce the same degree of activation when pH falls from approximately 7 to 6 (Fig. 22.1). For this reason it is at least plausible that a reduction in the sensitivity of the contractile proteins to calcium does in fact represent a major formal and material cause of the early pump failure of the ischemic heart.

A direct role for ATP lack in causing the loss of contractility in the ischemic myocardium, as discussed earlier in this chapter and in Chapter 11, is unlikely. This conclusion is based not only on evidence that ATP concentrations in the ischemic myocardium remain well above those needed to saturate the ATP-binding site of myosin, but also on the likelihood that should a marked fall in ATP concentration occur, it would affect known ion pumps in a manner that leads to rigor and not the marked weakness seen in the acutely ischemic myocardium (Table 22.1). In the case of longstanding ischemia, however, (e.g., after 40–60 min of total ischemia), ATP lack probably represents the efficient cause of cell death, the formal and material causes being most likely related to loss of membrane integrity and a resultant massive influx of calcium.

Final Cause of Rapid Loss of Contractility

The reduction in myocardial contractility caused by coronary occlusion, while clearly detrimental to the body as a whole, has certain advantages to the ischemic area of the myocardium. By reducing mechanical activity, the most costly of the ATP-utilizing functions, this early pump failure of the ischemic heart conserves chemical energy for other energy-consuming reactions that are important in the preservation of myocardial integrity, thereby delaying the development of necro-

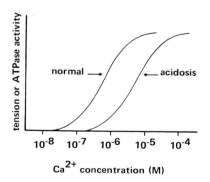

FIG. 22.1. Acidosis decreases the Ca^{2+} sensitivity of the contractile proteins, so a higher than normal level of ionized Ca^{2+} is needed to achieve a given degree of actin-myosin interaction in the acidotic heart.

sis. Furthermore, if excitation-contraction coupling were not quickly attenuated, the ischemic myocardium would soon deplete its high-energy phosphate stores, thereby producing a state of rigor. This state is not fully reversible, nor is it possible to re-establish perfusion once contracture develops (Chapter 11). In contrast, loss of contractility due to failure of excitation-contraction coupling is probably fully reversible, at least in its very early states (less than 40–60 min of total ischemia). Thus the ischemic regions of the heart protect themselves by curtailing their contribution to the pumping action of the heart. At the same time, of course, this compensatory mechanism reduces cardiac work and in so doing leads to the signs and symptoms of heart failure described in Chapter 21.

To the degree that the foregoing analysis of the final cause of the early pump failure of the ischemic heart is correct, attempts to improve the mechanical performance of the ischemic regions of the heart may increase cell damage. These considerations have led many investigators to advocate the use of agents that reduce the work of the heart in patients with *acute myocardial infarction:* the syndrome produced when blood flow to a region of the heart is suddenly compromised to such an extent that a portion of the myocardium becomes irreversibly damaged (infarcted). Unfortunately, the methods currently available do not permit precise measurement of the size of a myocardial infarct in living patients, so that evaluation of these theoretical considerations and their more practical therapeutic implications has not yet been completed in the cardiac patient. Simple relief of pain, for example, can be interpreted to mean either that an intervention has benefited the ischemic area or that it has hastened cell death. This is true because it is the "partly dead" cells that give rise to such symptoms as cardiac pain (angina pectoris) and arrhythmias. Thus relief of symptoms does not constitute *prima facie* evidence that the state of the ischemic myocardium has been improved.

DISORDERS OF RATE AND RHYTHM

Approximately half of the deaths caused by ischemic heart disease result from disordered cardiac rate and rhythm. In many cases these arrhythmias represent a terminal event in a clinical course characterized primarily by marked loss of contractile function. In such cases they arise when the pumping action of the heart is severely impaired, so that blood pressure falls to the extent that coronary arterial blood flow cannot provide for adequate perfusion of the regions of myocardium that are supplied by nonoccluded coronary arteries. In these cases, therefore, the arrhythmias represent a terminal event. While the mechanisms responsible for these terminal arrhythmias are of considerable theoretical interest, their correction is of only passing significance to a patient in whom cardiac contractile function is so severely compromised that even when rhythm is normal life is impossible. When this group of patients is omitted from consideration, a large group remains in whom disordered cardiac rate and rhythm either cause a less severely weakened heart to lose its ability to sustain life, or in whom the arrhythmia alone is the life-threatening event.

In patients who sustain an acute myocardial infarction (i.e., the ischemic necrosis of a large portion of the myocardium, usually of the left ventricle), changes in cardiac rate and rhythm are common. These arrhythmias can be grouped into three classes: sinus tachycardia, sinus bradycardia and the development of AV block, and premature systoles and tachycardia.

Sinus Tachycardia

Sinus tachycardia in patients with acute myocardial infarction can be the result of a number of factors, including excessive sympathetic activity provoked by the pain and anxiety associated with the myocardial infarction, or a reflex response to a fall in blood pressure (hypotension) caused by loss of myocardial function. Sinus tachycardia can also be part of the systemic response to the fever and release into the bloodstream of products of necrosis that accompany myocardial infarction. Dilatation of the right atrium, as occurs when the heart begins to fail, can cause sinus tachycardia by stretching the cells of the SA node.

The accelerated sinus rate initiated by pain and anxiety, and the reflex sinus tachycardia caused by hypotension are mediated by catecholamines released from the sympathetic nervous system and, to a lesser extent, from the adrenals. In these situations, therefore, the mechanism for the sinus tachycardia is basically that described in Chapter 19 *(Sympathetic Neurotransmitters)*. Increased sympathetic tone also contributes to the sinus tachycardia caused by fever and products of necrosis, although both of the latter also have direct, but poorly understood effects to accelerate the sinus pacemaker. While sinus tachycardia can exacerbate the signs and symptoms of heart failure in patients with acute myocardial infarction, this arrhythmia is not usually considered to be a consequence of a primary disorder of cardiac function. For this reason treatment of sinus tachycardia in patients with acute myocardial infarction is usually not directed to the arrhythmia itself but to those conditions which produce it, e.g., relief of pain and reduction of fever.

Sinus Bradycardia and AV Block

A slowed sinus rate in patients with acute myocardial infarction is usually vagal in origin, although examples of the sick sinus syndrome (Chapter 16) sometimes occur in this setting. Whether the vagal slowing commonly seen in acute myocardial infarction is due to an abnormal increase in vagal tone, a heightened sensitivity of the heart to normal vagal tone, or both cannot be determined in most cases. In such patients, however, it is likely that the mechanism for the slowing of sinus rate is that described in Chapter 19 *(Parasympathetic Neurotransmitters)*.

Sinus bradycardia in patients with acute myocardial infarction is commonly caused by the administration of pain-killing drugs, notably the opiates which have the ability to increase vagal tone. Such drugs may also act directly to slow the sinus pacemaker. Unlike the sinus tachycardias associated with acute myocardial infarction, where treatment is usually directed to the underlying abnormalities that produce reflex acceleration of pacemaker activity in the SA node, severe sinus bradycardia must itself be treated, usually by parasympathetic blocking agents or, in resistant cases, by insertion of an electrical pacemaker.

AV block in patients with acute myocardial infarction can arise either from direct damage to the fibers of the AV node and AV bundle or from a reflex depression of AV conduction that accompanies the heightened vagal tone described in the preceding paragraph. Distinction between these two types of patient is extremely important, for they differ considerably in their response to therapy and their prognosis. When the AV conduction system is structurally damaged in the ischemic heart, the prognosis is much worse than when AV block is due to reflex depression of conduction in the AV node. Patients exhibiting the former type of AV conduction disturbance are more prone to sudden death due to asystole. Recognition of these patients is important, for the implantation of an artificial electrical pacemaker can restore ventricular rate when the AV block is mild and prevent death should AV conduction fail suddenly. In contrast, AV block due to vagal depression of the AV node usually responds well to parasympathetic blocking agents and is furthermore almost always a transient complication of the early period following acute myocardial infarction.

Careful examination of the ECGs in patients with AV block complicating myocardial infarction, coupled with the use of the intracardiac electrogram, has in recent years permitted these two classes of AV conduction abnormalities to be differentiated with considerable accuracy. In the following paragraphs the "typical" findings in each type of AV block are described in terms of the principles set forth in previous chapters. These descriptions, intended primarily to illustrate the application of current physiological knowledge of the conduction system, should not be construed as attempts to define their actual clinical pictures; for this the reader is referred to standard textbooks of medicine or cardiology.

The distinction between AV block due to anatomical lesions of the AV conduction system and that which results from vagal depression of the AV node can be made with a reasonable degree of precision from the clinical ECG in cases of second-degree AV block exhibiting 3:2, 4:3, etc. AV conduction. When AV block is of the Mobitz type II variety (i.e., where P-R intervals do not lengthen before a dropped beat; Fig. 16.12), it is likely that the patient is suffering from an anatomical lesion in the AV conduction system. This correlation can be understood if it is assumed that when atrial impulses are conducted to the ventricles they do so by passage through a region of severely injured conduction tissue that is able either to conduct (usually with a delay) or not to conduct, but because of its small size the lesion does not allow the degree of the delay (i.e., the P-R interval) to vary significantly. Thus failure of AV conduction in the case of Mobitz type II AV block is not usually preceded by further prolongation of the P-R interval. In the case of second-degree AV block due to vagal suppression of AV nodal conduction, on the other hand, the Wenckebach phenomenon is usually seen; i.e., a dropped beat is preceded by a progressive increase in P-R interval (Fig. 16.11). This situation differs from that described above, for when

AV block occurs in the AV node itself, the abnormal conduction delay results from an exaggeration of the normal property of decremental conduction. For this reason AV block due to vagal depression of conduction in the AV node typically exhibits the features, and thus the sensitivity, to autonomic nervous system control characteristic of Mobitz type I AV block (Chapter 16). It should be stressed that these distinctions cannot be made from the ECGs in patients with first-degree AV block, 2:1 second-degree AV block, or third-degree (complete) AV block.

Analysis of intracardiac electrograms is extremely useful in confirming the diagnosis of the nature of the conduction delay in patients with Mobitz type I or type II AV block. When AV block is due to an anatomical lesion in the AV conduction system, conduction through the AV node and into the bundle of His is usually normal as such lesions are most commonly located more distally in the AV bundle. Thus the intracardiac electrogram shows a normal A-H interval but a prolonged H-V interval (Fig. 16.13). In contrast, where the conduction delay is in the AV node, the A-H interval is prolonged while the H-V interval is normal. The intracardiac electrogram can also be used to determine the location of the conduction delay in patients with first-degree AV block or second-degree AV block with 2:1 AV conduction; again the distinction is made on the basis of whether the A-H or the H-V interval is prolonged. Similarly, in third-degree AV block, the finding of a normal A-H interval not followed by evidence of ventricular activation (a V deflection) indicates that the site of conduction delay is located distally in the AV conduction system, suggesting an anatomical lesion. When in complete AV block the A deflections are not followed by an H deflection (and where commonly a constant and normal H-V interval is seen before each beat of ventricular origin), it is likely that the arrhythmia is due to reflex depression of conduction within the AV node itself. It should be emphasized that these rules apply in the majority of cases but do not provide a completely accurate guide as to either the nature of the lesion or the prognosis in any individual patient.

Premature Systoles and Tachycardias

There are a number of mechanisms by which an interruption of coronary blood flow can lead to premature systoles and tachycardias. Some of these arise from reflex changes, most commonly increased sympathetic tone that results from pain, anxiety, low blood pressure, etc. (see above). Most of these arrhythmias, however, arise from abnormalities in the ischemic areas of the myocardium. These abnormalities in turn are most commonly sequelae of partial membrane depolarization during diastole. The dependence of the cardiac cell on a continuing supply of oxygen, and the resulting marked curtailment of ATP production when coronary blood flow is interrupted, can inhibit the sodium pump and so is probably directly responsible for a fall in intracellular potassium. The depolarizing effects of reduced $[K^+]_i$ are magnified by the accumulation of this ion in the extracellular space around the ischemic cell, so that resting potential falls toward zero. In the most severely affected regions of the ischemic heart, the membrane potential falls to levels that completely abolish any ability to either initiate or propagate a sodium-dependent action potential. In contrast, the slow inward current is inactivated less by partial membrane depolarization so that slow responses (Chapter 17) can arise in ischemic regions of the heart. For this reason the less severely ischemic areas around the region of complete myocardial necrosis are most likely to give rise to premature systoles and tachycardias. These "marginal areas" exhibit slowly rising, low-amplitude action potentials (slow responses) because of these effects of partial depolarization, which inactivate the opening of the fast channel. As the marginal areas around an infarcted area of the ventricles may remain in a viable but depressed state for hours, days, or even longer after a single occlusive event in the coronary arterial tree, the risk of serious arrhythmia can persist in such patients. Similarly, reduction in coronary blood flow, in the absence of a major coronary occlusion and resulting myocardial infarction, can provoke arrhythmias in areas of moderately ischemic myocardium that exhibit decremental conduction. Indeed, even when coronary arterial blood supply remains constant, although at a reduced level, an increase in cardiac work can cause a decline in resting membrane potential by causing energy demands to exceed the ability of the moderately ischemic myocardium to produce ATP.

Shortening of action potential duration also occurs in the ischemic heart. This effect accompanies partial membrane depolarization, whose ability to produce premature systoles and tachycardias is discussed below. Unlike the partial membrane depolarization in the ischemic heart, which can be attributed to inhibition of the sodium pump in the energy-starved myocardium, the mechanism responsible for abbreviation of the action potential is poorly understood. To some extent, shortening of the action potential plateau reflects the impaired opening of the slow channel described earlier in this chapter in terms of its effect of reducing myocardial contractility. Accumulation of potassium in the extracellular space surrounding the myocardial cells, by its effect of accelerating repolarization (Chapter 19), can represent an additional factor that may contribute to abbreviation of the action potential in ischemic regions of the myocardium. The ability of the resulting disparity between action potential durations in adjacent regions of the heart to cause re-entrant arrhythmias was discussed in Chapter 17.

Yet another mechanism that may cause premature systoles and tachycardias to develop in the ischemic heart is apparent when the effects of the partial membrane depolarization just described are considered in light of the description of the re-entrant arrhythmias due to conduction abnormalities (Chapter 17). The slowing of conduction velocity caused by inactivation of the fast channel when there is partial membrane depolarization (Chapter 17), and the emergence of "slow responses" when membrane potential falls to approximately -50 mV, lead to decremental conduction and unidirectional block. These conduction abnormalities, in turn, provide a setting which predisposes to the development of re-entrant premature systoles and tachycardias. Ischemia may also slow conduction by increasing the resistance of the intercalated disc (Chapter 16). These mechanisms operate primarily in the marginal areas around a myocardial infarction because membrane potential falls to zero in the central regions of the infarct, which therefore is completely inexcitable.

The implications of these concepts of arrhythmogenesis have already been touched on, and it should be re-emphasized that it is the *partial* depression of excitability in the ischemic ventricle that sets the stage for the development of premature systoles and the much more dangerous tachycardias. Not only do these considerations provide an explanation for the greatest incidence of such arrhythmias soon after the onset of a myocardial infarction, they also indicate several principles of therapy in such patients. Thus on theoretical grounds, effective therapeutic measures include not only interventions intended to improve conduction, but also the administration of agents whose main actions are to impair conduction. The ability of the latter to depress conduction in the so-called "marginal" areas around an acute myocardial infarct and to inhibit excitability in depressed areas in the chronically ischemic heart can abolish potential sites for the development of these arrhythmias.

At the present time, measures directed to the prevention and therapy of arrhythmias in patients with ischemic heart disease are based almost entirely on empiric observation because little is known of the way in which ischemia alters the properties of the cardiac sarcolemma and the ionic currents this membrane controls. Also, knowledge of the action of different antiarrhythmic agents on specific ionic currents in the heart is so new, and thus so scanty, that few attempts have yet been made to evaluate the effects of agents that act on abnormal ionic currents in the ischemic heart. These aspects of cardiac physiology and pharmacology are advancing extremely rapidly, however, and represent a very promising area for future research.

BIBLIOGRAPHY

Challoner, D. R., and Steinberg, D. (1966): Oxidative metabolism of myocardium as influenced by fatty acids and epinephrine. *Am. J. Physiol.,* 211:897–902.

Katz, A. M. (1973): Effects of ischemia on the contractile process of heart muscle. *Am. J. Cardiol.,* 32:456–460.

Morgan, H. E., editor (1976): The cellular basis of ischemia and infarction. *Circulation (Suppl. I),* 53:I-3–I-44.

Schwartz, A., Wood, J. M., Allen, J. C., Bornet, E. P., Entman, M. L., Goldstein, M. A., Sordahl, L. A., and Suzuki, M. (1973): Biochemical and morphologic correlates of cardiac ischemia. I. Membrane systems. *Am. J. Cardiol.,* 32:46–61.

See also bibliographies to Chapters 3 and 4, and the textbooks of cardiology cited at the end of Chapter 20.

Subject Index

A-bands, of sarcomere, 11
Aberrant conduction, 318–319, 337; *see also*
   Interval-duration relationship
Acceptor control of oxidative phosphorylation,
   67–68
Accessory conduction pathways, 261–262
   in paroxysmal supraventricular tachycardia,
    341
   in pre-excitation, 326–327
Acetate, *see* Acetyl-CoA
Acetyl-CoA
   and fatty acid metabolism, 49, 55
   formation of, 49, 55
   oxidation by tricarboxylic acid cycle, 56–58
Acetylcholine, *see* Vagal stimulation
Acidosis
   and calcium binding to troponin, 179
   in heart failure, 415, 416–417
   in ischemic heart, 421, 425, 426–427
   and lactic acid accumulation, 32
   negative inotropic actions of, 179
   and phosphofructokinase activity, 40
Actin, 12, 90, 95–98
   ATP hydrolysis by, 96
   binding by myosin, 92
   biological properties of, 97
   F-actin, 96
   G-actin, 96
   interactions with myosin, 93–94, 97, 104,
    109, 111–113, 114–116
   and length-tension relationship, 128–130
   molecular characteristics of, 96
   organization in sarcomere, 97–98
   in thin filament, 97–98, 101
   tropomyosin bound to, 98–99, 107–108
   troponin components bound to, 100, 108–
    109
Action potential, 229–256; *see also* Depolarization; Repolarization
   acetylcholine affecting, 362–364
   antiarrhythmic agents affecting, 375–377
   in atrium, 253
   in AV node, 253–254, 364, 370
   calcium levels affecting, 359–362
   catecholamines affecting, 368–370
   and conduction velocity, 299; *see also* Decremental conduction
   duration affected by membrane-stabilizing
    agents, 376
   early repolarization phase in, 241–242
   and full recovery time, 248
   interval-duration relationship in, 249–250
   ionic movements during, 139, 245–247
   in ischemic heart, 425–426, 432
   and membrane permeability, 233, 236
   plateau phase in, 242–243
   potassium levels affecting, 355–358
   in Purkinje fibers, 229, 235–250, 254–255

and QRS complex, 267, 285
and refractory periods, 247–249
in SA node, 250–253, 367
in specific regions of heart, 250–255
and supernormal period, 248
upstroke of, *see* Depolarization
in ventricle, 255
Active points of muscle
   tension in, 87, 117, 167
   two states of, 86–87, 167
Active state, 123–126
   in cardiac muscle, 134
Actomyosin, 97, 101–104, 105–106
   actin-myosin interactions in, 169–173; *see*
    also Contractility
   affecting contractility, 169–172, 178–195
   calcium regulating, 178–195
   plasticizing effects of ATP, 102, 113, 114,
    180
   potassium affecting, 180
   sarcomere length affecting, 129
   active complex in, 114
   ATPase activity of, *see* Calcium, and acto-
    myosin
   physicochemical changes in, 89, 101–104
   rigor complex in, 115–116, 117; *see also*
    Rigor
   and maximum isometric tension, 167–170
Acute myocardial infarction, *see* Ischemic
   heart
Acyl carnitine formation, 54
Acyl-CoA, 53–54
   transfer into mitochondria, 54
Adenosine diphosphate, *see* ADP
Adenosine monophosphate, *see* AMP
Adenosine triphosphate, *see* ATP
Adenylate cyclase, *see* AMP, cyclic, production of
Adenylate kinase, and adenine nucleotide concentrations, 41
ADP
   affecting hexokinase, 39
   affecting oxidative phosphorylation, 67–68
   affecting phosphofructokinase, 40–41, 71
   affecting tricarboxylic acid cycle, 58
   in ischemic heart, 421, 426
β-Adrenergic agonists, *see* Catecholamines
β-Adrenergic antagonists, *see* Antiarrhythmic
   drugs; β-Blocking agents
Aerobic glycolysis, *see* Glycolysis, aerobic
Afterload
   and contraction in heart muscle, 200
   and contraction in skeletal muscle, 197–198
   and work performance, 73–74
Aging, myosin ATPase activity and myocardial contractility in, 176, 177
A-H interval, *see* Electrocardiogram, intracardiac

434